Textbook of Dental Anatomy
A Practical Approach

System requirement:

- Operating System—Windows XP or above
- Web Browser—Internet Explorer 8 or above, Google Chrome, Mozilla Firefox
- Essential plugins—Java and Flash player
  - Facing problems in viewing content—It may be your system does not have java enabled.
  - If Videos do not show up—It may be the system requires flash player or need to manage flash setting. To learn more about flash setting click on the link in the help section.
  - You can test java and flash by using the links from the help section of the CD/DVD.

Accompanying CD/DVD Rom is playable only in computer and not in DVD player.
CD/DVD has Autorun function—It may take few seconds to load on your computer. If it does not works for you then follow the steps below to access the contents manually:

- Click on my computer
- Select the CD/DVD drive and click open/explore—This will show list of files in the CD/DVD
- Find and double click file—"Launch.html"

For more information about troubleshoot of Autorun click on: http://support.microsoft.com/kb/330135

DVD Contents

Textbook of Dental Anatomy A Practical Approach

Jayalakshmi Kumaraswamy BDS MDS
Professor
Department of Oral Pathology and Microbiology
Vydehi Institute of Dental Sciences
Affiliated to Rajiv Gandhi University of Health Sciences
Bengaluru, Karnataka, India

JAYPEE

JAYPEE BROTHERS MEDICAL PUBLISHERS (P) LTD

New Delhi • London • Philadelphia • Panama

Jaypee Brothers Medical Publishers (P) Ltd

Headquarters

Jaypee Brothers Medical Publishers (P) Ltd
4838/24, Ansari Road, Daryaganj
New Delhi 110 002, India
Phone: +91-11-43574357
Fax: +91-11-43574314
Email: jaypee@jaypeebrothers.com

Overseas Offices

J.P. Medical Ltd
83 Victoria Street, London
SW1H 0HW (UK)
Phone: +44-2031708910
Fax: +02-03-0086180
Email: info@jpmedpub.com

Jaypee-Highlights Medical Publishers Inc.
City of Knowledge, Bld. 237, Clayton
Panama City, Panama
Phone: +1 507-301-0496
Fax: +1 507-301-0499
Email: cservice@jphmedical.com

Jaypee Medical Inc.
The Bourse
111 South Independence Mall East
Suite 835, Philadelphia, PA 19106, USA
Phone: +1 267-519-9789
Email: jpmed.us@gmail.com

Jaypee Brothers Medical Publishers (P) Ltd
17/1-B Babar Road, Block-B, Shaymali
Mohammadpur, Dhaka-1207
Bangladesh
Mobile: +08801912003485
Email: jaypeedhaka@gmail.com

Jaypee Brothers Medical Publishers (P) Ltd
Bhotahity, Kathmandu, Nepal
Phone: +977-9741283608
Email: kathmandu@jaypeebrothers.com

Website: www.jaypeebrothers.com
Website: www.jaypeedigital.com

Inquiries for bulk sales may be solicited at: jaypee@jaypeebrothers.com

Textbook of Dental Anatomy: A Practical Approach

First Edition: **2014**

ISBN: 978-93-5090-839-6

Printed at : Samrat Offset Pvt. Ltd.

Dedicated to

My family, who inspired the dream,
My teachers, who nurtured the dream
and
The students, who are yet to dream.

Preface

The subject of Dental Anatomy is the basic foundation in dentistry. When a student enters the BDS Course, he/she should have the knowledge of teeth present, morphology of teeth and functions of teeth, because throughout the career, it is helpful as a dental practitioner, whether it is restoring or replacing teeth. Morphology of teeth also helps in identification of developmental anomalies, which may be correlated to any other skeletal abnormalities, hormonal disturbances, etc. For this reason, a simplified and easily understandable morphology of teeth is included in this textbook and also focused on ground section of teeth, how to identify the natural teeth and different dentition casts.

As it is said that "Reading is the exercise to brain as physical activity to the body". A dental practitioner should attain the knowledge of subject and also should possess practical skill. To understand the anatomy of teeth, one must know teeth carving. The most outstanding feature of this textbook is that a very simplified carving technique is described stepwise with diagrammatic illustrations and photographs for easy understanding and learning.

"I hear, I forget, I see, I remember, I do, I understand". Let us follow this phrase and understand the morphology of teeth by carving. One uniqueness of this textbook is that an Interactive DVD-ROM is attached to it, in which a live demonstration of carving technique for teeth is provided, so that the student can visualize and learn the carving technique. Demonstration of carving for permanent maxillary central incisor, permanent maxillary canine, permanent maxillary first premolar and permanent maxillary first molar is provided in the Interactive DVD-ROM. The carving of remaining permanent teeth and deciduous teeth can be followed by using the same technique.

All attempts have been made for the benefit of learners, i.e. undergraduates and postgraduates—the budding teachers and practitioners.

Jayalakshmi Kumaraswamy

Acknowledgments

I thank ..... for coming up with a lovely textbook, Wheeler's Dental Anatomy and the knowledge I gained from it.

I thank my husband, Dr Ravi Kumar H, children Anish Kumar and Ananya Kumar, for their time, patience and sacrifices they had to make. I extend my thanks to my family and relatives, for the constant support.

It is my pleasant privilege and honor to express my sincere gratitude and heart filled thanks to my teacher and guide Dr S Hemavathy, Professor and Head, Department of Oral Pathology and Microbiology, Government Dental College, Bengaluru, for timely support, efficient guidance and above all for being a constant source of inspiration to me.

My special thanks to Dr K Karpagaselvi, Professor and Head, Department of Oral Pathology and Microbiology, Vydehi Institute of Dental Sciences and Research Center, Bengaluru, who kind heartedly allowed me to utilize the facilities available in the department. I would also like to thank the staff in the department, Dr Archana Patil, Dr Veena N, Dr Srinivas, Dr Lokesh, Dr Jeevan, Dr Vinod Kumar, Mrs Dorothy Anitha, Mrs Jamuna Rani and Ms Priyadarshini, for their support, cooperation and making this venture a success.

I am grately indebted to Dr Archana Patil, Dr Srinivas and Dr Lakshmi Krishnan, for taking out time for this book and proofreading. I would like to acknowledge with extreme gratitude, the unstinted support provided by Dr Jaya Naidu, Professor and Dr Shubha, Lecturer Staff, Department of Pedodontics, Vydehi Institute of Dental Sciences and Research Center, Bengaluru, for the photographs of deciduous dentition.

I extend my special thanks to postgraduate students, Dr Lakshmi Krishnan and Dr Sushma R, for recording of carving demonstration, capturing of photographs of casts and helping out in refining illustrations and also thank Dr Raghunandan, Dr Harish, Dr Akshatha and Dr Divya, for their timely help and support.

The many rough drafts and the final copy of the manuscript were typed by Mrs Nagarathna, to whom special thanks are due. I thank Mr Bhaskar, for editing the illustrations.

I owe a deep sense of gratitude to the management of Vydehi Institute of Dental Sciences and Research Center, Bengaluru, for their support.

I also gratefully acknowledge the contributions made by all the talented professional staff of M/s Jaypee Brothers Medical Publishers (P) Ltd, New Delhi, India, for translating my imagination and efforts into this book.

Most of all, I thank God, for all the kindness and mercy bestowed upon me.

I would be appreciated if the readers come out with feedback and will thus give me the opportunity to learn more and more feedback from the reader will be well appreciated and will contribute to the betterment of future editions.

Textbook of Dental Anatomy: A Practical Approach is today a reality due to the combined efforts and mending support from various quarters, which together makes the experience of bringing out this book a memorable journey.

Contents

CHAPTER

1

Introduction

Dental Anatomy is a subject in which, through the knowledge of basic sciences, a practical skill may be obtained for a dental practitioner. Morphology of teeth helps and guides us to identify developmental anomalies, which may be one of the features of clinical condition and also helps to provide skills for restoring a tooth or replacing a tooth.

An attempt is made to simplify the morphology of teeth and carving technique. A simpler carving technique is provided in this textbook for dental students.

PRINCIPLES OF CARVING TECHNIQUE

a. A modified pen grasp should be used to hold a lecron carver (Fig. 1.1)
b. Wax block should be smoothened before carving is proceeded.
c. Direction of carving should be in one direction only.
d. Uniform pressure should be applied during carving.
e. Finishing is done by removing the excess wax and also by carving the surface uniform.
f. After finishing, polishing should be done by using a pellet of cotton or a piece of soft cloth. A pellet of cotton is preferable to polish the minor details of teeth. Polishing should also follow the carving, otherwise the carved features will be lost.

Modified pen grasp used in carving: the right thumb and index finger will hold the carver, the middle finger placed near the carving edge which will control the carving. The ring finger and little finger will support the wax block (Fig. 1.1).

NOMENCLATURE

Certain terms should be known to understand dental anatomy. The term maxillary means upper jaw, mandibular means lower jaw. Primary means belonging to the first stage of any process. The term deciduous means not permanent, transitory.

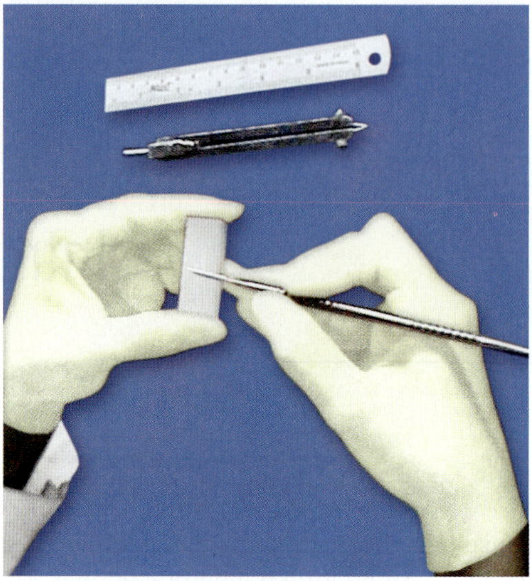

Fig. 1.1: Modified pen grasp

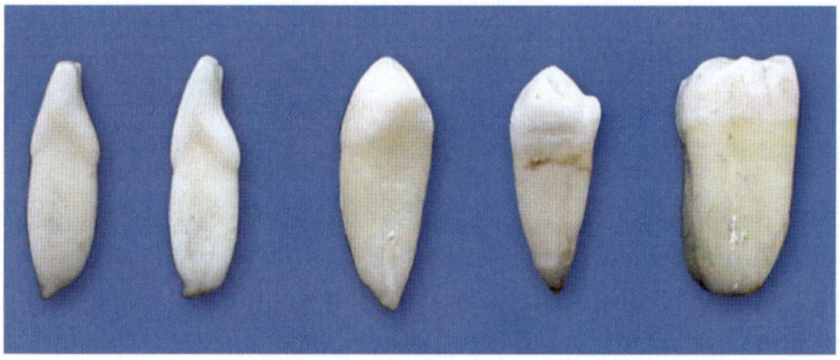

Fig. 1.2: Photograph showing crown and root of various permanent mandibular teeth
(*Courtesy*: Department of Oral Pathology, Vydehi Institute of Dental Sciences, Bangalore)

Deciduous teeth commonly called as milk tooth is defined as "One of the temporary teeth of a mammal that are replaced by permanent teeth."

The term succedaneous can be used to describe a successor dentition. The term permanent dentition suggests it is permanent (Fig. 1.2).

THE CROWN AND ROOT (FIGS 1.2 AND 1.3)

Each tooth has a crown and root portion. The crown is covered with enamel and the root portion is covered with cementum. The junction of crown and root is cervical line. The hard tissues of a tooth are enamel, dentin and cementum. The soft tissue of a tooth is pulp.

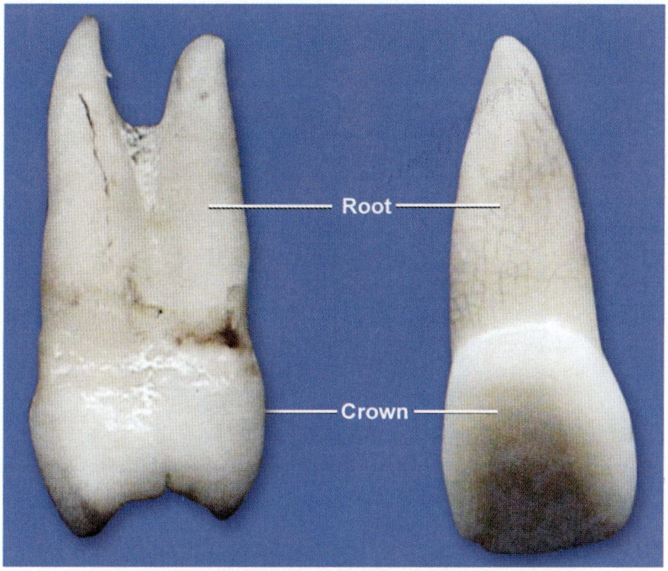

Fig. 1.3: Crown and root
(*Courtesy*: Department of Oral Pathology, Vydehi Institute of Dental Sciences, Bangalore)

SURFACE

Anterior teeth are incisors and canines. Posterior teeth are premolars and molars. Surfaces of anterior teeth are:

a. Labial surface: Surface toward the lips
b. Mesial surface: Surface toward the midline
c. Distal surface: Surface away from the midline
d. Lingual surface: Surface toward the tongue
e. Palatal surface: Surface toward the palate

Surfaces of posterior teeth are:

a. Buccal/facial surface: Surface toward the cheek
b. Mesial surface: Surface toward the midline
c. Distal surface: Surface away from the midline
d. Lingual surface: Surface toward the tongue
e. Palatal surface: Surface toward the palate

ANATOMICAL LANDMARKS OF TOOTH[1,2]

Cusp: A cusp is an elevation or mound on the crown portion of a tooth making up a divisional part of the occlusal surface (Fig. 1.5).

Tubercle: A tubercle is a smaller elevation on some portion of the crown produced by an extra formation of enamel.

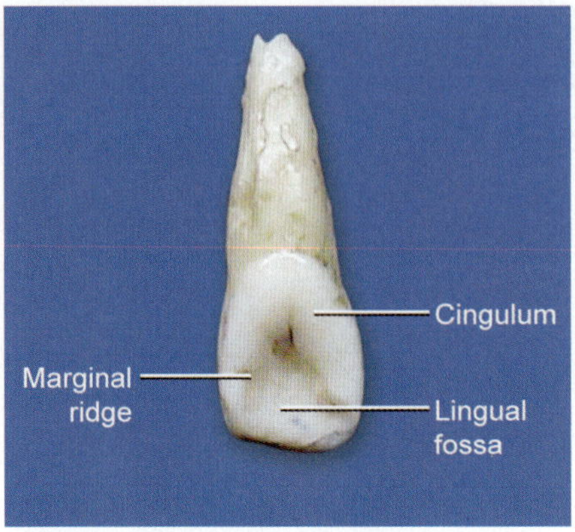

Fig. 1.4: Cingulum, ridge and fossa

(*Courtesy*: Department of Oral Pathology, Vydehi Institute of Dental Sciences, Bangalore)

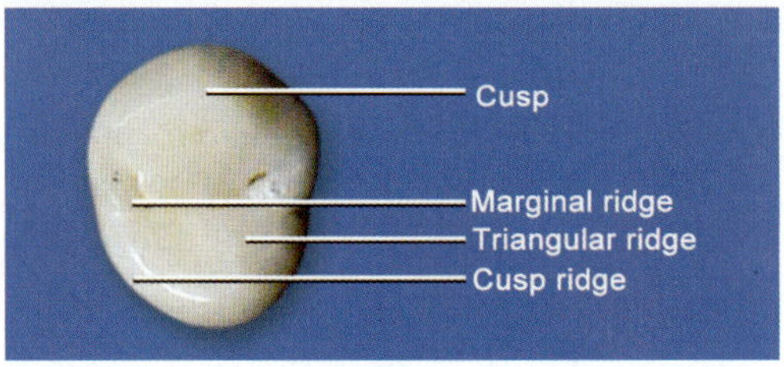

Fig. 1.5: Ridges and cusp

(*Courtesy*: Department of Oral Pathology, Vydehi Institute of Dental Sciences, Bangalore)

Cingulum: A cingulum or girdle, is the lingual lobe of an anterior tooth and makes up the bulk of the cervical third of the lingual surface (Fig. 1.4).

Ridge: A ridge is any linear elevation on the surface of a tooth and is named according to its location (e.g. buccal, incisal, marginal, etc.) (Figs 1.4 and 1.5).

Marginal ridges are those rounded borders of the enamel that form the mesial and distal margins of the occlusal surfaces of premolars and molars and mesial and distal margins of the lingual surfaces of the incisors and canine.

Triangular ridges descend from tips of the cusps of molars and premolars toward the central part of the occlusal surface. They are named after the cusps to which they belong. When a buccal and lingual triangular ridge join, they form a transverse ridge. A transverse ridge is the union of two triangular ridges transversely crossing the surface of a posterior tooth.

Oblique ridge: The oblique ridge is a ridge obliquely crossing the occlusal surfaces of maxillary molars and formed by the union of triangular ridge of distobuccal cusp and distal cusp ridge of mesiolingual cusp.

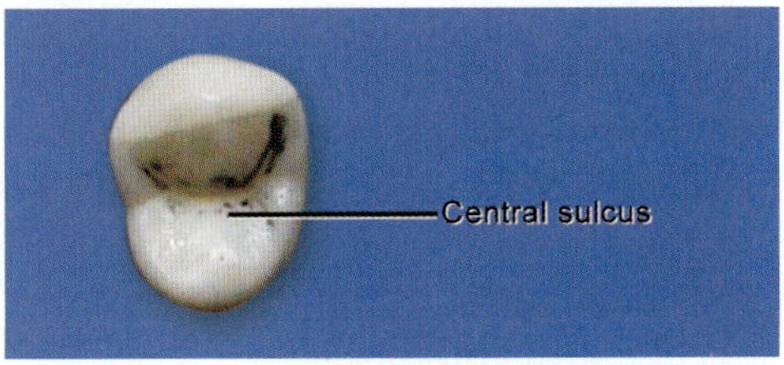

Fig. 1.6: Sulcus

(*Courtesy*: Department of Oral Pathology, Vydehi Institute of Dental Sciences, Bangalore)

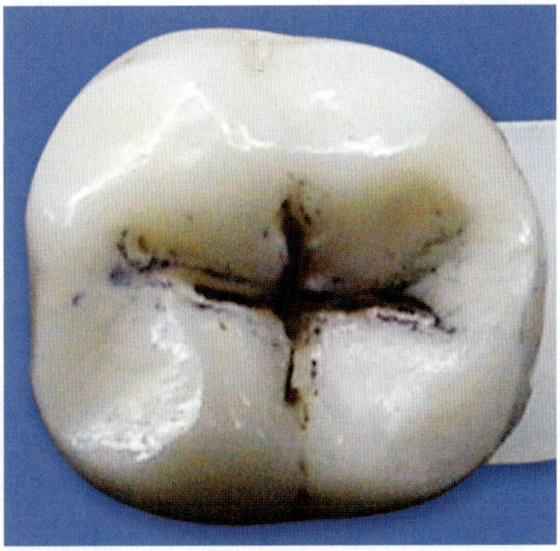

Fig. 1.7: Photograph showing grooves and pits

(*Courtesy*: Department of Oral Pathology, Vydehi Institute of Dental Sciences, Bangalore)

Fossa (Fig. 1.4): A fossa is an irregular depression or concavity; they are named according to the location. Lingual fossae are seen on lingual surface of incisors and central fossae on occlusal surface of molars. Triangular fossae are found on premolars and molars on the occlusal surface, mesial or distal to marginal ridges.

Sulcus: A sulcus is a long depression or valley on the surface of a tooth between ridges and cusps, the inclines of which meet at an angle. Sulcus has a developmental groove at the junction of its inclines (Fig. 1.6).

Groove (Fig. 1.7): A developmental groove is a shallow groove or line between the primary parts of the crown or root. A supplementary groove is also a shallow linear depression on surface of a tooth, radiating from the developmental groove, but does not mark the junction of primary parts.

Different types of developmental grooves are seen such as: central developmental groove, mesial developmental groove, distal developmental groove, buccal developmental groove, lingual developmental groove, etc.

Pits (Fig. 1.7): Pit is a small pinpoint depression located at the junction of developmental grooves or at terminals of these grooves. Types are—central pit, distal pit and mesial pit.

Lobe: A lobe is one of the primary sections of formation in the development of crown. Cusps and mamelons are representative of lobes. A mamelon is any one of the three rounded protuberances found on the incisal ridges of newly erupted incisor teeth.

Division into thirds of crown and root for descriptive purpose and easy understanding.[1,2] The crown and root are divided into thirds. Cervical third, middle third and incisal/occlusal third of crown. Cervical third, middle third and apical third of root (Fig.1.8).

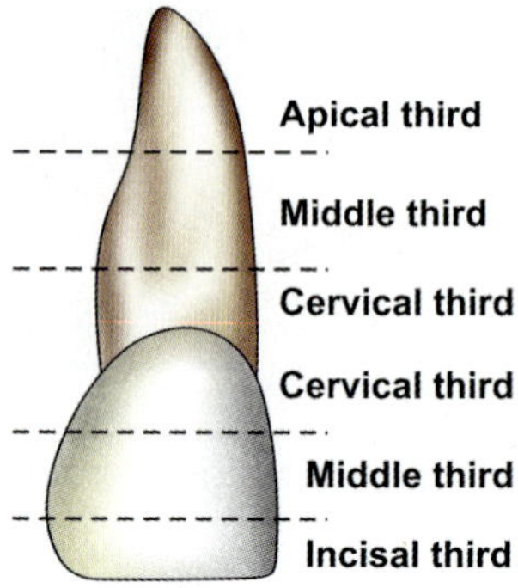

Fig. 1.8: Division of crown into thirds

LINE ANGLES AND POINT ANGLES[1,2]

A line angle is formed by the junction of two surfaces. The line angles of anterior teeth are (Fig. 1.9):

- Mesiolabial
- Distolabial
- Mesiolingual
- Distolingual
- Labioincisal
- Linguoincisal

The line angles of posterior teeth are (Fig. 1.10):

- Mesiobuccal
- Distobuccal
- Mesiolingual
- Distolingual
- Labio occlusal
- Linguo occlusal

A point angle is formed by the junction of three surfaces. The point angles of anterior teeth are (Fig. 1.11):

- Mesiolabio incisal
- Distolabio incisal
- Mesiolingual incisal
- Distolingual incisal

The point angles of posterior teeth are (Fig. 1.11):

- Mesiobucco occlusal
- Distobucco occlusal
- Mesiolingual occlusal
- Distolingual occlusal

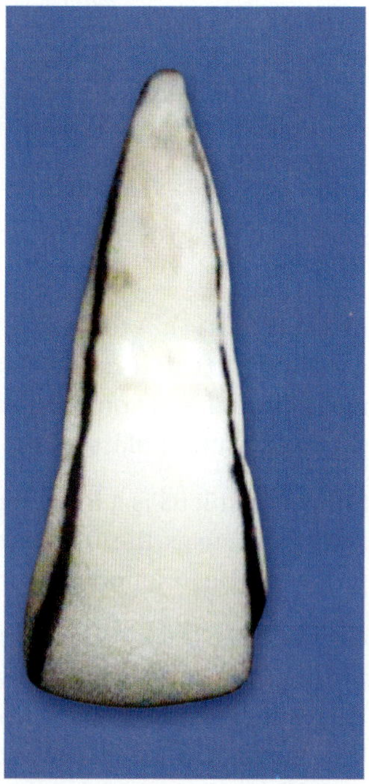

Fig. 1.9: The ink marking is to represent line angles on the crown as well as on the root of a anterior tooth

(*Courtesy*: Department of Oral Pathology, Vydehi Institute of Dental Sciences, Bangalore)

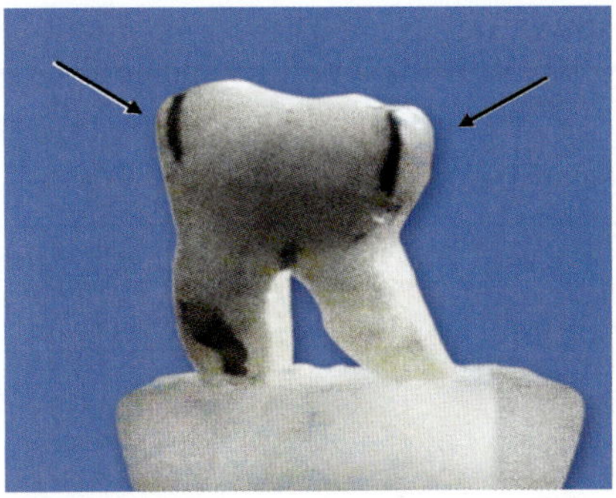

Fig. 1.10: Photograph showing mesiolingual and distolingual line angles of posterior tooth (ink markings)

(*Courtesy*: Department of Oral Pathology, Vydehi Institute of Dental Sciences, Bangalore)

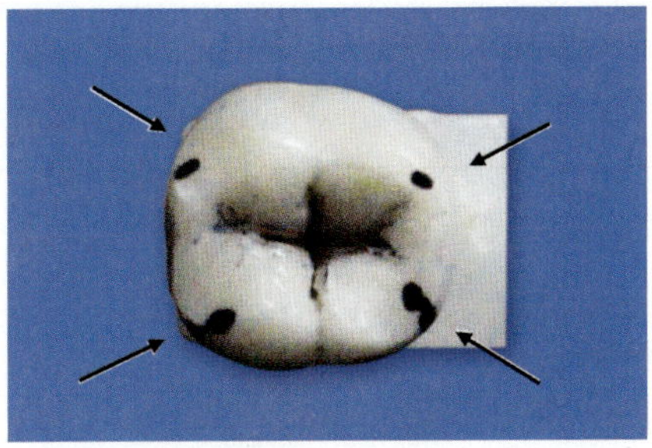

Fig. 1.11: The ink dot markings in the picture showing point angles described in text

(*Courtesy*: Department of Oral Pathology, Vydehi Institute of Dental Sciences, Bangalore)

CHRONOLOGIES OF HUMAN DENTITION[2]

Many early labels and charts disagreed on timing of chronological events. One of the altered and widely used table by Schour and Massler and presents a long history of subsequent development and compilations (Table 1.1).

Table 1.1: Chronology of human dentition

Dentition	Tooth	First evidence of calcification (Weeks *in utero*)	Crown completed (Months)	Eruption (Months)	Root completed (Years)
Primary (upper)	i1	14(13–16)	1½	10(8–12)	1½
	i2	16(14$^2/_3$–16½)[b]	2½	11(9–13)	2
	C	17(15–18)[b]	9	19(16–22)	3¼
	M1	15½(14½–17)	6	16(13–19) (14–18)	2½
	M2	19(16–23½)	11	29(25–33)	3
Primary (lower)	i1	14(13–16)	2½	8(6–10)	1½
	i2	16(14^2/2–)	3	13(10–16)	1½
	C	17(16–)	9	20(17–23)	3¼
	M1	15½(14½–17)	5½	16(14–18)	2¼
	M2	18(17–19½)	10	27(23–31) (24–30)	3
Permanent (upper)	i1	3–4	4–5	7–8	10
	i2	10–12	4–5	8–9	11
	C	4–5	6–7	11–12	13–15
	P1	1½–1¾	5–6	10–11	12–13
	P2	2–2¼	6–7	10–12	12–14
	M1	at birth	2½–3	6–7	09–10
	M2	2½–3	7–8	12–13	14–16
	M3	7–9	12–16	17–21	18–25

Contd..

Contd..

Dentition	Tooth	First evidence of calcification (Weeks *in utero*)	Crown completed (Months)	Eruption (Months)	Root completed (Years)
	L1	3–4	4–5	6–7	9
	L2	3–4	4–5	7–8	10
	C	4–5	6–7	9–10	12–14
Permanent	P1	1¾–2	5–6	10–12	12–13
(lower)	P2	2¼–2½	6–7	11–12	13–14
	M1	at birth	2½ –3	6–7	9–10
	M2	2½–3	7–8	11–13	14–15
	M3	8–10	12–16	17–21	18–25

REFERENCES

1. Woelfel JB, Scheid RC. Dental Anatomy. Williams & Wilkins. 1997.
2. Ash, Nelson. Wheelers Dental Anatomy, Physiology & Occlusion. 8th edition. Elsevier. 2003.

CHAPTER

2

Dental Formula and Tooth Numbering Systems

The denomination and number of all mammalian teeth are expressed by formulae that are used to differentiate the human dentition from that of other species. The denomination of each tooth is often represented by the initial letter in its name (e.g. I for incisor, C for canine, P for premolar, M for molar); each letter is followed by a horizontal line and the number of each type of tooth is placed above the line for maxillary (Upper jaw) and below the line for mandibular (Lower jaw). The formulae include one side only with the number of teeth in each jaw being the same for humans.[1,2]

The dental formula for the deciduous teeth is as follows:[2]

$$I\ \frac{2}{2} \qquad C\ \frac{1}{1} \qquad M\ \frac{2}{2} = 10$$

This formula is read as: Incisors, two maxillary and two mandibular. Canines, one maxillary and one mandibular. Molars, two maxillary and two mandibular, that is 10 total on one side, right or left.

The dental formula for permanent teeth is as follows:[2]

$$I\ \frac{2}{2} \qquad C\ \frac{1}{1} \qquad P\ \frac{2}{2} \qquad M\ \frac{3}{3} = 16$$

Premolars: Two maxillary and two mandibular, and third molar, one maxillary and one mandibular is added to this formula.

TOOTH NUMBERING SYSTEMS[1,2]

Several systems are in use in the world, but only a few are considered here. Different tooth numbering systems were introduced in order to help in identification of teeth and to record data. Each system has its own advantages and disadvantages, so there is no system that is universally accepted by the dental profession.

ZSIGMONDY/PALMER SYSTEM[1,2]

The symbolic system for permanent dentition was introduced by Adolf Zsigmondy of Vienna in 1861 and then modified for the primary dentition in 1864. Palmer published the symbolic system in 1870. This symbolic system is referred as Zsigmondy/Palmer notation system.

The Zsigmondy/Palmer notation for permanent dentition is a four quadrant system as follows:

8 7 6 5 4 3 2 1	1 2 3 4 5 6 7 8
8 7 6 5 4 3 2 1	1 2 3 4 5 6 7 8

Beginning with the central incisors, the teeth are numbered 1 through 8 in each arch, e.g. the left maxillary second premolar is designated as 5 and for right mandibular canine as 3.

And for deciduous dentition, the Palmer notation system as given below:

E D C B A	A B C D E
E D C B A	A B C D E

The notation is given beginning with central incisors, the teeth are given alphabets A through E in each arch, e.g. the mandibular left lateral incisor is designated as B and for maxillary right first molar is D.

Disadvantage:[2] This system presents difficulty where the appropriate font is not available for keyboard recording of Zsigmondy/Palmer symbolic notation.

The American Dental Association System (The Universal System)[1,2]: This system was introduced in 1968. In the universal system for the permanent dentition, the maxillary teeth are numbered from 1 through 16, beginning with the right third molar upto left third molar. Beginning with the mandibular left third molar upto right third molar, the teeth are numbered 17 through 32; thus, the right maxillary first molar is designated as 3, the maxillary left central incisor as 9 and the left mandibular first molar as 19. The following universal notation designates the entire permanent dentition:

1	2	3	4	5	6	7	8	9	10	11	12	13	14	15	16
32	31	30	29	28	27	26	25	24	23	22	21	20	19	18	17

The universal system for deciduous dentition is as follows:

A	B	C	D	E	F	G	H	I	J
T	S	R	Q	P	O	N	M	L	K

The maxillary teeth beginning with the right second molar use the letters A through J; for the mandibular teeth letters K through T are used, beginning with the left mandibular second molar. For example, the left maxillary second molar is designated as J and right mandibular lateral incisor is designated as Q.

Advantage:[2] Acceptable to computer language since the universal system is designated with a unique number, leading to less confusion than with the Palmer notation.

Disadvantage:[2] Difficult to remember each designated tooth.

Federation Dentaire Internationale System (Two Digit System):[1,2] This two digit system was proposed by FDI in 1971 for both primary and permanent dentitions and was adopted by World Health Organization (WHO) and accepted by other organizations such as International Association for Dental Research (IADR). The FDI system for permanent dentition is as follows:

		Upper right									Upper left				
18	17	16	15	14	13	12	11	21	22	23	24	25	26	27	28
48	47	46	45	44	43	42	41	31	32	33	34	35	36	37	38
		Lower right									Lower left				

The first digit indicates the quadrant (1 to 4) and the second digit indicates the tooth within a quadrant: 1 to 8 for permanent teeth. The number 45 refers to mandibular right second premolar and the number 27 refers to maxillary left second molar.

The number 27 should be pronounced as two-seven not twenty seven.

The FDI system for deciduous teeth is as follows:

55	54	53	52	51	61	62	63	64	65
85	84	83	82	81	71	72	73	74	75

Number 5 indicates maxillary right, 6 indicates maxillary left, 7 indicates mandibular left and 8 indicates mandibular right quadrants. The second number of the two digit system is the tooth, e.g. 74 refers to mandibular left first molar.

Advantage:[2] Every tooth has a unique number.

The other systems include: Viktor Haderup of Denmark[2,3] in 1891 devised a variant of the eight-tooth quadrant system in which plus (+) and minus (-) were used to differentiate between upper and lower quadrants, and between right and left quadrants (e.g. +1 = upper right central incisor; -1 = lower left central incisor). Primary teeth were numbered as upper right (05 + to 01+), lower left (-01 to -05). This system is followed in European countries.[3]

REFERENCES

1. Woelfel JB, Scheid RC. Dental Anatomy. Williams & Wilkins. 1997.
2. Ash, Nelson. Wheelers Dental Anatomy, Physiology & Occlusion. 8th edn. Elsevier. 2003.
3. Available from: http://knol.google.com/k/dr-charles-m/tooth-numbering-system-teeth-numbering/3mflbd6iv8g1u/40.Version 10.knol.2010may4.

CHAPTER

3

The Permanent Incisors

The **maxillary central incisor** is located in the anterior maxillary jaw and is usually the most visible of all teeth in the mouth. It is located mesial to the maxillary lateral incisor. As with all incisors, their function is for shearing or cutting food during mastication.[1,2] There are no cusps on the teeth. Instead, the surface area of the tooth used in shearing is called an incisal ridge or incisal edge.[2] Formation of these teeth begin at 14 weeks in utero for the deciduous dentition and 3 to 4 months of age for the permanent dentition.[3]

Incisors (from *Latin incidere,* "to cut") are the first kind of tooth in anterior region of heterodont mammals. They are located in the premaxilla above and mandible below.[4]

The aggregate of cells which eventually form a tooth are derived from the ectoderm of the first branchial arch and the ectomesenchyme of the neural crest.[3] As in all cases of tooth development, the first hard tissue to begin forming is dentin, with enamel appearing immediately afterwards.[3]

THE PERMANENT MAXILLARY CENTRAL INCISOR

Morphology

The maxillary incisors are four in number. The maxillary central incisors are present on either side of the maxilla.[1] They are larger than lateral incisors. Major function is cutting the food during the process of mastication and also helps in speech and esthetics.[1,2] These incisors consist of incisal ridge and incisal edge.[2] Incisal ridge is a rounded portion which merges with the mesio-and distoincisal angles and the labial and lingual surfaces.[2] Incisal edge terms an angle formed by the merging of two surfaces.[2] It is formed by the junction of the linguoincisal surface and the labial surface. Edge is seen when occlusal wear has occurred.[2]

Labial Aspect[1,2] (Fig. 3.1)

Outline

Crown: The mesial outline of the crown is slightly convex, almost straight from cervical line till the mesioincisal angle. The mesial contact area is present at mesioincisal angle, which is sharp. The distal outline of the crown is more convex from the cervical line till the distoincisal angle. The distoincisal angle is rounded. The incisal outline is regular and straight in a mesiodistal direction. The cervical line shows curvature: the convexity is facing toward the root apex and concavity is facing toward the incisal ridge.

Root: The root outline is regular and gradually tapers toward the root apex.

Surface

Crown: The cervical third of the labial surface is convex, whereas the middle third and incisal third is flat.

Root: The surface of the root is smooth and convex throughout. Root apex is blunt and rounded.

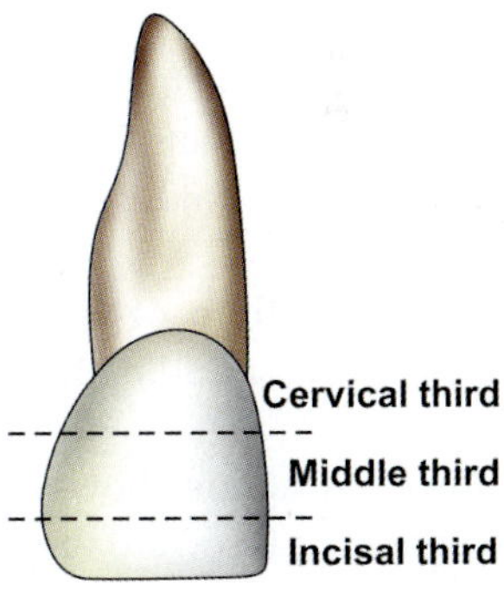

Fig. 3.1: Permanent maxillary right central incisor, labial aspect

Lingual Aspect[1,2] (Fig. 3.2A)

Outline

The crown and root outline is similar to labial aspect.

Surface

The cervical third shows convexity due to presence of cingulum. Confluent with the cingulum, mesial marginal ridge and distal marginal ridge is present.

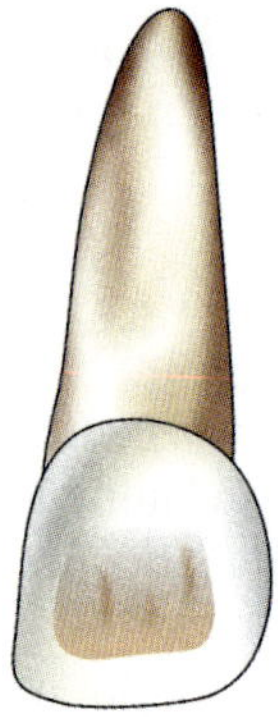

Fig. 3.2A: Permanent maxillary right central incisor, lingual aspect

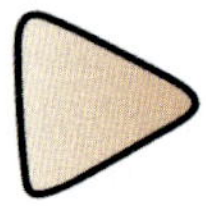

Fig. 3.2B: Cross section of roof at cervix showing triangular form with rounded angles

Outlining the lingual fossa, linguoincisal ridge is seen. A shallow concavity is present below the cingulum, i.e. lingual fossa (Fig. 3.2A). Both the crown and the root taper lingually, making the lingual portion of the root appear narrower than the labial portion. A cross section of root shows triangular form, the base is toward the labial aspect and apex is toward the lingual aspect (Fig. 3.2B).

Mesial Aspect[1,2] (Figs 3.3 and 3.4)

Outline

Crown: The mesial outline is wedge shaped; base is toward the cervical line and apex toward the incisal ridge. Labial outline of the mesial aspect—at the cervical third is convex, middle third and incisal third is straight till the incisal edge (Fig. 3.3).

Lingual outline of the mesial aspect—cervical third is convex (because of cingulum), middle third is concave and incisal third is slightly convex (Fig. 3.3).

The cervical line shows curvature—the convexity is towards the incisal edge and concavity is toward the root apex.

Root: The root outline is regular and gradually tapers toward the root apex. Root apex is blunt and rounded.

Surface

The crown and root surface is slightly convex and smooth.

A very important characteristic feature of this tooth is that when a line drawn through the centre of the crown and root from mesial aspect of the tooth, the line will bisect the apex of the root, crest of curvature of cervical line and the incisal ridge (Fig. 3.4). This feature is also present on distal aspect.

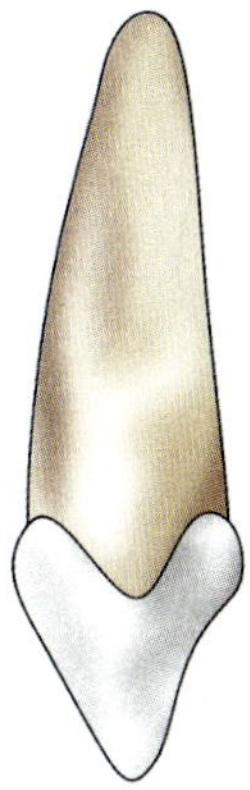

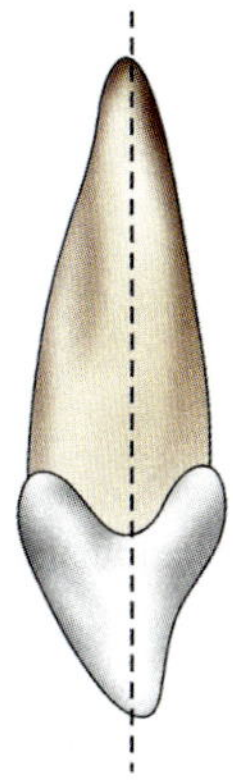

Figs 3.3 and 3.4: Permanent maxillary right central incisor, mesial aspect

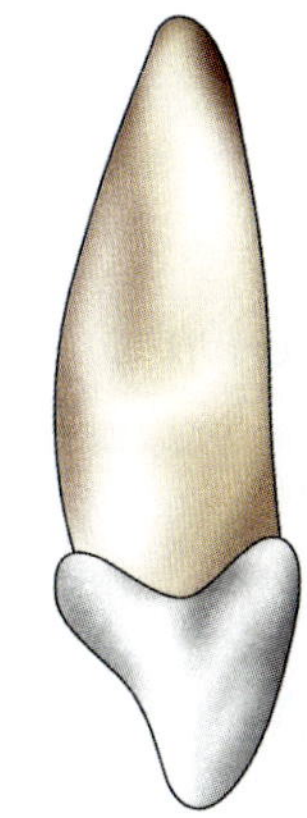

Fig. 3.5: Permanent maxillary right central incisor, distal aspect

Distal Aspect[1,2] (Fig. 3.5)

Both crown and root outline appear similar to mesial aspect except for the following differences.

1. Curvature of cervical line is less by 1 mm than on the mesial aspect.
2. Crown appears thicker because of the slope of the labial surface distolingually, much of lingual surface is seen from the distal aspect.

Incisal Aspect[1,2] (Fig. 3.6)

Dimension: The mesiodistal width is greater than the labiolingual width.

Outline

The labial outline towards the cervical third is convex. The lingual outline is tapered towards the cingulum. The cingulum of the crown makes up the cervical

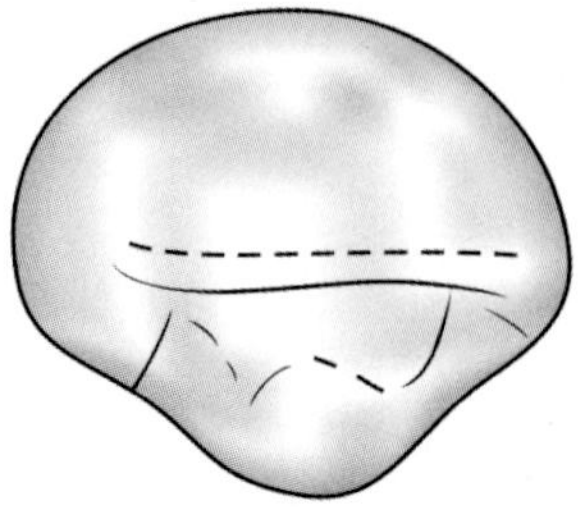

Fig. 3.6: Permanent maxillary right central incisor, incisal aspect

portion of the lingual surface. The mesiolabial and distolabial line angles are prominent from the incisal aspect. The incisal ridge is straight from incisal aspect.

Carving Technique

Measurements (in mm)

Cervico-incisal length of crown	-	10.5
Length of root	-	13.0
Mesiodistal dimension of crown	-	8.5
Mesiodistal dimension of crown at cervix	-	7.0
Labiolingual width of crown	-	7.0
Labiolingual width of crown at cervix	-	6.0
Curvature of cervical line - mesial aspect	-	3.5
Curvature of cervical line - distal aspect	-	2.5

Step 1: Smoothen the wax block. Mark the four aspects on the wax block, i.e. labial, lingual, mesial and distal denoting by their starting letters as **'La'** for labial, **'Li'** for lingual, **'M'** for mesial **'D'** for distal for anterior teeth for both maxillary and mandibular teeth, i.e. permanent maxillary right and left central and lateral incisor, permanent maxillary right and left canine, permanent mandibular right and left central and lateral incisor and permanent mandibular right and left canine. Always carve the crown and root together for anterior teeth.

Step 2: After marking the aspects, turn toward the labial aspect, draw a midline on the labial aspect. (*Note:* Markings on the wax block should be superficial). Mark the crown length, root length and also the mesiodistal width of crown and mesiodistal width of crown at cervix (See Fig. 3.7A).

Step 3: Draw the labial outline on the wax block (Fig. 3.7B).

Step 4: Carve according to the outline removing the excess wax. As a beginner, when removing the excess wax carve out only 0.5 mm at one time and the pressure applied should be uniform and carving in one direction only. When it is posed from labial aspect, the mesial and distal outline should appear parallel throughout the surface of the block (See Fig. 3.7C).

Step 5: Extend the length of crown and root from labial aspect to mesial, distal and lingual aspect.

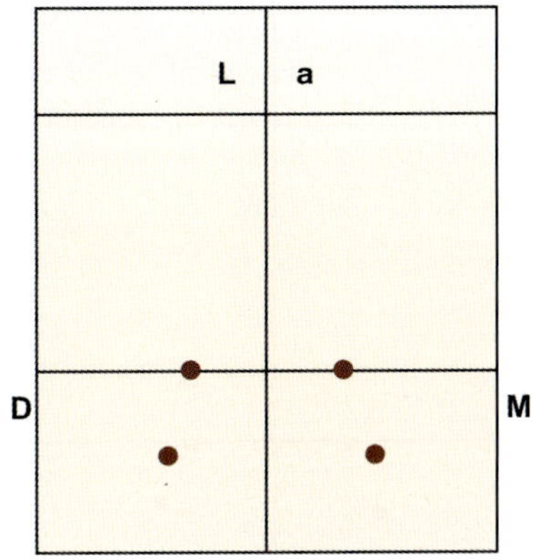

Fig. 3.7A: Step 2

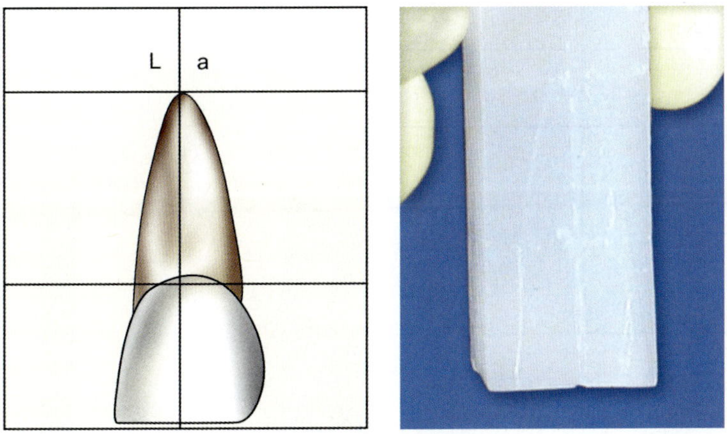

Fig. 3.7B: Step 3

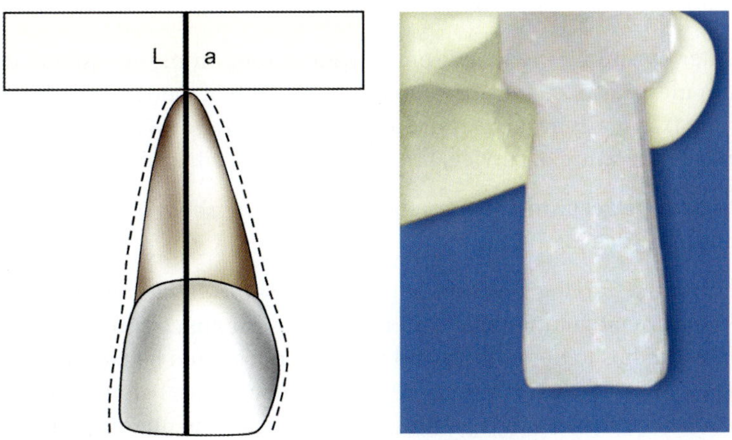

Fig. 3.7C: Step 4

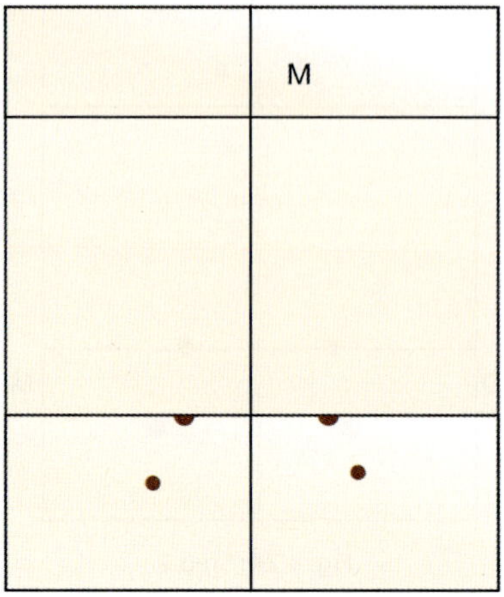

Fig. 3.7D: Step 6

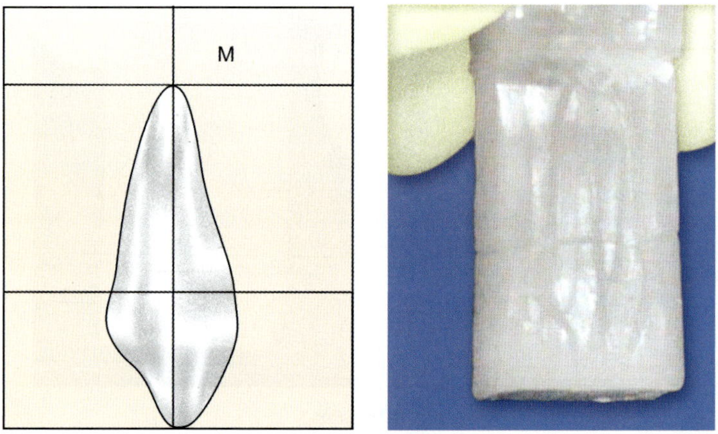

Fig. 3.7E: Step 6

Step 6: After extending the length of crown and root on mesial aspect, draw a midline on mesial aspect, mark the labiolingual width of crown and labiolingual width at cervix. Now draw the mesial outline (Figs 3.7D and 3.7E). Ensure that the root apex, the curvature of cervical line and the incisal edge fall in one line.

Step 7: Now carve according to mesial outline, leaving about 0.5 mm excess wax than the outline (See Fig. 3.7F).

Step 8: Turn the carving towards lingual aspect, the tooth will appear as in (Fig. 3.7G). Here cingulum width and the root width appear broader. Now the cingulum width has to be reduced and also the root should be tapered lingually from labial aspect (Fig. 3.7H). Carve the ridges and fossa just below the cingulum, carve a concavity (fossa) leaving about 1 mm of wax at the margins for marginal ridges and at the incisal ridge for linguoincisal ridge. Once the lingual fossa is

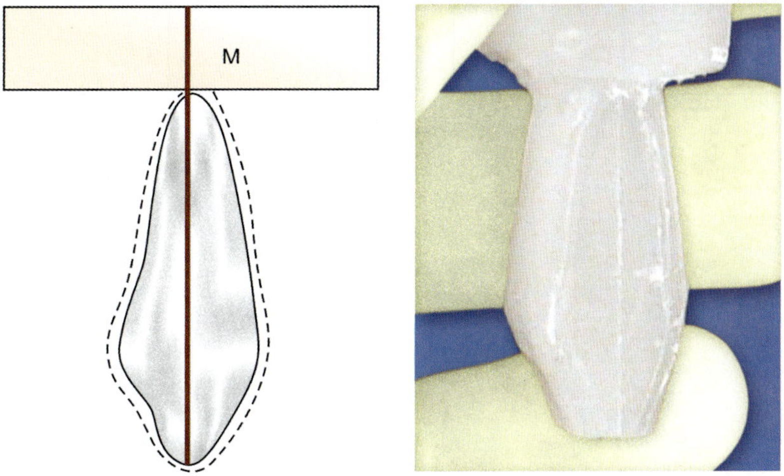

Fig. 3.7F: Step 7

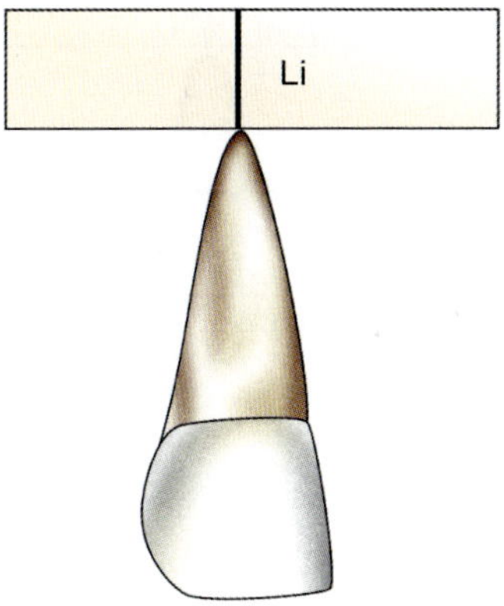

Fig. 3.7G: Step 8

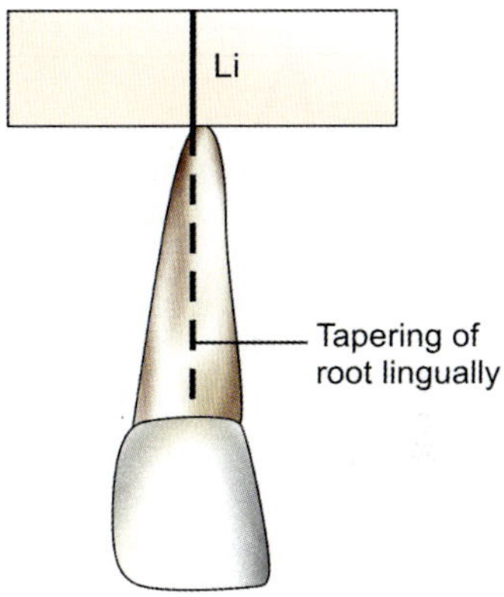

Fig. 3.7H: Step 8

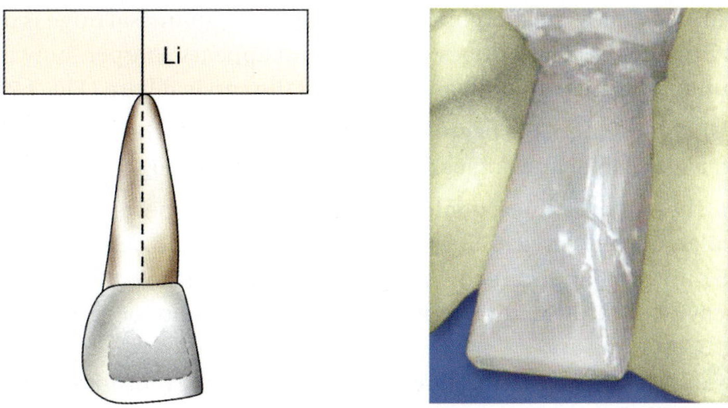

Fig. 3.7I: Step 8

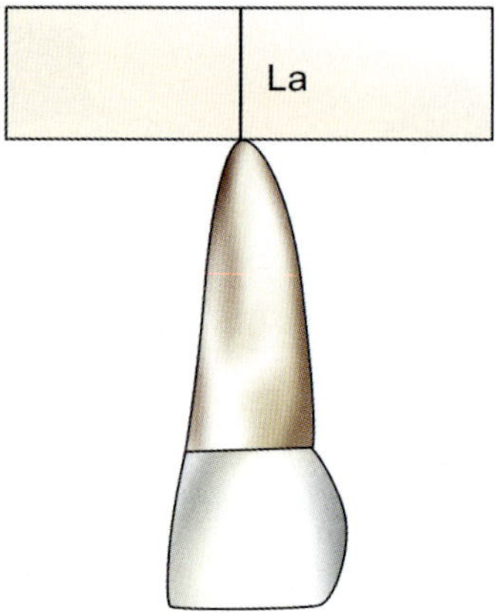

Fig. 3.7J: Step 9

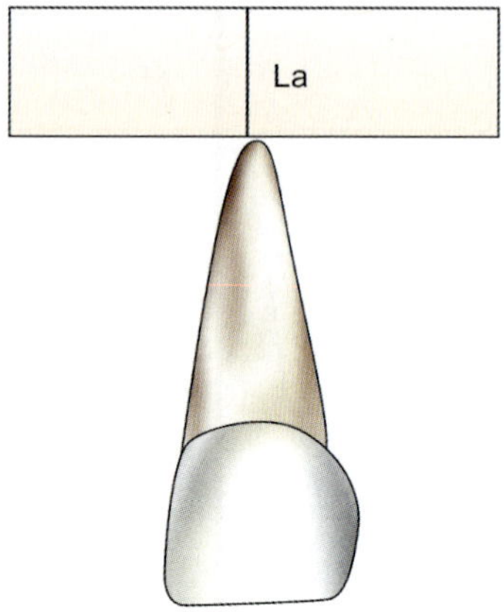

Fig. 3.7K: Step 10

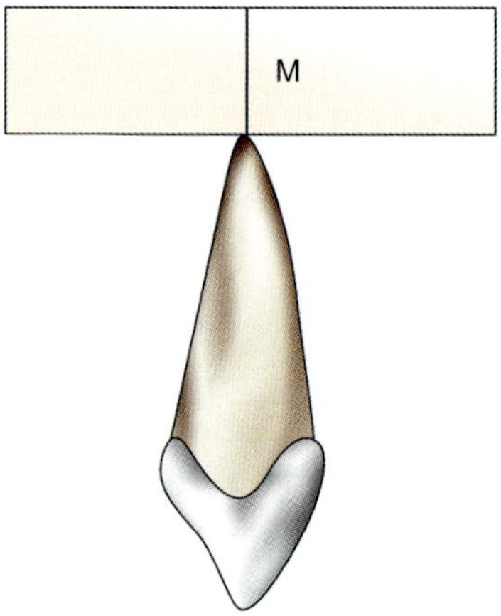

Fig. 3.7L: Step 10

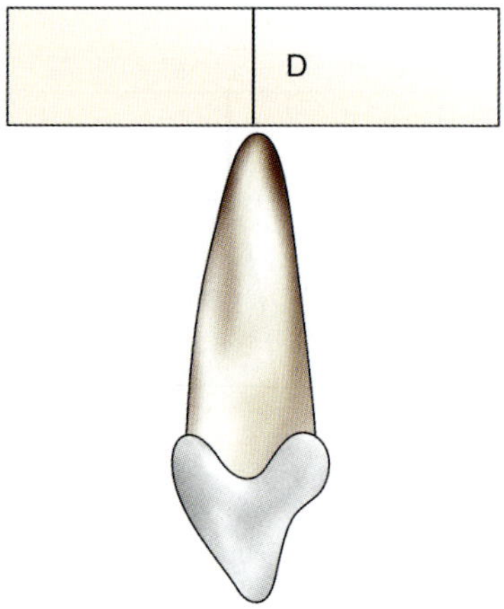

Fig. 3.7M: Step 10

carved, automatically the marginal ridges and the linguoincisal ridge is obtained. After carving the fossa and ridges the cingulum appears sharper, now round off the cingulum to appear smooth and convex at the cervical $^1/_3$rd (Fig. 3.7I).

Step 9: Once the lingual aspect is carved, turn towards the labial aspect then round off all the labial line angles of crown and root (See Fig. 3.7J).

Step 10: The cervical line should be drawn on all aspects. Labially draw a semicircular/curved cervical line (Fig. 3.7K). Mesially the curvature of cervical line is 3.5 mm (see Fig. 3.7L) showing the convexity facing toward the incisal edge and concavity toward the root apex. Distally the curvature of cervical line is 2.5 mm (Fig. 3.7M).

Lingually draw a curved cervical line, the convexity facing root apex and concavity toward the incisal ridge (Fig. 3.7N).

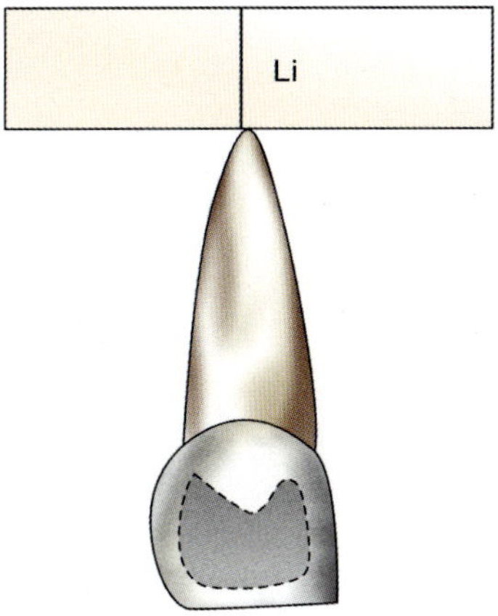

Fig. 3.7N: Step 10

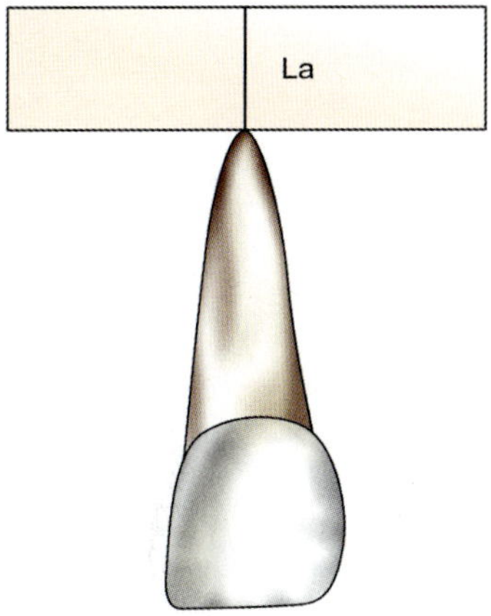

Fig. 3.7O: Step 12

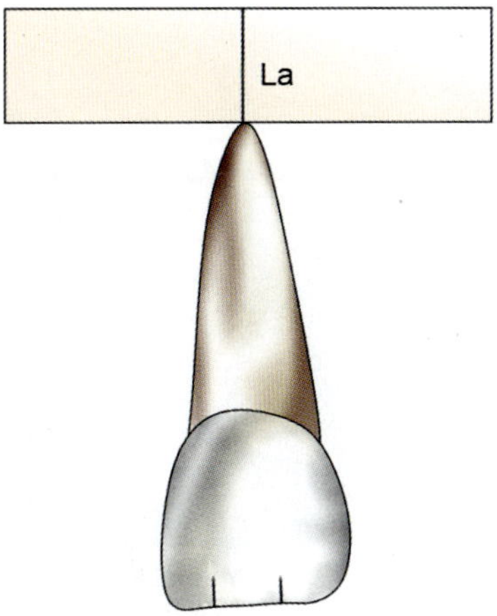

Fig. 3.7P: Step 12

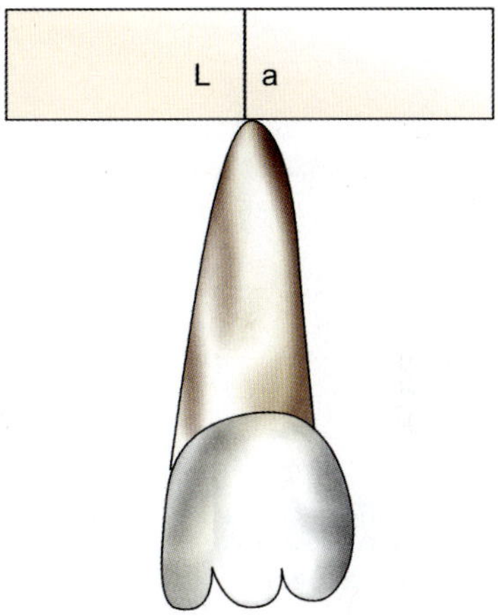

Fig. 3.7Q: Carved central incisor

Step 11: Finishing has to be done by removing the excess wax, complete tooth surface should be carved smooth.

Step 12: Carve the mamelons on the incisal ridge. To carve mamelons draw two equal vertical lines on the incisal $^1/_3$rd (Fig. 3.7O), deepen the two lines and round off the two lines. So as to appear as three rounded protuberances on the incisal ridge (Fig. 3.7P).

Step 13: Before polishing, the distoincisal angle should be rounded and the mesioincisal angle should be carved sharper. Polishing should be done according to the direction of carving otherwise by rough polishing the minor details of the tooth may be lost. Figures 3.7Q, 3.7R and 3.8 is a carved central incisor.

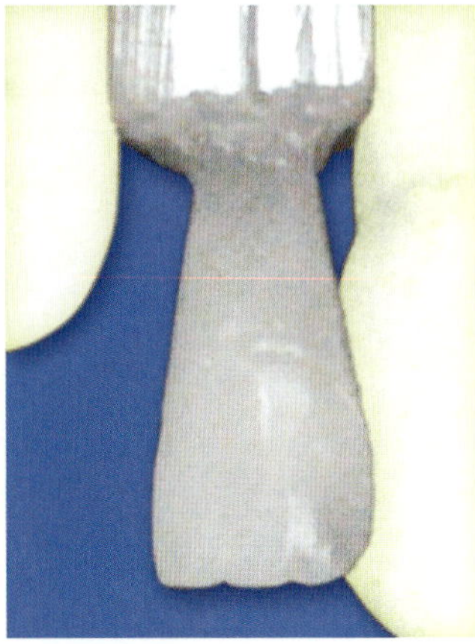

Fig. 3.7R: Step 13

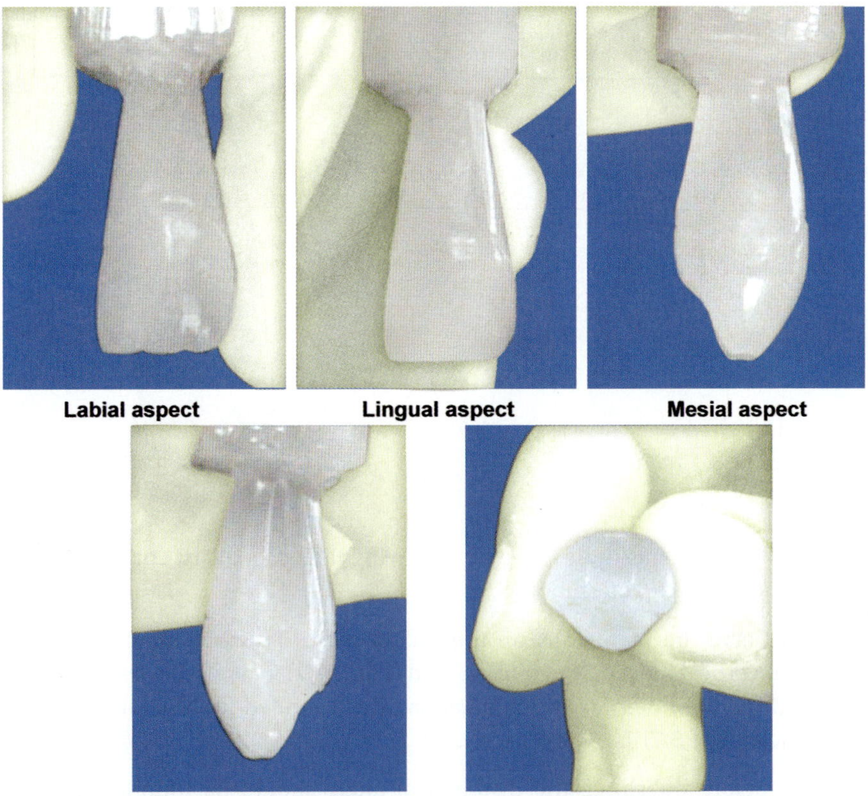

Fig. 3.8: Carved permanent mandibular canine

REFERENCES

1. Woelfel JB, Scheid RC. Dental Anatomy. Williams & Wilkins. 1997.
2. Ash, Nelson. Wheelers Dental Anatomy, Physiology & Occlusion. 8th edition. Elsevier. 2003.
3. Antonio Nanci. Ten Cate's Oral Histology. 6th edition. Elsevier. 2005.
4. www.wikipedia.com.

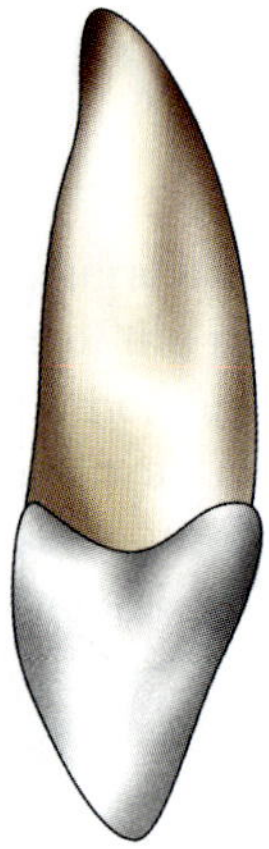

Fig. 3.12: Permanent maxillary left lateral incisor, distal aspect

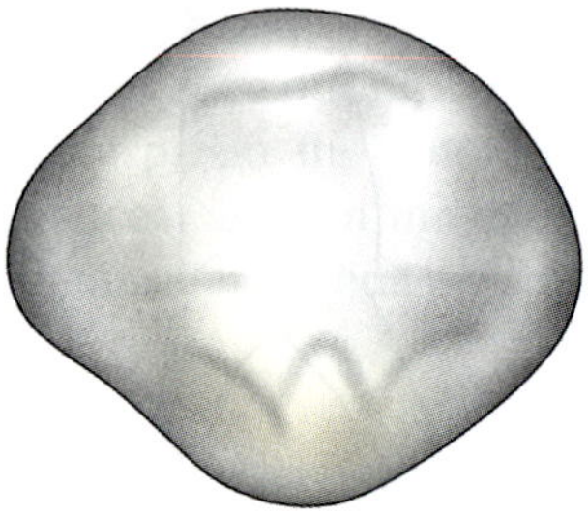

Fig. 3.13: Permanent maxillary left lateral incisor, incisal aspect

The differences from mesial aspect are:

a. Crown appears thicker distally because of the well development of the distal marginal ridge.
b. Curvature of cervical line is less by 1 mm than on the mesial aspect.
c. A developmental groove runs on the root distally throughout the length of the root.

Incisal Aspect[1,2] (Fig. 3.13)

Dimension: The labiolingual width is greater than the mesiodistal width.

Outline and Surface: The labial outline is more curved because of the convex labial surface, whereas the lingual outline shows concavity and convexity; the concavity is due to lingual fossa and convexity is due to cingulum. The incisal ridge is curved from incisal aspect.

Carving Technique

Measurements (in mm)

Cervico-incisal length of crown	-	9.0
Length of root	-	13.0
Mesiodistal diameter of crown	-	6.5
Mesiodistal diameter of crown at cervix	-	5.0
Labiolingual diameter of crown	-	6.0
Labiolingual diameter of crown at cervix	-	5.0
Curvature of cervical line - mesial	-	3.0
Curvature of cervical line - distal	-	2.0

The carving technique is similar to permanent maxillary central incisor. The morphology and measurements of permanent maxillary lateral incisor should be followed. The permanent incisors carving steps may be followed as illustrated diagrammatically in Figures 3.14A to 3.14K and 3.15.

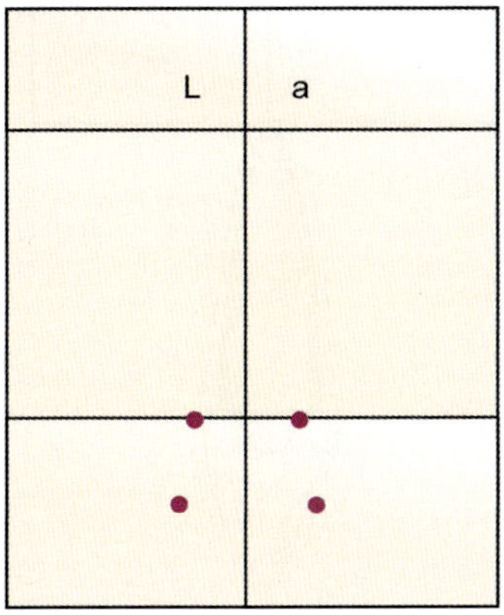

Fig. 3.14A: Step 1—Mark the length of crown, root, mesiodistal width of crown and at cervix

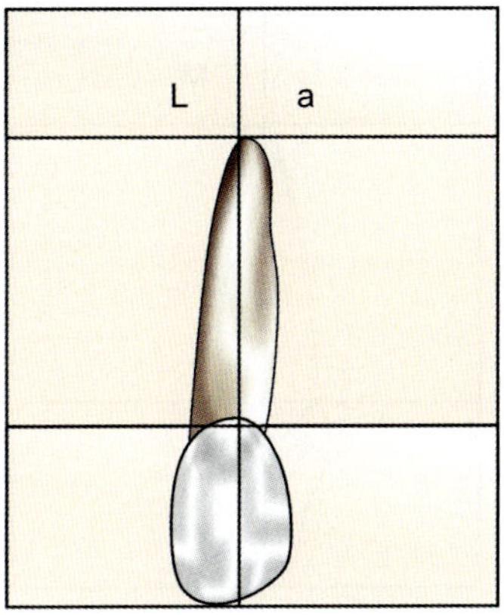

Fig. 3.14B: Step 2—Draw the labial outline

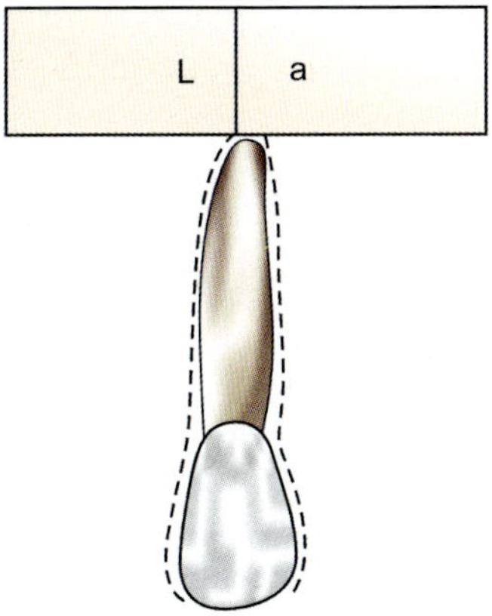

Fig. 3.14C: Step 3—Carve according to the labial outline leaving about 0.5 mm wax extra

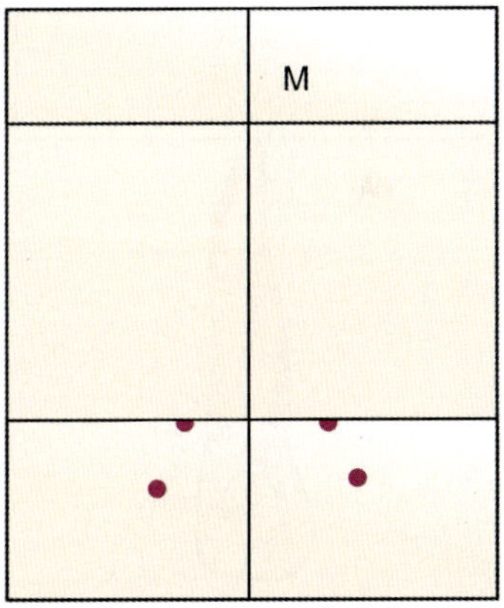

Fig. 3.14D: Step 4—Mark the labiolingual width of crown and labiolingual width at cervix on mesial aspect

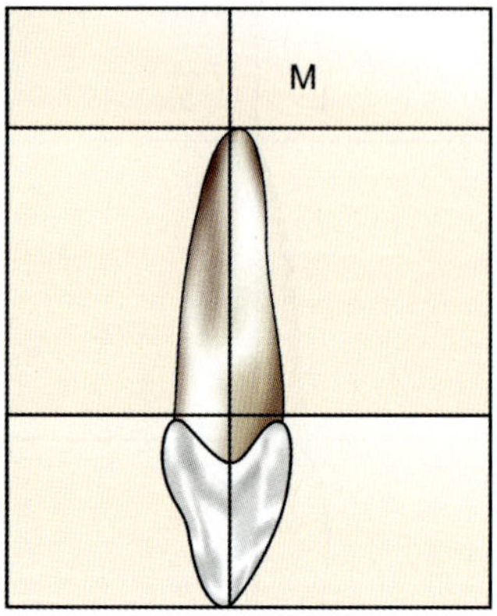

Fig. 3.14E: Step 5—Draw the mesial outline of crown and root

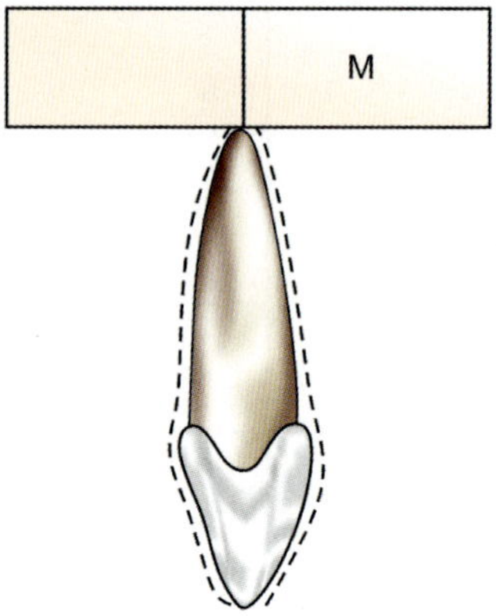

Fig. 3.14F: Step 6—Carve according to the outline leaving about 0.5 mm of wax extra

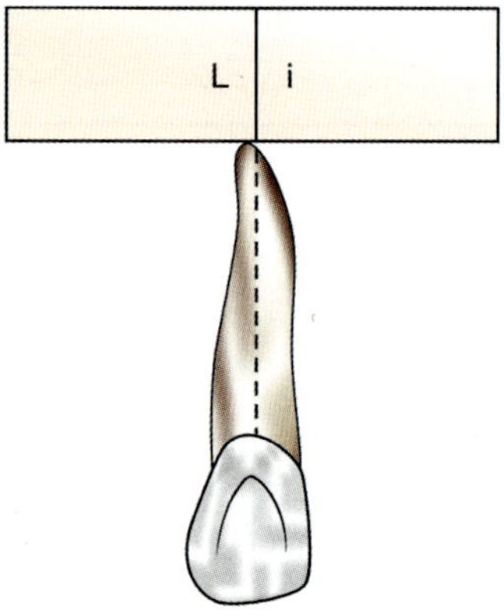

Fig. 3.14G: Step 7—Carve the cingulum, lingual fossa, lingual ridge, marginal ridges and taper the root lingually

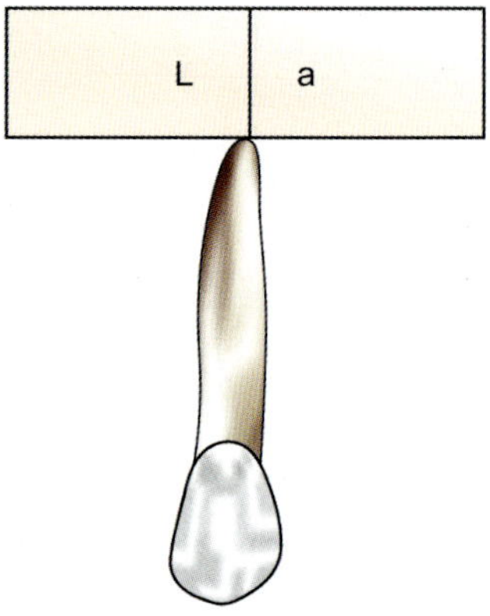

Fig. 3.14H: Step 8—Carve the incisal ridge, round off the labial line angles of crown and root

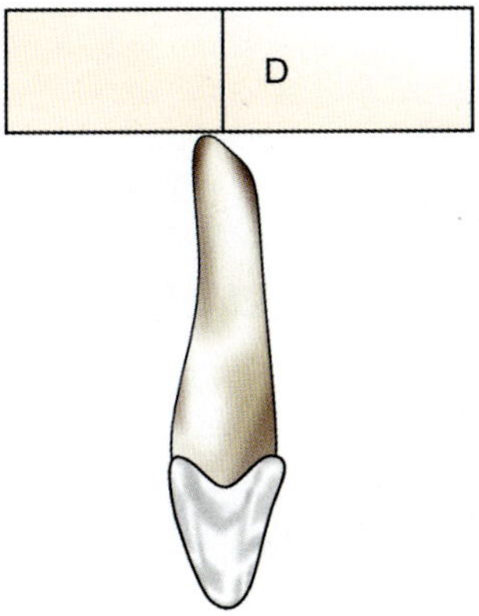

Fig. 3.14I: Step 9—Draw the cervical line on distal aspect

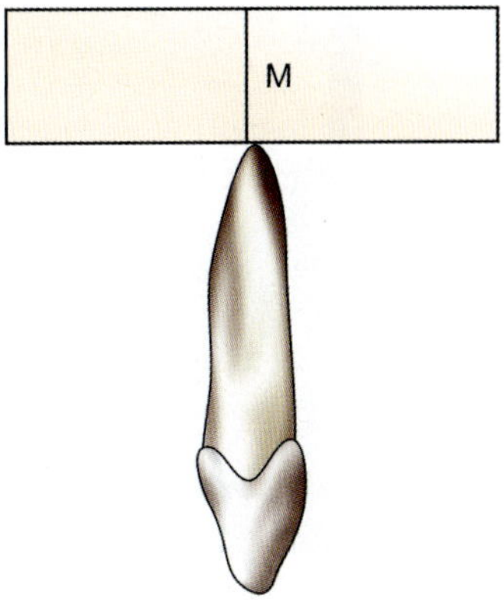

Fig. 3.14J: Step 10—Draw the cervical line on mesial aspect

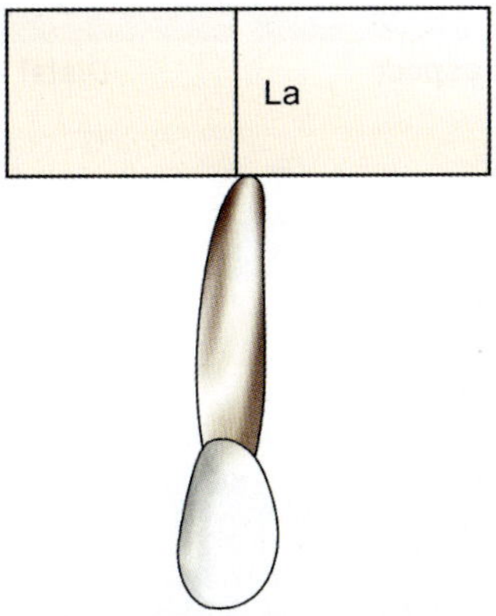

Fig. 3.14K: Carved permanent maxillary lateral incisor

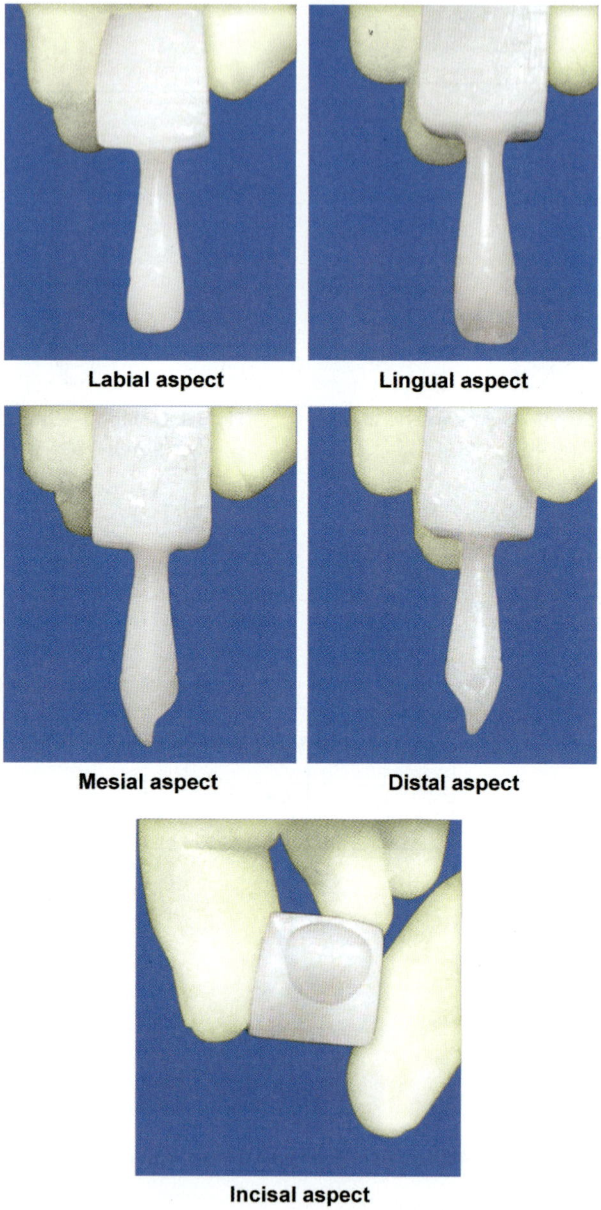

Fig. 3.15: Permanent maxillary lateral incisor

REFERENCES

1. Woelfel JB, Scheid RC. Dental Anatomy. Williams & Wilkins. 1997.
2. Ash, Nelson. Wheelers Dental Anatomy, Physiology & Occlusion. 8th edition. Elsevier. 2003.
3. www.wikipedia.com

THE PERMANENT MANDIBULAR CENTRAL INCISOR

Morphology

Labial Aspect[1,2] (Fig. 3.16)

Outline

Crown: The mesial outline of the labial aspect from mesioincisal angle drops straight down till the cervical line and is along with the mesial outline of the root. The mesioincisal angle is sharp. The distal outline of the labial aspect from distoincisal angle also drops straight down but near the cervical third a slight convergence is present toward the cervical line.

The cervical line curves—the convexity is present toward the incisal ridge.

The incisal outline is straight and is perpendicular to the long axis of the tooth. This is a characteristic feature of this tooth and serves as an identification feature.

Root: The mesial outline of the root is straight and distal outline curves slightly. Both the outlines gradually taper toward the root apex.

Surface

Crown: The cervical third of the crown shows convexity, the middle and incisal third is flat.

Root: Smooth surface and convexity is seen throughout the length of root.

Lingual Aspect[1,2] (Fig. 3.17)

Outline

The outline of the crown and root is similar to that of labial aspect.

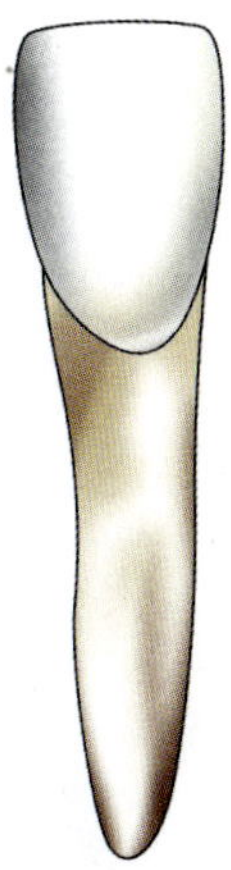

Fig. 3.16: Permanent mandibular right central incisor, labial aspect

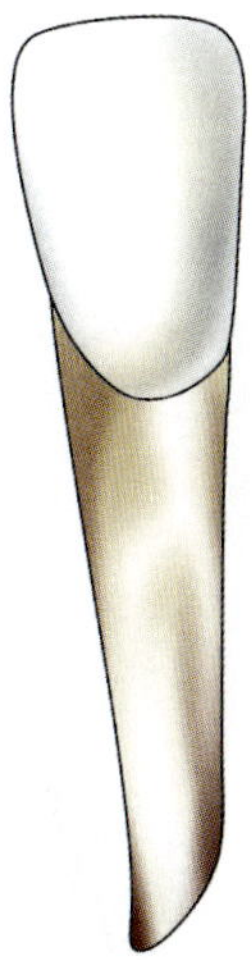

Fig. 3.17: Permanent mandibular right central incisor, lingual aspect

Surface
Both the crown and root taper toward the lingual aspect.

Crown: A less prominent cingulum is present at the cervical third of the crown. Marginal ridges are prominent at incisal third with a shallow lingual fossa present at the incisal third.

Root: Surface of the root is smooth and the root tapers lingually.

Mesial Aspect[1,2] (Fig. 3.18)

Outline
Crown: The labial outline at the cervical third is convex, the middle and incisal third is straight sloping rapidly till the incisal edge. The incisal edge is lingually placed. The cervical third of the lingual outline is slightly concave and incisal third is straight. The curvature of the cervical line is about 3.0 mm; the convexity facing the incisal edge and concavity is toward the root apex.

Root: The root outline is regular, uniform and straight toward a blunt root apex.

Surface
Crown: The surface of the crown is convex and smooth at the incisal third, flat at the middle third cervical to contact area.

Root: The root surface is broad and flat. Developmental depression is present with increased depth at the junction of middle and apical third of the root.

Distal Aspect[1,2] (Fig. 3.19)

Outline
The outline of the crown and root is similar to mesial aspect.

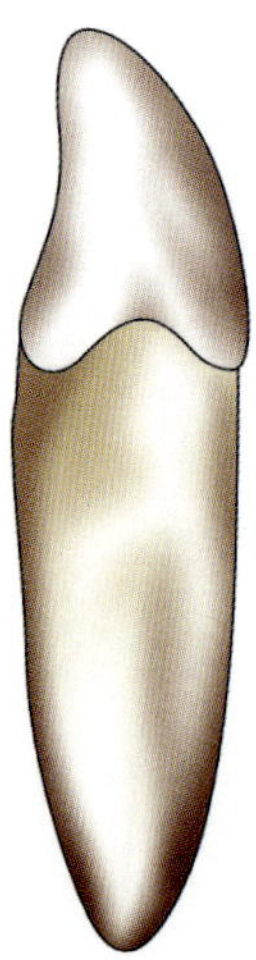

Fig. 3.18: Permanent mandibular right central incisor, mesial aspect

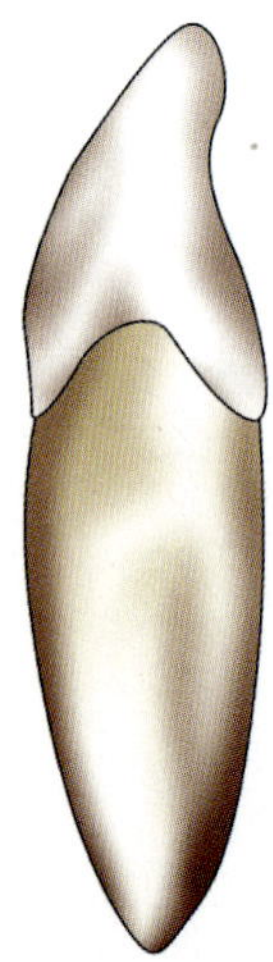

Fig. 3.19: Permanent mandibular right central incisor, distal aspect

Differences from mesial aspect are:

a. Curvature of cervical line is less by 1 mm than the mesial aspect.
b. Cervical third of crown surface shows slight concavity.
c. Developmental depression on the root surface is more deeper compared to the mesial aspect and also a developmental groove is present on this aspect.

Incisal Aspect[1,2] (Fig. 3.20)

Dimension: The labiolingual diameter is greater than the mesiodistal diameter of the crown. The labial portion is wider than the lingual portion mesiodistally. The lingual outline shows concavity and convexity.

The incisal ridge is straight and is perpendicular to the long axis of the tooth labiolingually which is the characteristic feature of this tooth.

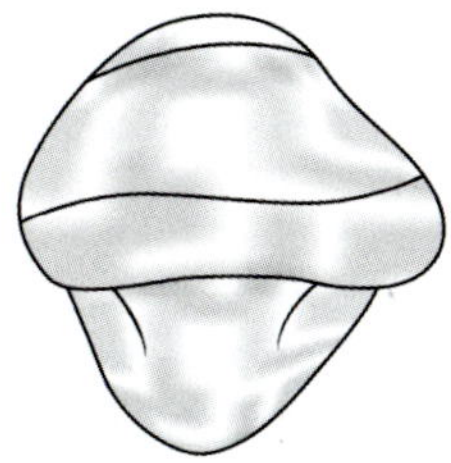

Fig. 3.20: Permanent mandibular right central incisor, incisal aspect

Carving Technique

Measurements (in mm)

Cervico-incisal length of crown	–	9.0
Length of root	–	12.5
Mesiodistal diameter of crown	–	5.0
Mesiodistal diameter of crown at cervix	–	3.5
Labiolingual diameter of crown	–	6.0
Labiolingual diameter of crown at cervix	–	5.3
Curvature of cervical line - mesial	–	3.0
Curvature of cervical line - distal	–	2.0

The technique of carving can be followed similar to permanent maxillary central incisor. The following diagrams illustrate the steps in carving (Figs 3.21A to 3.21K). Figure 3.22 is a carved mandibular central incisor.

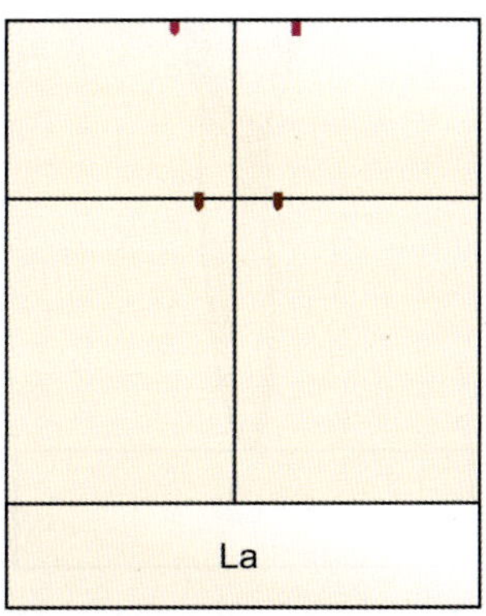

Fig. 3.21A: Step 1—Mark the length of crown, root, mesiodistal width of crown and at cervix

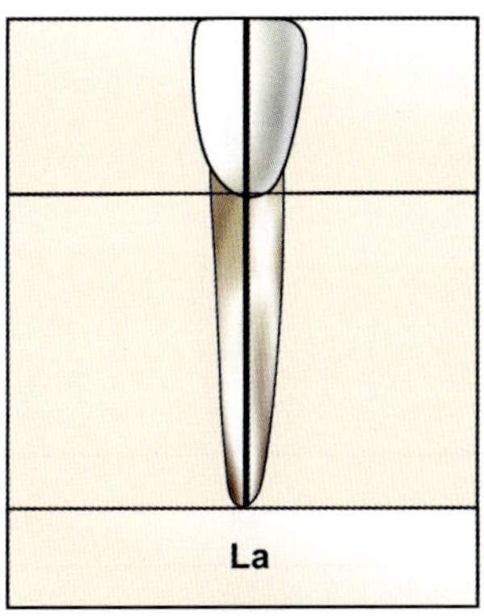

Fig. 3.21B: Step 2—Draw the labial outline

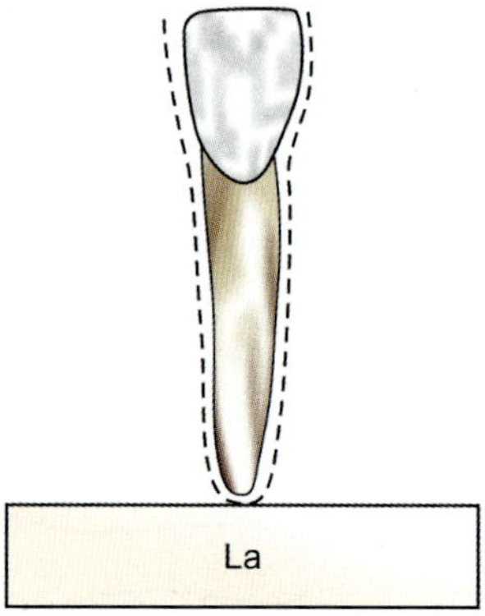

Fig. 3.21C: Step 3—Carve according to the labial outline leaving about 0.5 mm wax extra

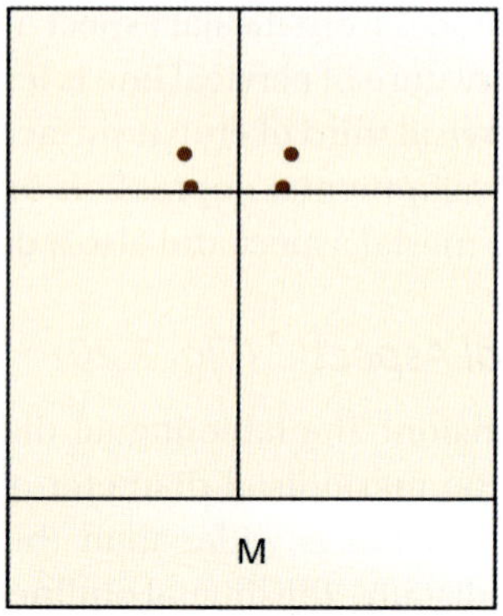

Fig. 3.21D: Step 4—Mark the labiolingual width of crown and labiolingual width at cervix on mesial aspect

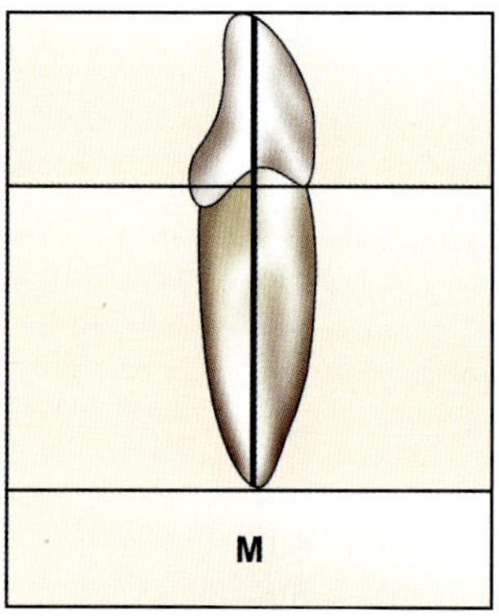

Fig. 3.21E: Step 5—Draw the mesial outline of crown and root

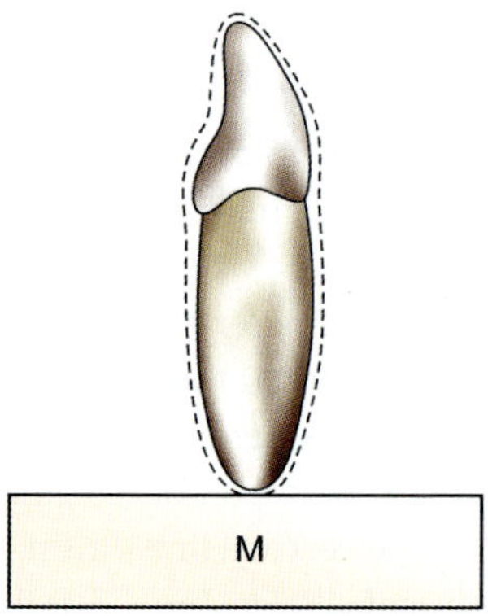

Fig. 3.21F: Step 6—Carve according to the outline leaving about 0.5 mm of wax extra

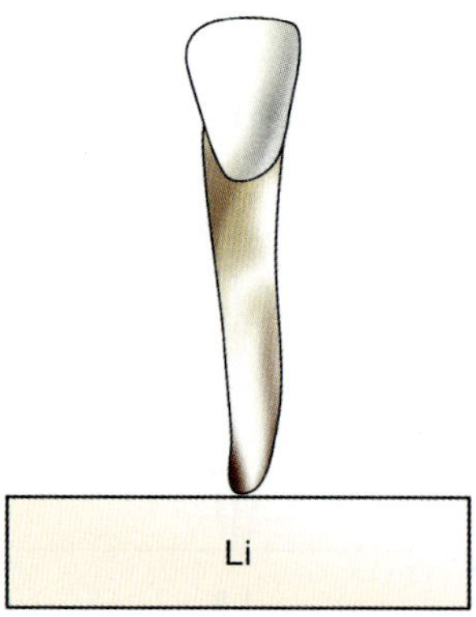

Fig. 3.21G: Step 7—Carve the cingulum, lingual fossa, lingual ridge, marginal ridges and taper the root lingually

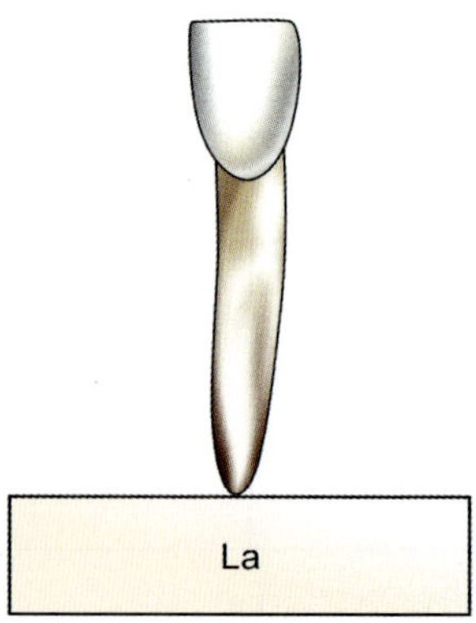

Fig. 3.21H: Step 8—Carve the incisal ridge, round off the labial line angles of crown and root

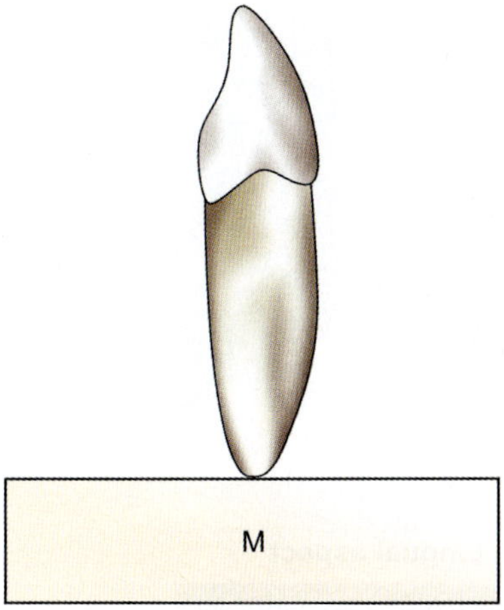

Fig. 3.21I: Step 9—Draw the cervical line on mesial aspect

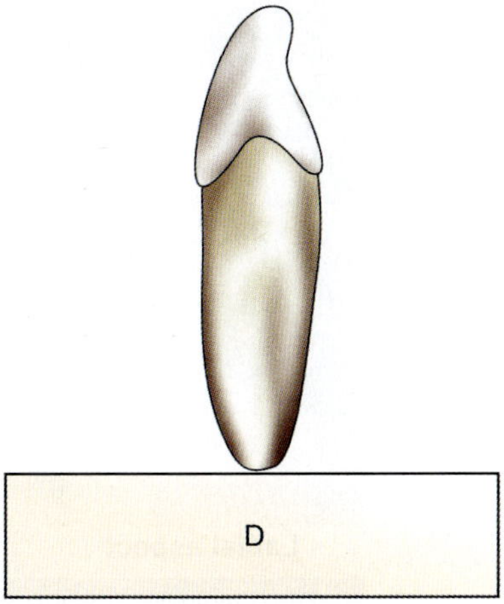

Fig. 3.21J: Step 10—Draw the cervical line on distal aspect

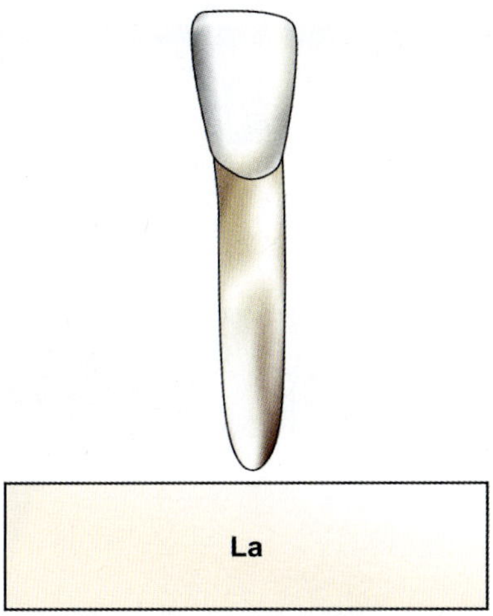

Fig. 3.21K: Carved permanent mandibular central incisor

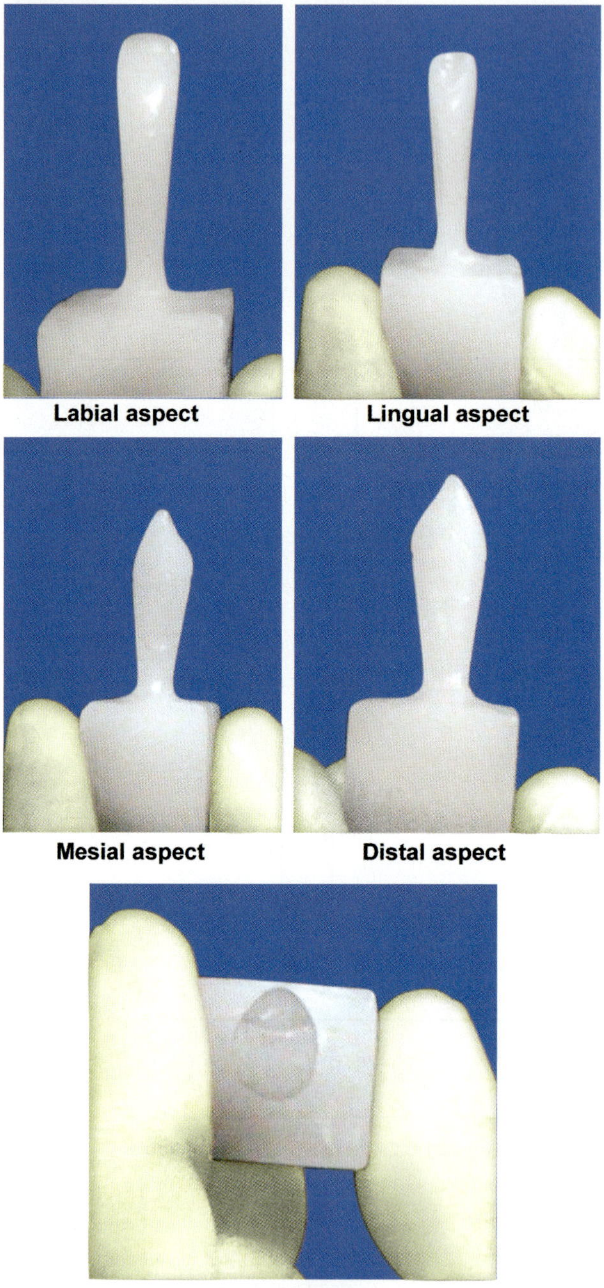

Fig. 3.22: Permanent mandibular central incisor

REFERENCES

1. Woelfel JB, Scheid RC. Dental Anatomy. Williams & Wilkins. 1997.
2. Ash, Nelson. Wheelers Dental Anatomy, Physiology & Occlusion. 8th edition. Elsevier. 2003.

THE PERMANENT MANDIBULAR LATERAL INCISOR

Morphology

Since the mandibular lateral incisor simulates the function of mandibular central incisor, the tooth closely resembles the mandibular central incisor except for some differences.[2]

Labial Aspect[1,2] (Fig. 3.23)

Outline

Crown: The mesial outline from cervical line till the mesioincisal angle is straight. The mesio-incisal angle is sharp. Mesial contact area is placed at the mesioincisal angle. The distal outline from cervical line; the cervical third is slightly concave, the middle third of distal outline is convex whereas the incisal third merges with the incisal outline, i.e. the incisal outline slopes downward toward the distal aspect in a cervical direction. The distal contact area is placed at the junction of middle and incisal third.

Root: The root gradually tapers toward the apex. The apex is distally tilted.

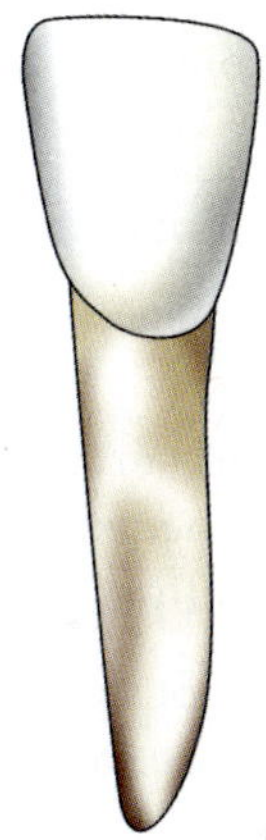

Fig. 3.23: Permanent mandibular left lateral incisor, labial aspect

Surface

Crown: The cervical third and middle third shows convexity.

Root: Root surface is smooth and convex.

Differences from permanent mandibular central incisor (Labial aspect):[2]

1. Incisal ridge in mandibular lateral incisor slopes downward toward the distal aspect in a cervical direction whereas the incisal ridge in mandibular central incisor is straight and perpendicular to the long axis of the tooth.
2. Distal contact area in mandibular lateral incisor is placed at the junction of middle and incisal third whereas in mandibular central incisor it is placed at the distoincisal angle.
3. Mesiodistal width of permanent mandibular lateral incisor is greater by 1 mm than the central incisor.

Lingual Aspect[1,2] (Fig. 3.24)

Outline: The outline of crown and root is similar to that of labial aspect.

Surface: Cervical third of the crown shows convexity, i.e. cingulum. Cingulum is not well developed as maxillary incisors. Marginal ridges are prominent at incisal third. A shallow concavity is seen at the incisal third, i.e. lingual fossa. The outlines and surfaces of the mandibular incisors are regular and symmetrical.

Mesial Aspect[1,2] (Fig. 3.25)

Outline

Crown: The cervical third of labial outline is convex. The middle and incisal third is straight sloping rapidly till the incisal edge. The incisal edge is lingually placed. The cervical third of lingual outline is slightly convex, middle third is slightly concave and the incisal third is straight. The curvature of cervical line is about 2 mm, the convexity is facing toward the incisal edge and concavity is toward the root apex.

Root: The root outline is regular, uniform and straight toward a blunt or pointed root end.

Surface

Crown: The surface of crown is convex and smooth at the incisal edge and becomes broader and flatter at the middle third cervical to contact area. Cervical third is slightly concave.

Root: The root surface is broad and flat. Developmental depression is present on the root surface and is deeper at the junction of middle and apical third.

Distal Aspect[1,2] (Fig. 3.26)

Outline: The outline of the crown and root is similar to mesial aspect.

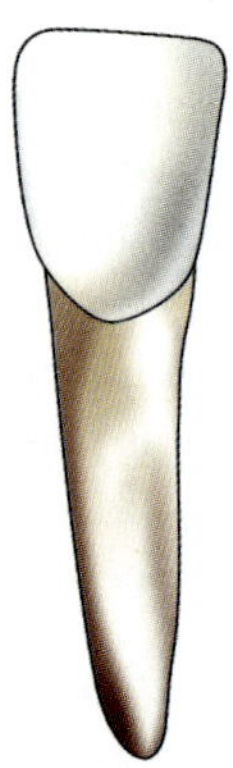

Fig. 3.24: Permanent mandibular left lateral incisor, lingual aspect

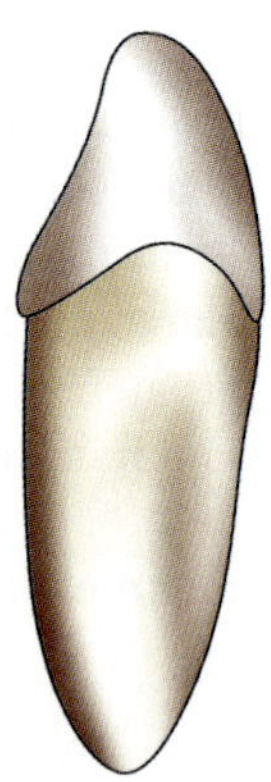

Fig. 3.25: Permanent mandibular left lateral incisor, mesial aspect

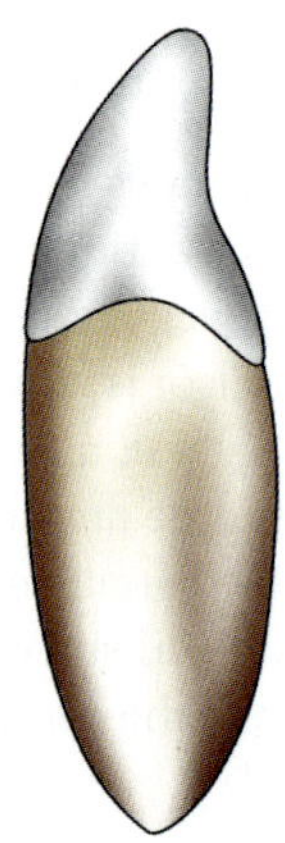

Fig. 3.26: Permanent mandibular left lateral incisor, distal aspect

Differences from mesial aspect are:

a. Distal side of the crown is shorter than the mesial side because of the sloping of the incisal ridge downwards toward the distal aspect in a cervical direction.
b. Distal contact area is placed more cervically.
c. Curvature of cervical line is less by 1 mm than the mesial aspect.
d. Developmental depression on the root surface is more deeper with a developmental groove.

Incisal Aspect[1,2] (Fig. 3.27)

Dimension: The labiolingual diameter is greater than the mesiodistal diameter. The labial outline is wider mesiodistally than the lingual outline. The lingual outline shows concavity.

Difference from permanent mandibular central incisor:[2]

The incisal edge is not at approximate right angles to a line bisecting the crown labiolingually from incisal aspect.

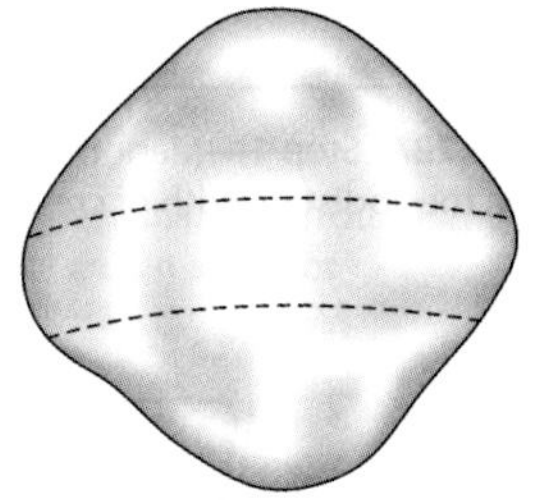

Fig. 3.27: Permanent mandibular left lateral incisor, incisal aspect

Carving Technique

Measurements (in mm)

Cervico-incisal length of crown	-	9.5
Length of root	-	14
Mesiodistal diameter of crown	-	5.5
Mesiodistal diameter of crown at cervix	-	4.0
Labiolingual diameter of crown	-	6.5
Labiolingual diameter of crown at cervix	-	5.8
Curvature of cervical line - mesial	-	3.0
Curvature of cervical line - distal	-	2.0

The technique for mandibular lateral incisor is similar to permanent maxillary central incisor but the dimensions and morphology should be followed. The following diagrams illustrate the steps in carving (Figs 3.28A to 3.28K). Figure 3.29 is a carved mandibular lateral incisor.

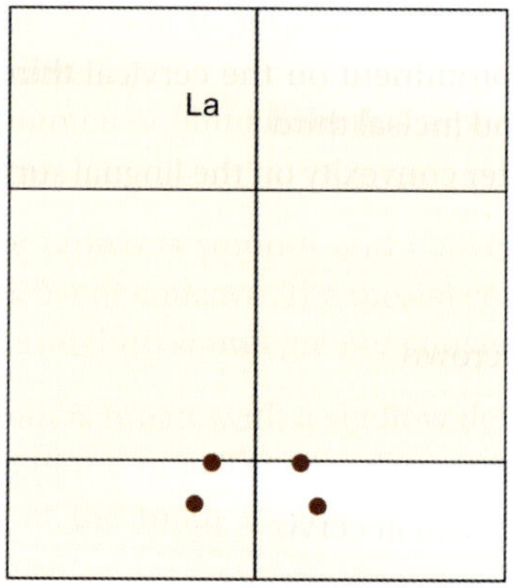

Fig. 4.6A: Step 1

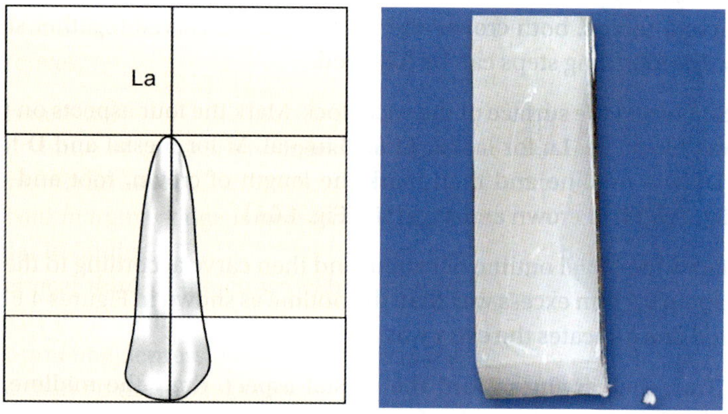

Fig. 4.6B: Step 2

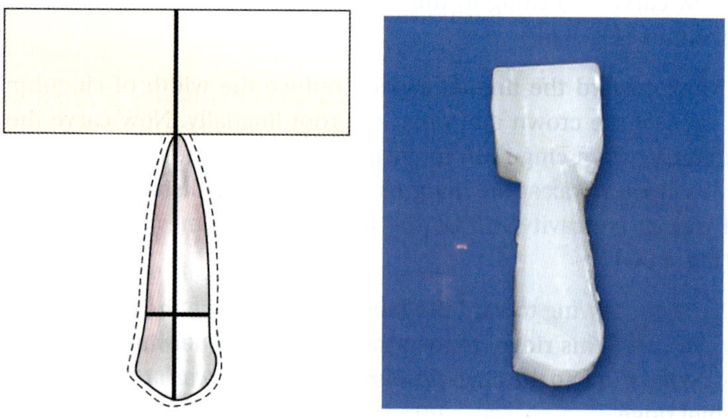

Fig. 4.6C: Step 2

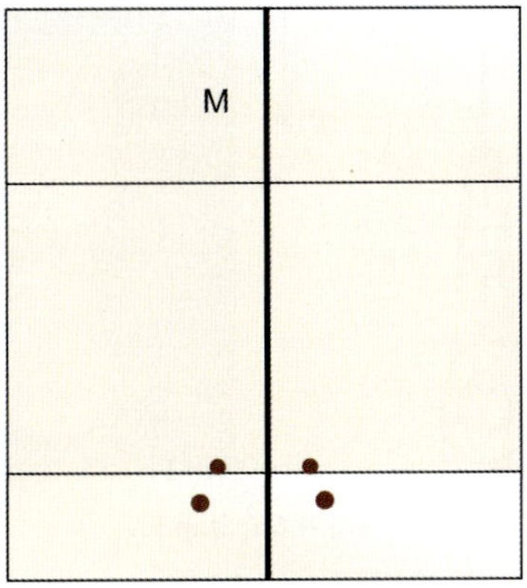

Fig. 4.6D: Step 3

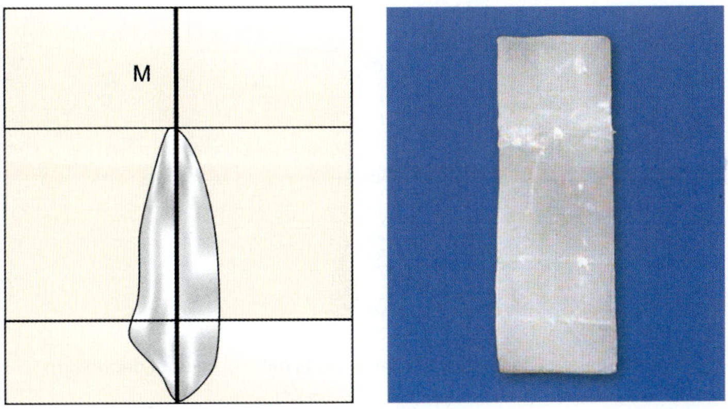

Fig. 4.6E: Step 3

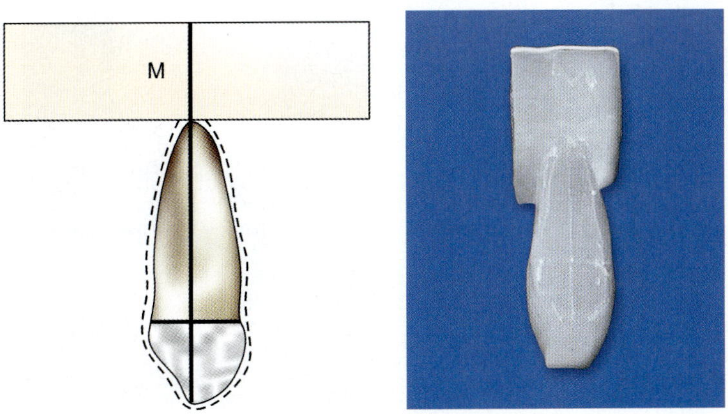

Fig. 4.6F: Step 4

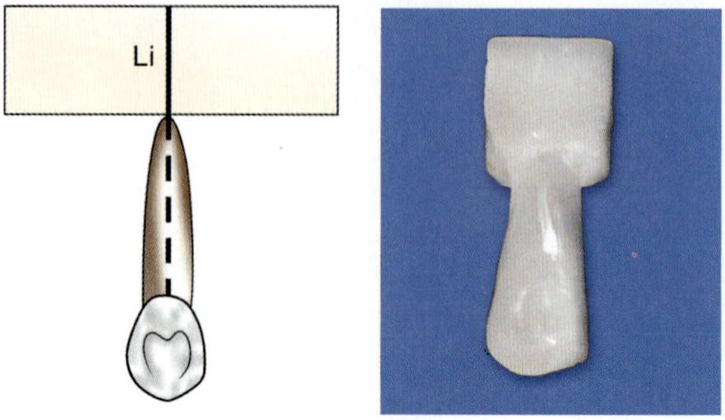

Fig. 4.6G: Step 5

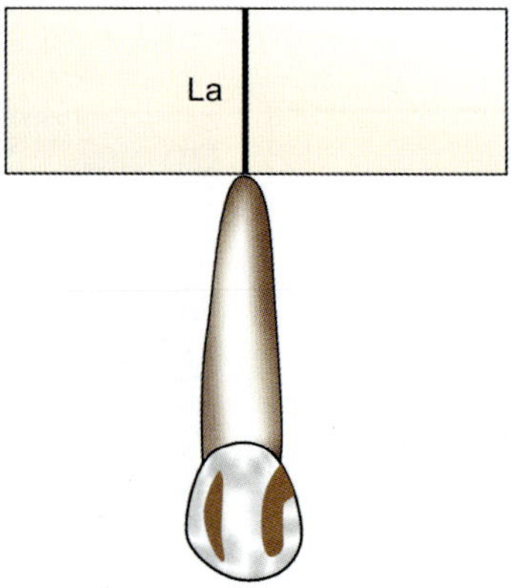

Fig. 4.6H: Step 6—shaded part represents developmental depression

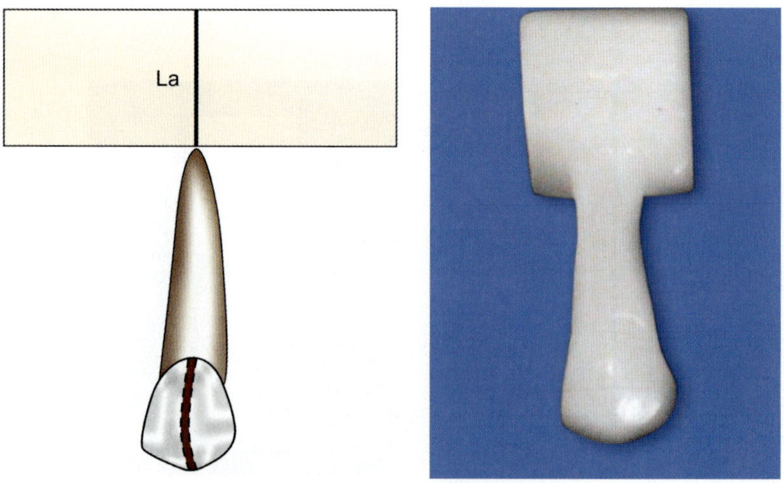

Fig. 4.7: Carved permanent maxillary canine

Deepen the wax lateral to the labial ridge, which will be the developmental depressions on the labial surface (Fig. 4.6H).

Draw the cervical line on all the aspects. For curvature of cervical line on mesial aspect, mark 2.5 mm and for curvature of cervical line on distal aspect, mark 1.5 mm. Keep a note on the mesial and distal contact area.

Step 7: Carve out any excess wax after measuring the dimensions again. Round off the labial line angles of crown and root. Extend the distal developmental depression of labial surface to cervical third surface of distal aspect. After this, do polishing with a pellet of cotton following the carving to avoid loss of the carved features (Fig. 4.7).

REFERENCES

1. Woelfel JB, Scheid RC. Dental Anatomy. Williams & Wilkins. 1997.
2. Ash, Nelson. Wheelers Dental Anatomy, Physiology & Occlusion. 8th edition. Elsevier. 2003.

THE PERMANENT MANDIBULAR CANINE

Since, the function is similar to permanent maxillary canine, morphology of permanent mandibular canine has close resemblance to maxillary canine.[2] The difference between every aspect is described.

Labial Aspect[1,2] (Fig. 4.8)

a. The mesiodistal dimension of mandibular canine is less by 1 mm than the maxillary canine.
b. The crown length is greater by 1 mm.
c. The mesial outline is straight along with the mesial outline of the root.
d. The mesial contact area is at mesioincisal angle.
e. Both the cusp ridges are straight, the distal cusp ridge being longer.
f. The distal contact area is present below the distoincisal angle.
g. The crown of mandibular canine appears to be bent over the root base.
h. The curvature of cervical line is similar to maxillary canine, i.e. the convexity is toward the root apex and concavity is toward the cusp tip.
i. The root length is less by 1 mm and the root apex is more pointed than the maxillary canine.
j. The labial ridge is thin, straight and extends from cusp tip to middle of cervical line.
k. The cusp tip of mandibular canine is more pointed than the maxillary canine.

Lingual Aspect[1,2] (Fig. 4.9)

The crown and root outline is similar to the labial aspect. The differences from maxillary canine are:
a. The crown and root tapering is more.
b. Cingulum is less prominent and smooth.
c. Marginal ridges are less pronounced.
d. Lingual fossa is shallow and is visible at the incisal third.
e. The lingual ridge is confined to the cusp tip of the crown.

Mesial Aspect[1,2] (Fig. 4.10)

Outline

Crown: The labial outline is less curved, i.e. the cervical third shows slight convexity. The lingual outline is similar to maxillary canine but is less prominent. The cusp tip is almost centered over the root. The curvature of cervical line is similar to maxillary canine.

Root: The root outline is similar to maxillary canine with a more pointed root apex.

Surface

Crown: The labiolingual width at the cervical third is less and appears thin compared to maxillary canine. The surface of the crown is more flat than the maxillary canine.

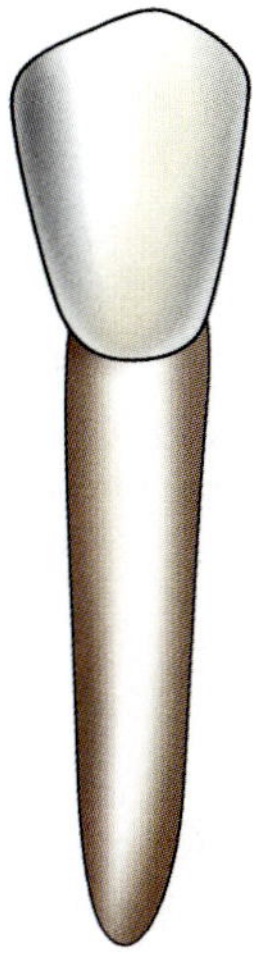

Fig. 4.8: Permanent mandibular right canine, labial aspect

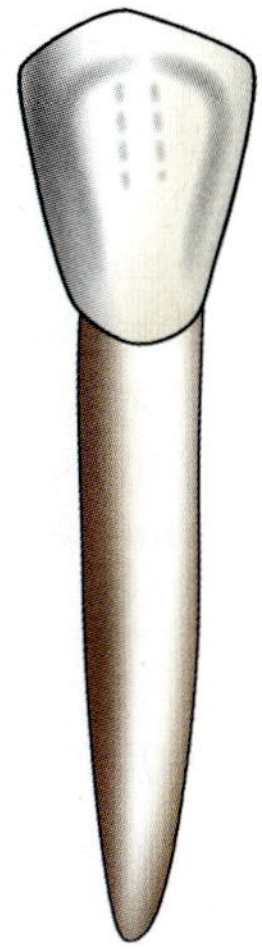

Fig. 4.9: Permanent mandibular right canine, lingual aspect

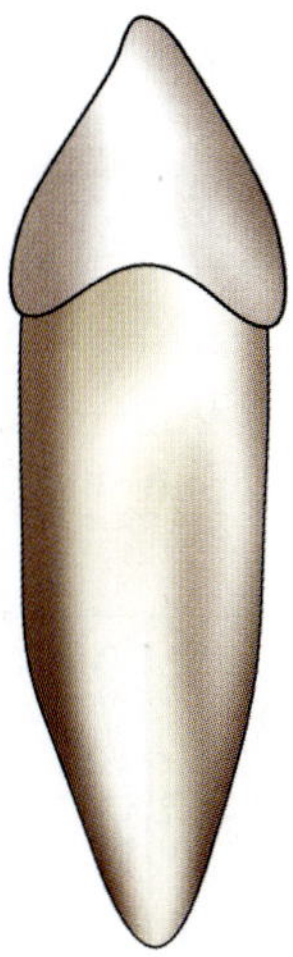

Fig. 4.10: Permanent mandibular right canine, mesial aspect

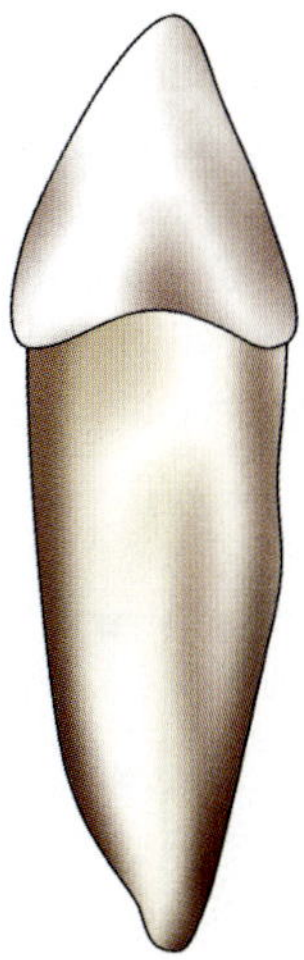

Fig. 4.11: Permanent mandibular right canine, distal aspect

Root: The developmental depression on the root is more deeper than the maxillary canine.

Distal Aspect[1,2] (Fig. 4.11)

The outline and surface of the crown and root is similar to mesial aspect. No marked difference is seen, except for the curvature of cervical line which is less by 1 mm and developmental depression on the root surface is much deeper than on the mesial aspect.

Incisal Aspect[1,2] (Fig. 4.12)

The incisal outline of mandibular canine is similar to maxillary canine, i.e. the labial outline is curved and the lingual outline shows convexity and concavity. The labiolingual width is greater than mesiodistal width.

It differs from the maxillary canine such that the cusp tip and mesial cusp ridges are lingually placed.

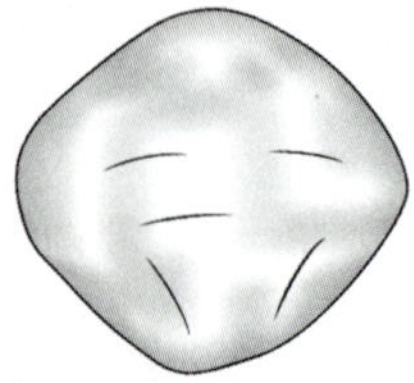

Fig. 4.12: Permanent mandibular right canine, incisal aspect

Carving Technique

The carving technique may be followed similar to that of maxillary canine. The following diagrams illustrate the steps in carving (Fig. 4.13A to 4.13I). Figure 4.14 is a carved permanent mandibular canine.

Measurements (in mm)

Cervico-incisal length of crown	–	11.0
Length of root	–	16.0
Mesiodistal diameter of crown	–	7.0
Mesiodistal diameter of crown at cervix	–	5.5
Labiolingual diameter of crown	–	7.5
Labiolingual diameter of crown at cervix	–	7.0
Curvature of cervical line - mesial	–	2.5
Curvature of cervical line - distal	–	1.0

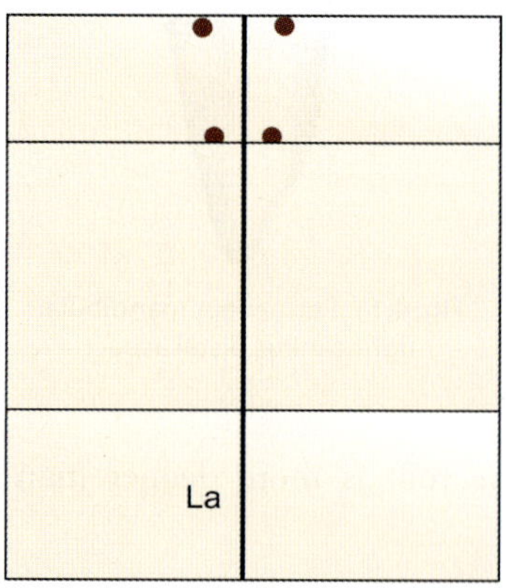

Fig. 4.13A: Step 1—Mark the crown length, root length, mesiodistal width of crown and at cervix

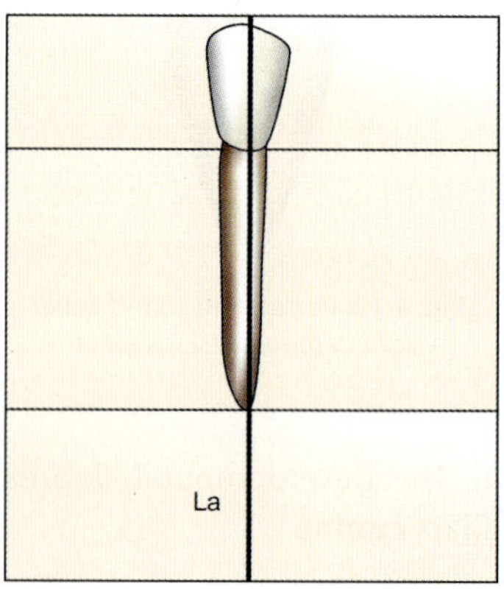

Fig. 4.13B: Step 2—Draw the labial outline

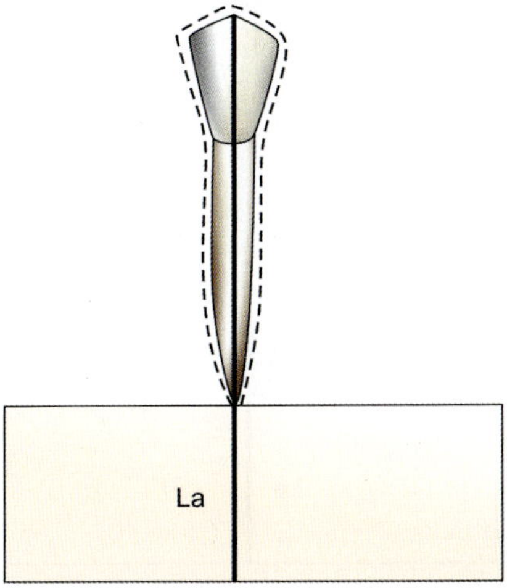

Fig. 4.13C: Step 3—Carve according to the labial outline leaving about 0.5 mm wax extra

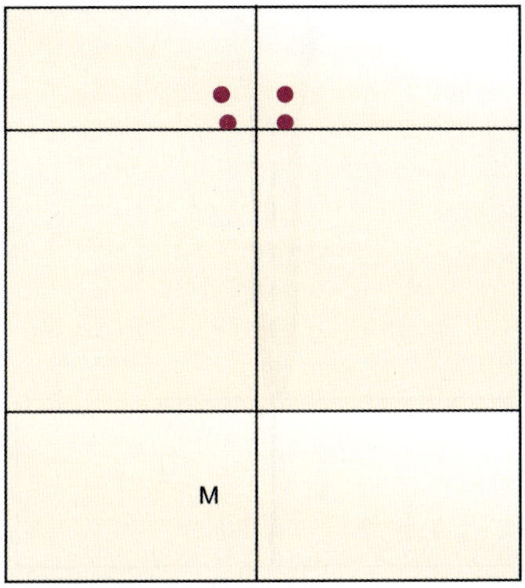

Fig. 4.13D: Step 4—Mark the labiolingual width of crown and labiolingual width at cervix on mesial aspect

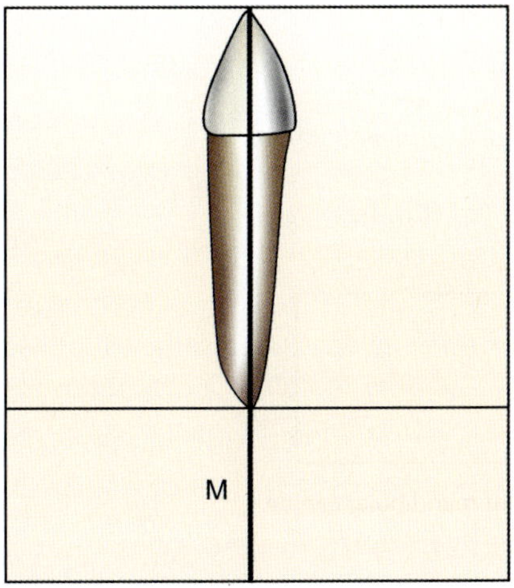

Fig. 4.13E: Step 5—Draw the mesial outline of crown and root

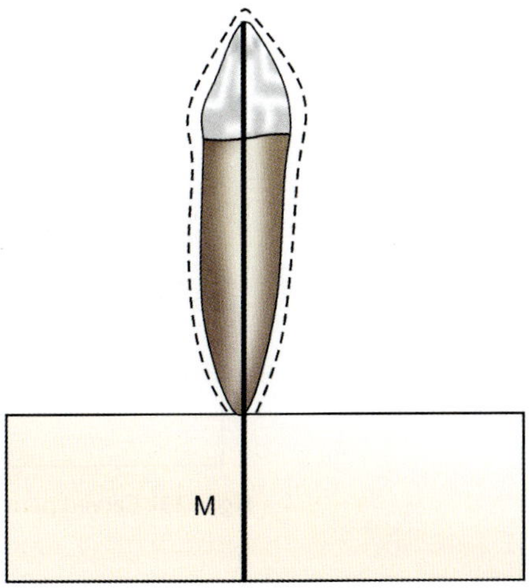

Fig. 4.13F: Step 6—Carve according to the outline leaving about 0.5 mm of wax extra

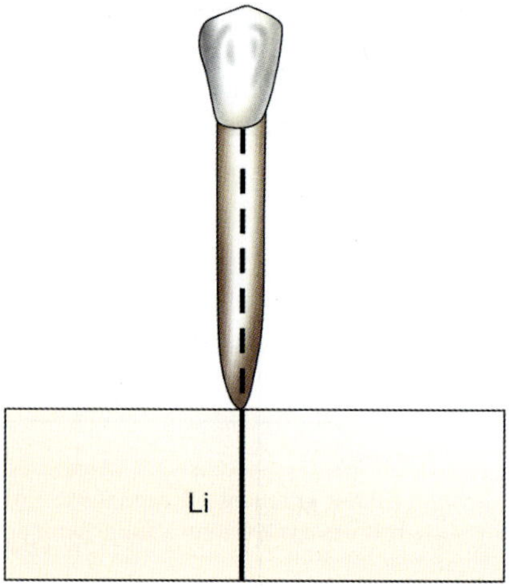

Fig. 4.13G: Step 7—Carve the cingulum, lingual fossa, lingual ridge, marginal ridges and taper the root lingually

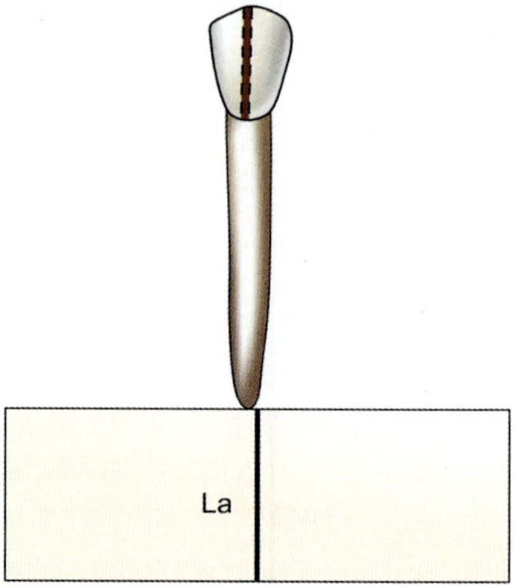

Fig. 4.13H: Step 8—Carve the labial ridge, round off the labial line angles of crown and root

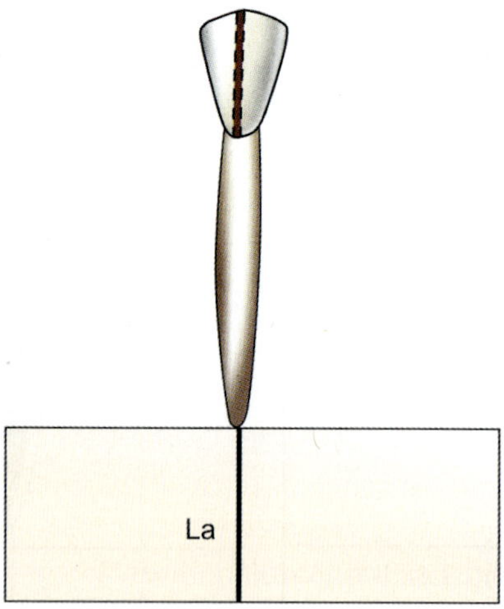

Fig. 4.13I: Carved permanent mandibular canine

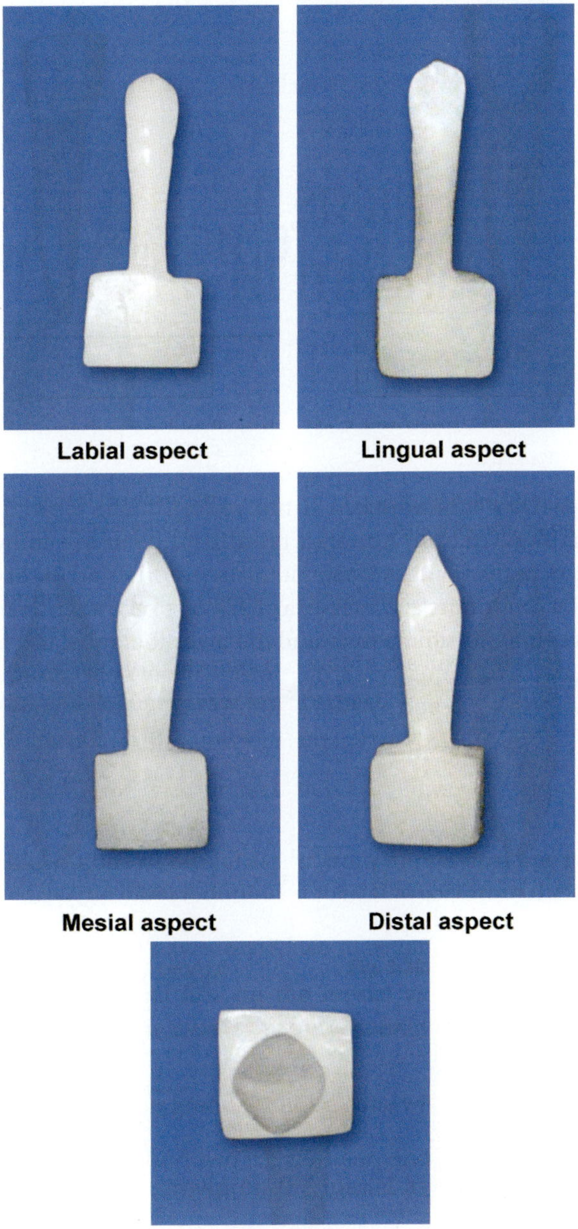

Fig. 4.14: Permanent mandibular canine

REFERENCES

1. Woelfel JB, Scheid RC. Dental Anatomy. Williams & Wilkins. 1997.
2. Ash, Nelson. Wheelers Dental Anatomy, Physiology & Occlusion. 8th edition. Elsevier. 2003.
3. www.wikipedia.com

CHAPTER

5

The Permanent Premolars

The **premolar** teeth or **bicuspids** are transitional teeth located between the canine and molar teeth.[1-3] In humans, there are two premolars per quadrant, making eight premolars total in the mouth.[3]

The premolars in humans are the maxillary first premolar, maxillary second premolar, mandibular first premolar, and the mandibular second premolar.[3]

THE PERMANENT MAXILLARY FIRST PREMOLAR

The **maxillary first premolar** is located laterally from both the maxillary canines of the oral cavity but mesial from both maxillary second premolars.[2] The function of this premolar is similar to that of canines in regard to tearing being the principal action during mastication. There are two cusps on maxillary first premolars, and the buccal cusp is sharp enough to resemble the prehensile teeth found in carnivorous animals.[3]

Morphology

The other synonym for this tooth is biscuspid teeth because of presence of two cusps. Maxillary first premolar develops from four lobes: three lobes for buccal cusp and one lobe for lingual cusp.

Buccal Aspect[1,2] (Fig. 5.1)

Outline

Crown: The shape of the crown is trapezoidal outline. The mesial outline is slightly concave at the cervical third. The middle third is convex, from here the outline is continuous with the mesial slope. The mesial slope is long and straight, sometimes it can be concave. The mesial contact area is placed occlusal to half of the crown length. The distal outline from the cervical line is straight. At the cervical third of the crown middle third shows convexity, from here the outline is continous with the distal slope. The distal slope is short and curved. The distal contact area is placed at same level as the mesial contact area, i.e. occlusal to half the crown length, but has a broader contact area.

The buccal cusp is longer than the lingual cusp. The curvature of cervical line shows convexity facing the root apex and concavity toward the cusp tip.

Root: The root outline gradually tapers toward a pointed root apex.

Surface

Crown: The buccal surface is convex. The middle buccal lobe is well developed giving rise to the buccal ridge. Adjacent to buccal ridge developmental depressions are seen mesially and distally.

Root: The root surface is convex and smooth throughout the length of root.

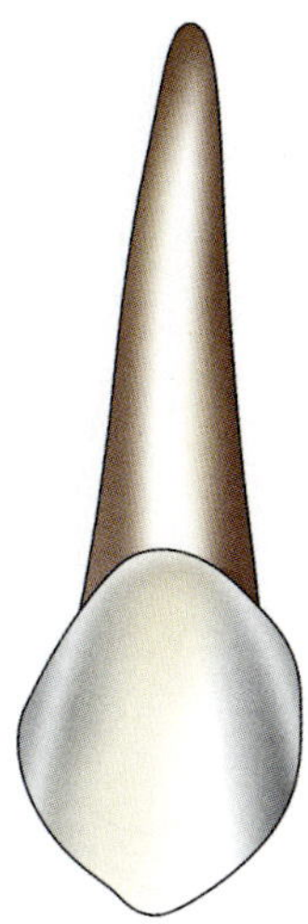

Fig. 5.1: Permanent maxillary right first premolar, buccal aspect

Lingual Aspect[1,2] *(Fig. 5.2)*

This outline is reverse of the buccal aspect.

Outline

Crown: Since the crown and root taper toward the lingual aspect and also the lingual cusp is shorter by 1 mm than the buccal cusp, part of the crown and root is seen from lingual aspect.

The mesial and distal outlines of lingual cusp is convex and are continuous with the mesial slope and distal slope. The cusp tip is more pointed than the buccal cusp tip. The cervical line is regular with slight convexity towards the root.

Root: The lingual outline of the root is regular and gradually tapers toward the blunt root apex.

Surface: The surface of the crown and root on the lingual aspect is more convex and smooth.

Mesial Aspect[1,2] *(Fig. 5.3)*

The crown from mesial aspect is trapezoidal in shape. Two cusps and two roots are seen from this aspect.

Outline

Crown: The buccal outline is convex from cervical line to the buccal cusp tip. Maximum convexity is located at the junction of cervical and middle third. The buccal cusp tip is located below the center of the buccal root. The lingual outline is smoothly convex from cervical line to the cusp tip. Crest of curvature is present at the center of middle third. The lingual cusp tip is in line with the lingual border

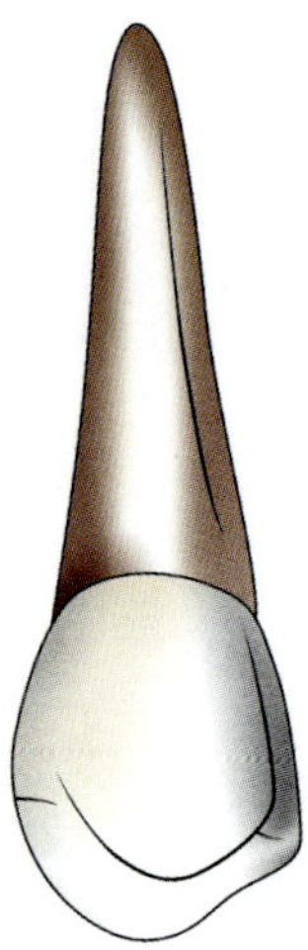

Fig. 5.2: Permanent maxillary right first premolar, lingual aspect

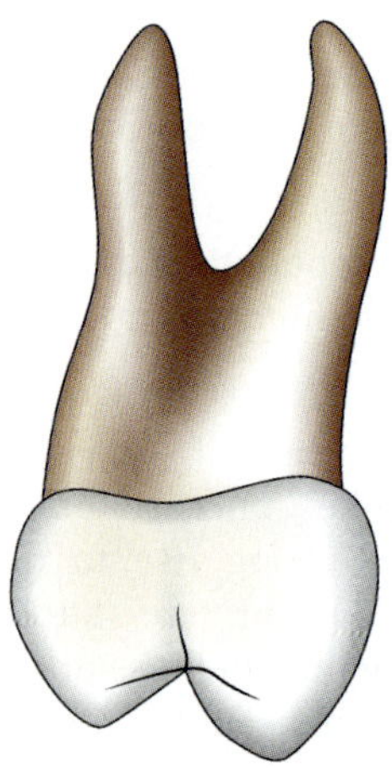

Fig. 5.3: Permanent maxillary right first premolar, mesial aspect

of the lingual root. Both the buccal and lingual cusp tip are present within the confines of the root trunk which is characteristic of all posterior maxillary teeth that is the measurement from the tip of the buccal cusp to the tip of the lingual cusp is less than the buccolingual measurement of the root at its cervical portion. The cusps of maxillary first premolar are long and sharp.

The cervical line outline may be regular or irregular and it is less compared to anterior teeth.

Root: Above the cervical line the buccal outline of the buccal root is straight with slight lingual inclination. At the middle third the outline is convex. The buccal root apex is blunt.

Cervical third of lingual outline is straight, middle third and apical third may show curvature. The lingual root apex is more pointed than the buccal root apex. The bifurcation is about half of the root length.

Surface

Crown: The mesial marginal ridge is placed at the junction of middle and occlusal third.

Characteristic features seen on mesial aspect:[2]

1. A well defined "*mesial marginal developmental groove*" in the enamel of the mesial marginal ridge. This marginal groove is continuous with the central groove on the occlusal surface of the crown, crossing the marginal ridge immediately lingual to the mesial contact area and terminates at a short distance cervical to the mesial marginal ridge on the mesial surface.
2. Presence of "*mesial developmental depression*" below the mesial contact area. This concavity is continuous apically beyond the cervical line, joins a deep developmental depression between the roots and ends at the root bifurcation. The mesial contact area is placed occlusal to half of the crown length.

Root: The mesial surface of the root portion is smoothly convex buccally and lingually except for the developmental depression present above the cervical line till the bifurcation.

Distal Aspect[1,2] *(Fig. 5.4)*

The crown and root are similar to mesial aspect. The distal contact area is placed occlusal to half of the crown length and is more broader.

Differences from mesial aspect:

1. The crown surface is convex at all points except for a small flattened area just cervical to contact area.

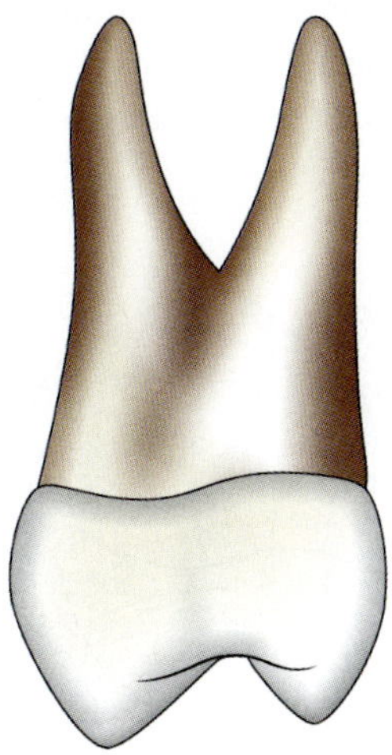

Fig. 5.4: Permanent maxillary right first premolar, distal aspect

2. The curvature of cervical line is less by 1 mm than on the mesial surface.
3. There is no deep developmental groove or developmental depression present on this aspect.
4. The root trunk is flat.

Occlusal Aspect[1,2] (Fig. 5.5)

The occlusal aspect is roughly hexagonal in shape. The six sides are mesiobuccal, mesial, mesiolingual, distobuccal, distal and distolingual (Fig. 5.6).

Dimensions (Fig. 5.6)

The buccolingual width is greater than the mesiodistal width.

The mesiolingual side is almost equal to distobuccal side, the distal and distolingual side is greater than the mesial and mesiolingual side. The distance from mesial crest (B) and buccal crest (A) is greater than the distance from buccal crest (A) to distal crest (C).

The distance from distal crest (C) and lingual crest (D) is greater than the distances from lingual crest (D) and mesial crest (B).

The width of buccal portion is greater than the lingual portion.

Ridges:

a. Mesiobuccal and distobuccal cusp ridges of buccal cusp are present.
b. Mesiolingual and distolingual cusp ridges of lingual cusp are also present.
c. Mesial marginal ridge and distal marginal ridge as well as.
d. Buccal triangular ridge and lingual triangular ridge are also seen.

Grooves:

a. Central developmental groove divides the occlusal surface buccolingually.
b. This central developmental groove extends distobucally giving rise to distobuccal developmental groove. It also runs mesially giving rise to mesial developmental groove. When this groove crosses the mesial marginal groove it is called as mesial marginal groove.

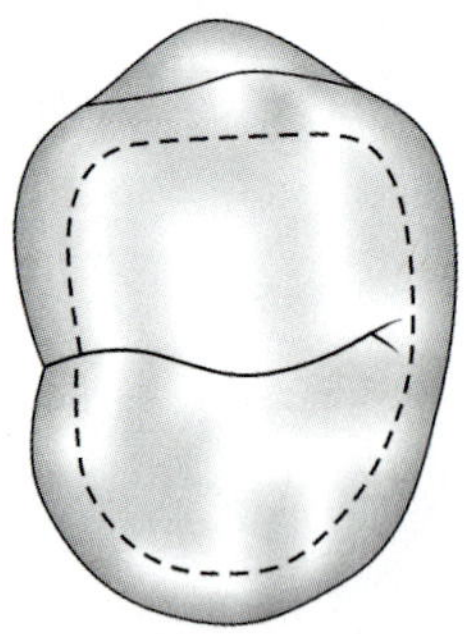

Fig. 5.5: Permanent maxillary right first premolar, occlusal aspect

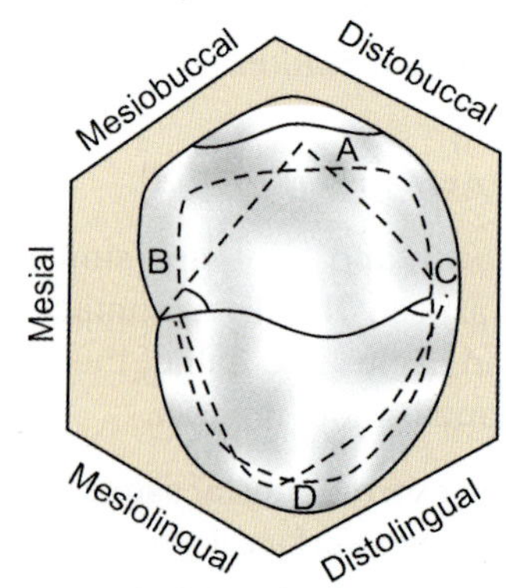

Fig. 5.6: Six sides on the occlusal aspect

Sulcus: The central sulcus harbors the central developmental groove.

Pits: Mesial and distal developmental pits are present where the groove branches mesially and distally.

Carving Technique

Measurements (in mm)

Cervico-occlusal length of crown	–	8.5
Length of root	–	14.0
Mesiodistal diameter of crown	–	7.0
Mesiodistal diameter of crown at cervix	–	5.0
Buccolingual diameter of crown	–	9.0
Buccolingual diameter of crown at cervix	–	8.0
Curvature of cervical line - mesial	–	1.0
Curvature of cervical line - distal	–	0.0

For posterior teeth always first carve the crown and then the root. Figure 5.8A and B is a carved maxillary premolar. The steps in carving for permanent maxillary first premolar are as follows:

Step 1: Smoothen the wax block. Mark the butt end to retain as base for carving. Mark the aspects, i.e. **B** for buccal aspect, **Li** for lingual aspect, **M** for mesial aspect and **D** for distal aspect.

Step 2: Mark the length of crown and length of root on all the four aspects.

Step 3: For carving all posterior teeth, i.e. maxillary and mandibular teeth, first carve the occlusal aspect and then proceed with other aspects; to carve the occlusal aspect, first mark the buccolingual width and mesiodistal width of crown on the other end of the butt end/base of the wax block as shown in Figure 5.7A.

Step 4: Draw the occlusal outline (Fig. 5.7B).

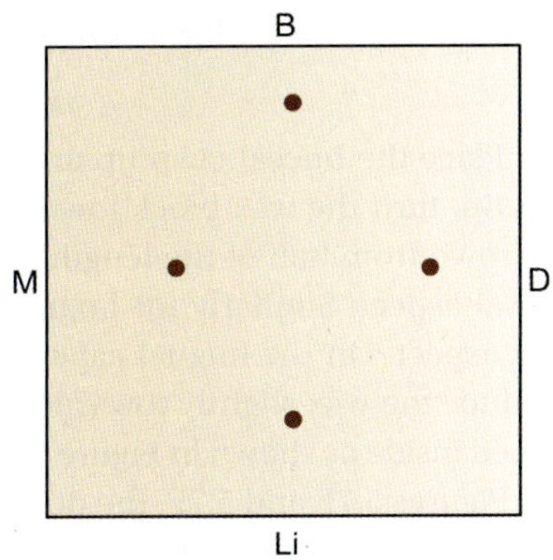

Fig. 5.7A: Step 3

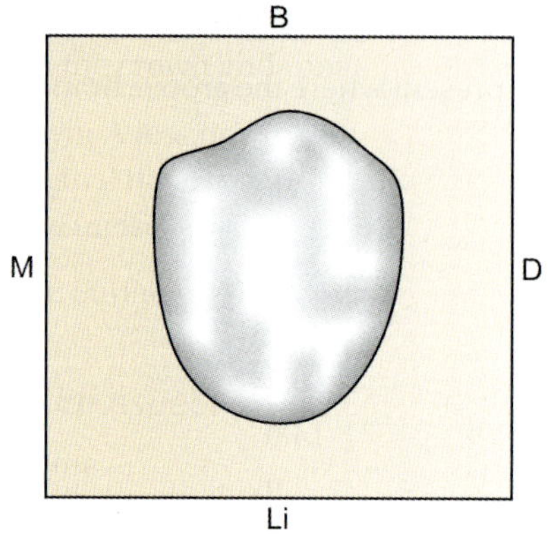

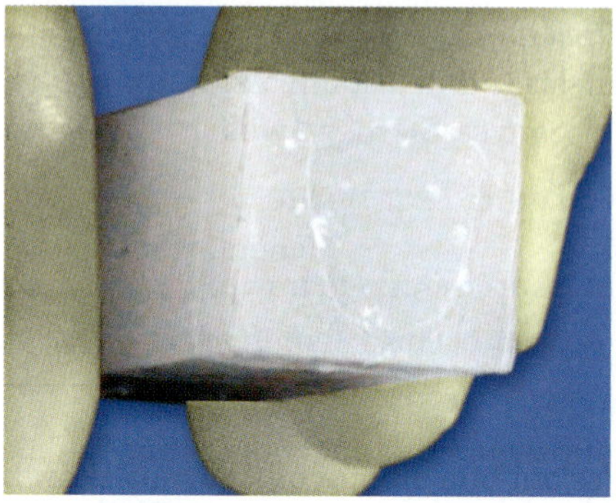

Fig. 5.7B: Occlusal outline, step 4

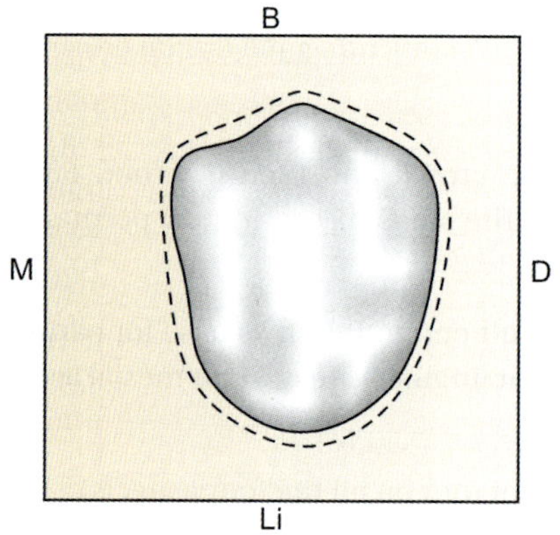

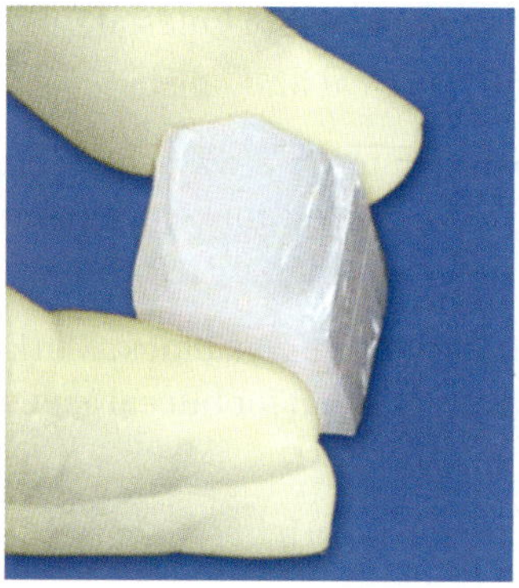

Fig. 5.7C: Step 5

Step 5 (Fig. 5.7C): After drawing the occlusal outline, carve according to this outline and leave about 0.5 mm of wax extra than the outline.

Step 6 (Fig. 5.7D): Now divide the occlusal aspect for cusps. To carve the two cusps, draw a line mesiodistally on the occlusal surface (buccal cusp is larger), deepen this line slightly.

Step 7 (Figs 5.7E and F): Place the buccal cusp tip and lingual cusp tip inside. To place the buccal cusp tip, turn the wax block toward the buccal aspect. On the buccal aspect of the crown from half of the length of crown reduce the wax slightly toward the occlusal aspect. Similarly for lingual cusp tip turn the wax block towards the lingual aspect. On the lingual aspect of the crown from half of the length of crown reduce the wax slightly toward the occlusal aspect. Now both the cusp tips are placed inside as shown in Figure 5.7G, if we see from either mesial or distal aspect. In Figures 5.7E and 5.7F, the doted lines indicate the wax removed and the direction of wax to be removed.

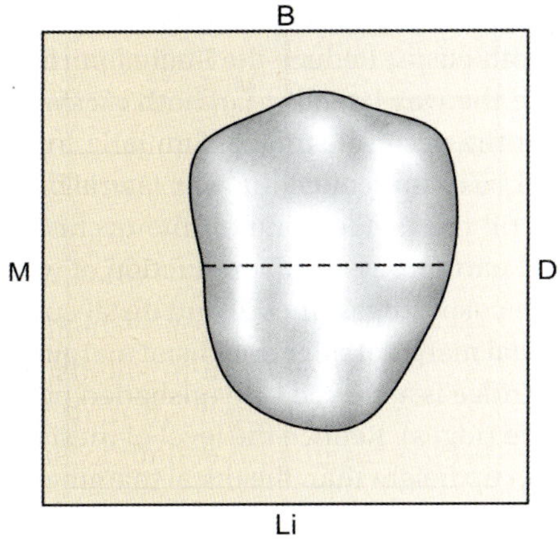

Fig. 5.7D: Step 6

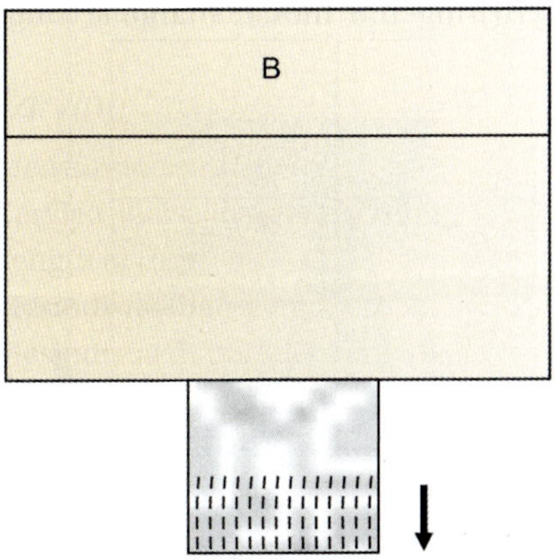

Fig. 5.7E: Step 7

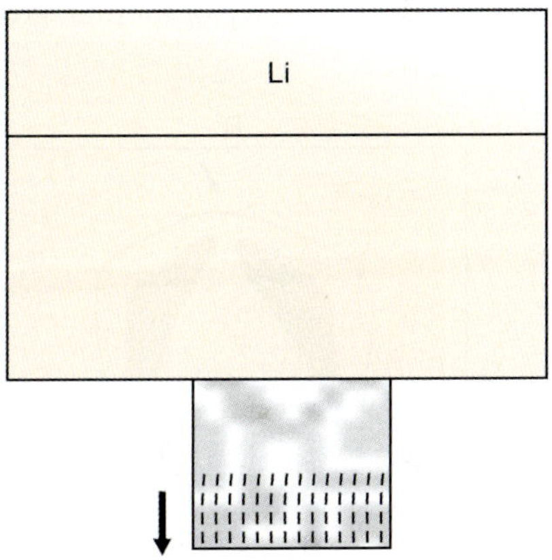

Fig. 5.7F: Step 7

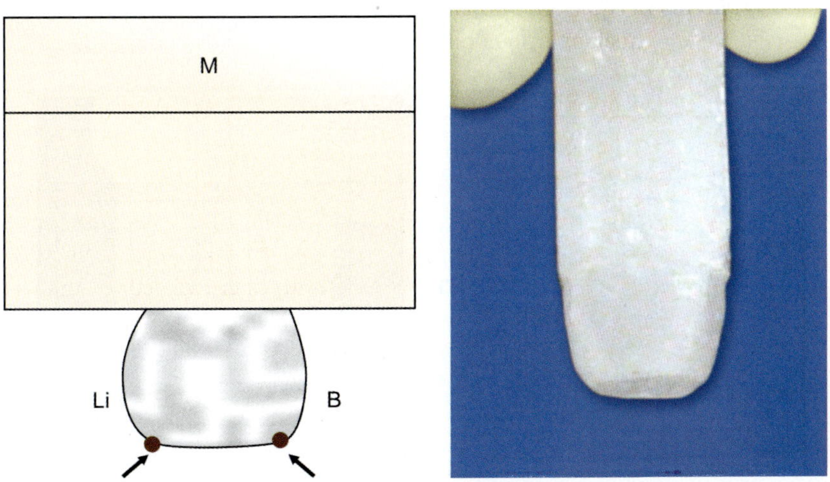

Fig. 5.7G: Step 7—Photograph showing lingual cusp tip placed inside

Step 8 (Fig. 5.7H): Turn the wax block towards the occlusal aspect. Carve the triangular ridges for both cusps. Reduce the lingual portion by 1 mm. From the buccal cusp tip reduce the wax laterally, i.e. both mesially and distally sloping till the divided line on the occlusal surface. Similarly for the lingual triangular ridge, from the lingual cusp tip reduce the wax laterally, i.e. both mesially and distally sloping down till the divided line on the occlusal surface as shown in (Fig. 5.7H), the shaded part represents the reduction of wax deeper. Once this is done automatically the cusps ridges (mesial and distal cusp ridges of buccal and lingual cusps), the mesial marginal ridge and distal marginal ridge and the buccal and lingual triangular ridge is achieved (the unshaded portion of the (Fig. 5.7H) represents all the above ridges). Reduce the level of mesial marginal ridge about 2 mm from buccal cusp tip height than the distal marginal ridge.

Step 9 (Fig. 5.7I): Once the ridges on the occlusal surface is carved, carve the central developmental groove deeper and then extend the groove mesially for mesial marginal developmental groove crossing the mesial marginal ridge

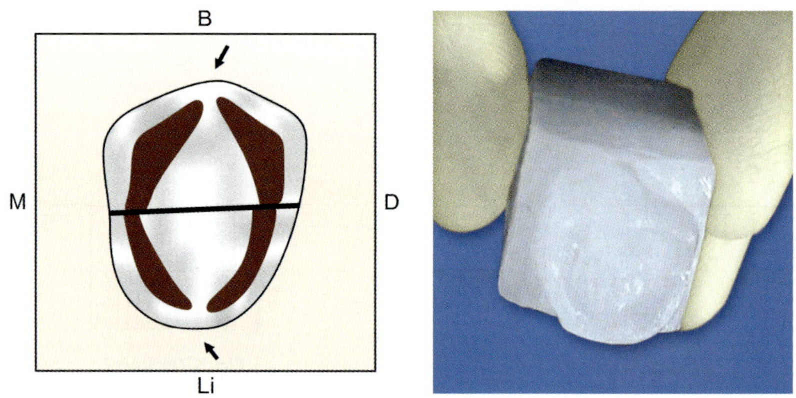

Fig. 5.7H: Step 8—Ridges on the occlusal surface

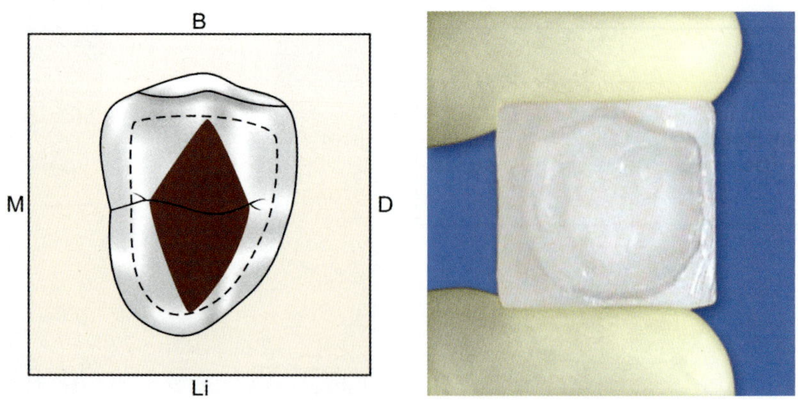

Fig. 5.7I: Step 9—Grooves and rigdes, the shaded parts are triangular ridges

and terminating on the mesial aspect of the crown and extend distobucally for distobuccal developmental groove on the occlusal surface. Carve pinpoint depressions where the groove branches mesially and distally for mesial and distal pits.

Step 10 (Fig. 5.7J): Once the occlusal aspect is carved, turn the wax block towards buccal aspect. Now carve the mesial slope which is long and straight then the distal slope which is short and curved. Carve the mesial and distal outline of buccal aspect. Carve the buccal ridge, for this reduce the wax deeper laterally (for developmental depressions mesial and distal to the buccal ridge) leaving the wax at the middle of the buccal surface from cervical line till the buccal cusp tip. The left over wax in the middle will serve as the buccal ridge.

Step 11 (Fig. 5.7K): Turn the carving toward mesial aspect, carve the buccal and lingual outline. Extend the mesial marginal developmental groove till the occlusal third. Carve the mesial developmental depression from the terminus of

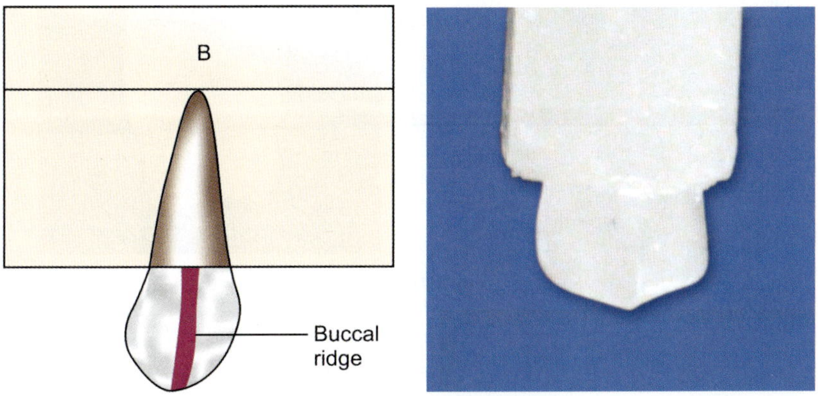

Fig. 5.7J: Step 10—Buccal aspect

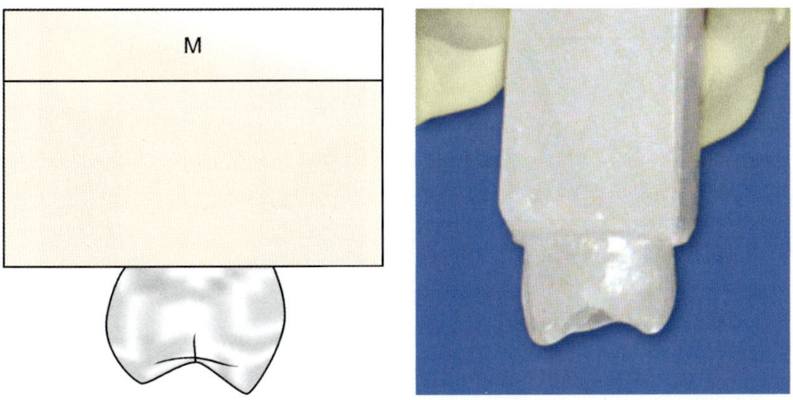

Fig. 5.7K: Step 11

groove till the cervical line. Very important point to be noted is that the cusp tips are placed inside as shown in Figure 5.7K and not flaring.

Step 12 (Fig. 5.7L): Turn the carving towards distal aspect, carve the buccal and lingual outline. Cervical third of distal aspect should be flattened.

Step 13 (Fig. 5.7M): Once the crown is completed, carve the roots, for this first turn the wax block toward the mesial aspect. Draw the root outline on the mesial aspect.

Step 14 (Fig.5.7N): After drawing the mesial outline of the root, carve according to the outline. Start bifurcating the root. Care should be taken while bifurcating,

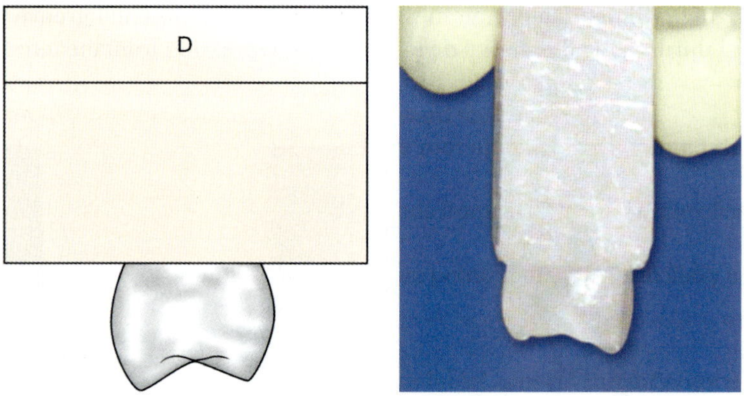

Fig. 5.7L: Step 12

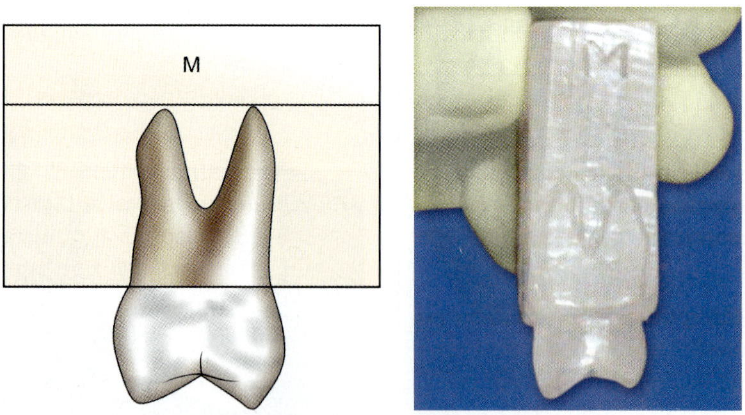

Fig. 5.7M: Step 13—Root outline on the mesial aspect

remove only minimal wax so as to avoid breakage of roots at this point. Extend the concavity present on the crown beyond the cervical line upto the bifurcation of the root.

Step 15 (Figs 5.8A and B): After this turn toward buccal and lingual aspect, carve the root outlines and then round off the roots. Measure the tooth, any excess wax can be removed. Round off all the line angles keeping the line angles more angular for maxillary first premolars.

Polish the tooth according to carving. For occlusal surface polish with a thin strand of cotton to avoid the loss of carved features. After polishing now taper the root apex (blunt) of buccal root and lingual root (pointed) and then do polishing for both root apices.

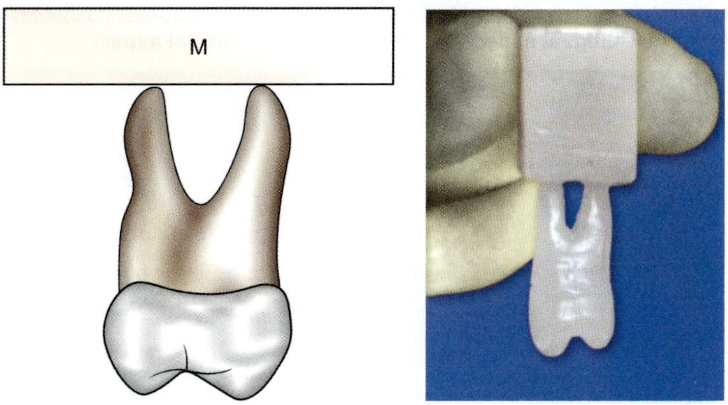

Fig. 5.7N: Step 14—Bifurcation of root

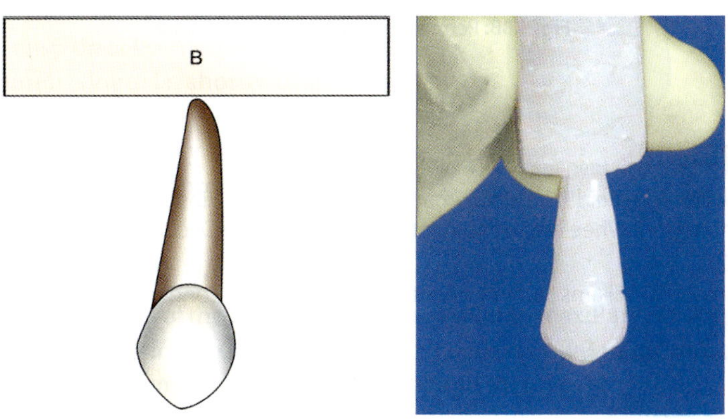

Fig. 5.8A: Carved permanent maxillary first premolar, buccal aspect

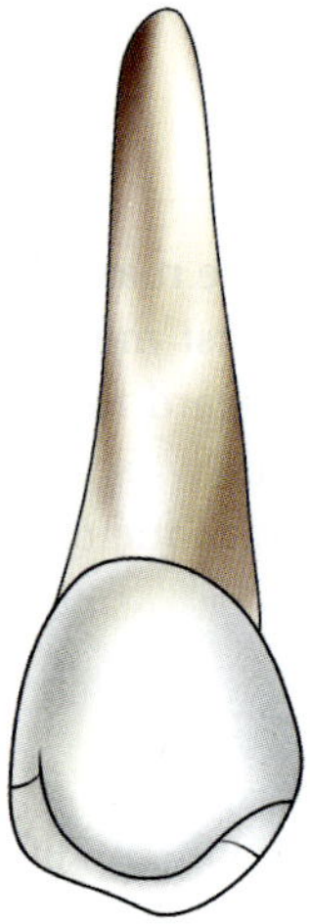

Fig. 5.10: Permanent maxillary right second premolar, lingual aspect

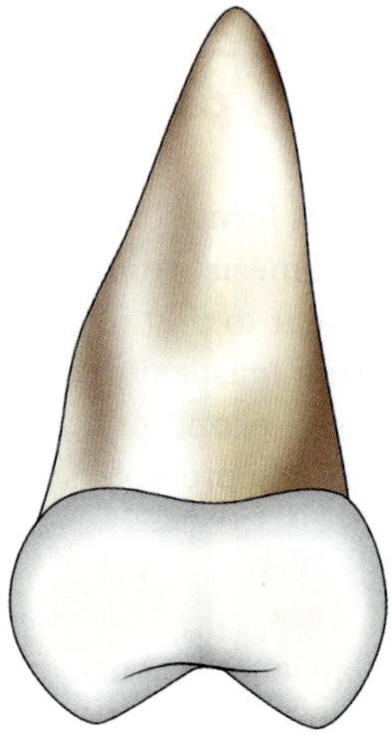

Fig. 5.11: Permanent maxillary right second premolar, mesial aspect

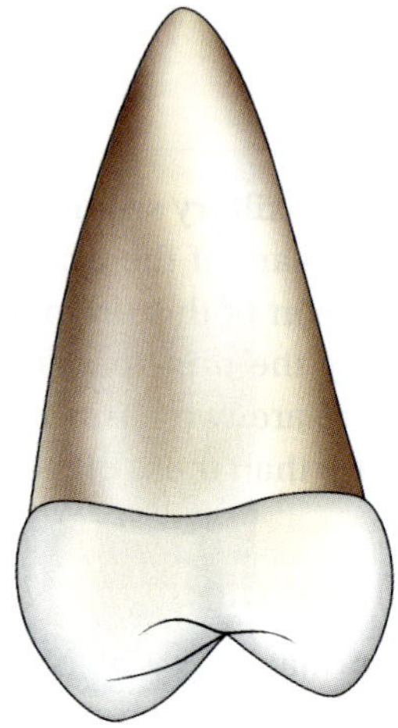

Fig. 5.12: Permanent maxillary right second premolar, distal aspect

Mesial Aspect[1,2] (Fig. 5.11)

The outline of the crown is almost similar to mesial aspect of maxillary first premolar.

The differences from maxillary first premolar are:

a. A single root is present. The labial outline of the root shows lingual inclination with blunt root apex.
b. Both buccal and lingual cusps are shorter by 1 mm than the maxillary first premolar cusps. Both the cusps height are at the same level.
c. The distance between the two cusps tips is greater which widens the occlusal surface labiolingually.
d. No developmental depression is present.
e. No developmental marginal groove is present.
f. A developmental groove is present on the root surface.
g. The surface of the crown and root is smooth and convex.

Distal Aspect[1,2] (Fig. 5.12)

The outline and surface of the crown and root is similar to mesial aspect.

The differences from mesial aspect are:

a. The curvature of cervical line is 0 mm.
b. Surface of the crown is more convex.
c. There is presence of developmental depression with a developmental groove on the root surface.

Occlusal Aspect[1,2] (Fig. 5.13)

Differences from maxillary first premolar:

a. The outline of the crown is more round or oval.
b. An irregular, shorter central developmental groove is present.
c. Multiple supplemental grooves radiating from central developmental groove. Because of these supplemental grooves the occlusal surface appears more wrinkled.

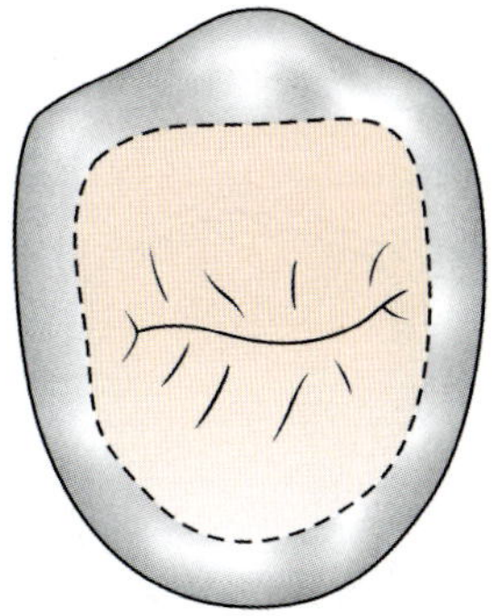

Fig. 5.13: Permanent maxillary right second premolar, occlusal aspect

Carving Technique

Measurements (in mm)

Cervico-occlusal length of crown	-	8.5
Length of root	-	14.0
Mesiodistal diameter of crown	-	7.0
Mesiodistal diameter of crown at cervix	-	5.0
Labiolingual diameter of crown	-	9.0
Labiolingual diameter of crown at cervix	-	8.0
Curvature of cervical line - mesial	-	1.0
Curvature of cervical line - distal	-	0.0

The detailed carving steps can be followed similar to permanent maxillary first premolar. The morphological features (Fig. 5.15) should be followed. First carve the crown and then the root (Figs 5.14A to 5.14O).

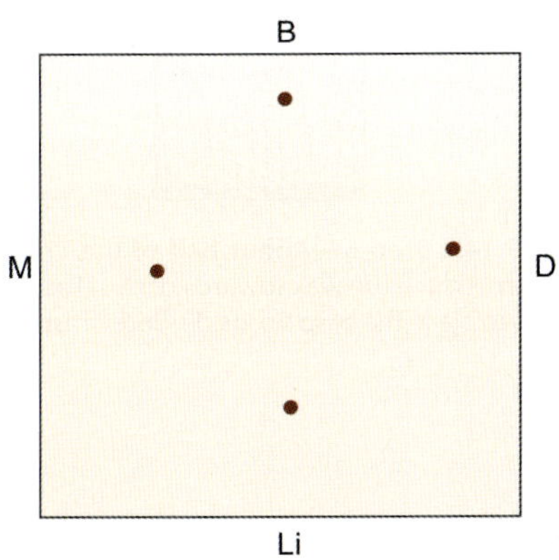

Fig. 5.14A: Step 1—Mark the buccolingual and mesiodistal width

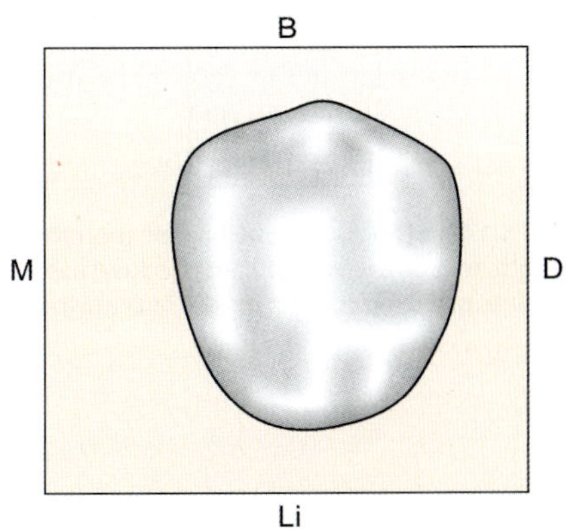

Fig. 5.14B: Step 2—Draw the occlusal outline

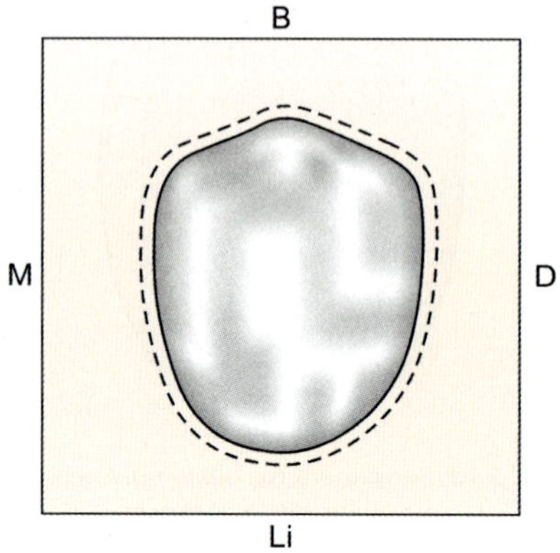

Fig. 5.14C: Step 3—Carve according to the outline leaving about 0.5 mm of wax extra

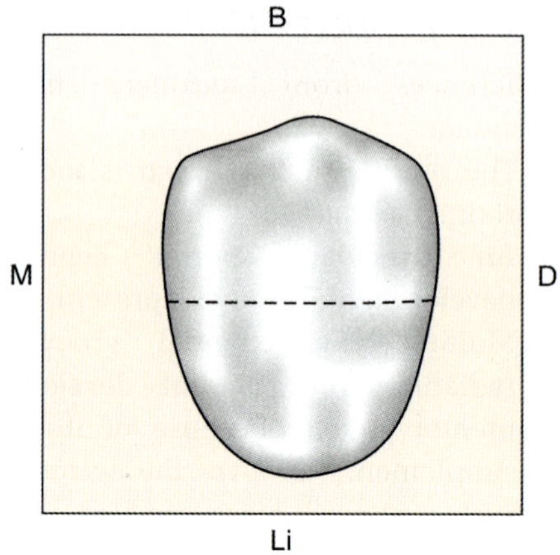

Fig. 5.14D: Step 4—Draw a midline to carve two cusps

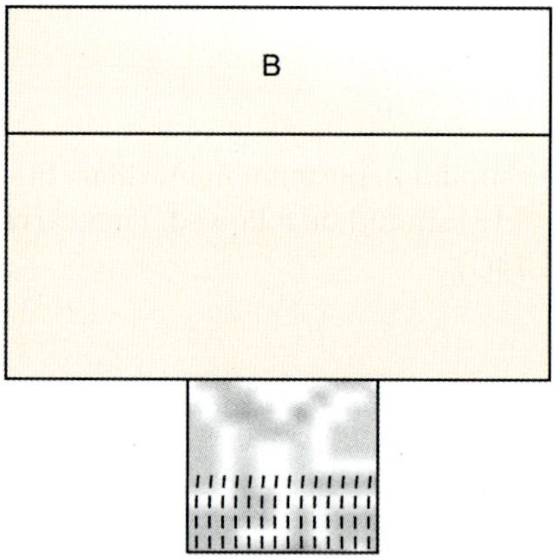

Fig. 5.14E: Step 5—About half of the crown length, reduce the wax towards occlusal aspect this is to place the cusp tip inside (buccal aspect)

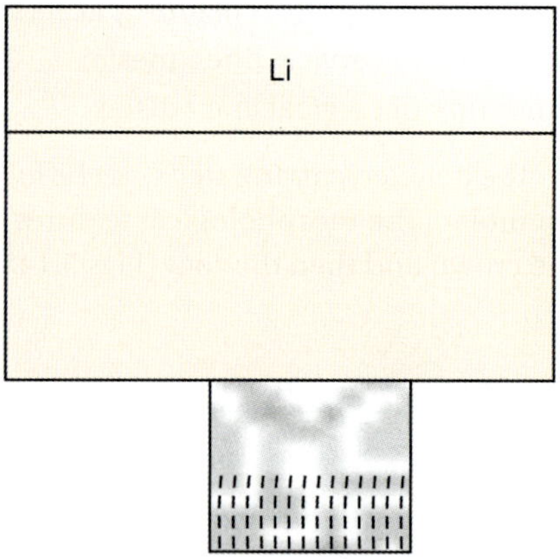

Fig. 5.14F: Step 6—About half of the crown length, reduce the wax towards occlusal aspect this is to place the cusp tip inside (lingual aspect)

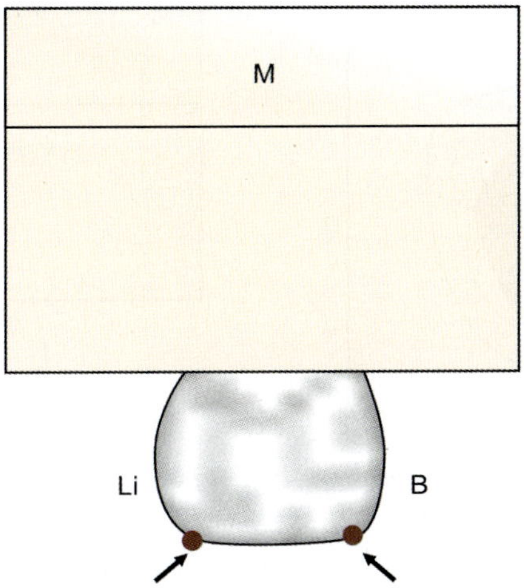

Fig. 5.14G: Step 7—The arrow mark pointing the buccal and lingual cusp tip placed inside from mesial aspect

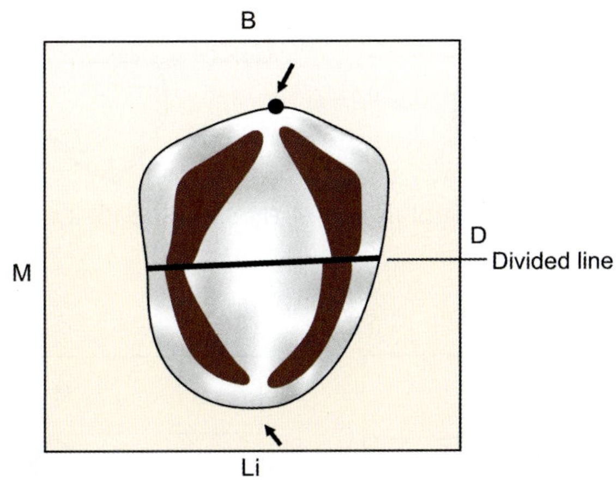

Fig. 5.14H: Step 8—The shaded part represents wax to be reduced so as to carve the buccal and lingual triangular ridges, marginal and cusp ridges of both cusps

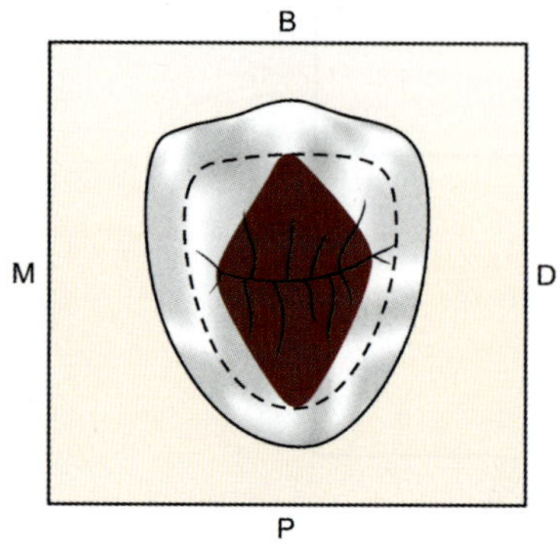

Fig. 5.14I: Step 9—Carve the grooves. The shaded parts are ridges

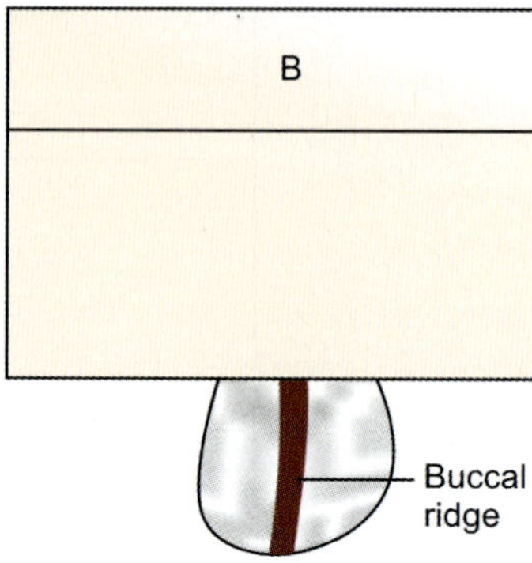

Fig. 5.14J: Step 10—Carve the buccal aspect outline and the buccal ridge

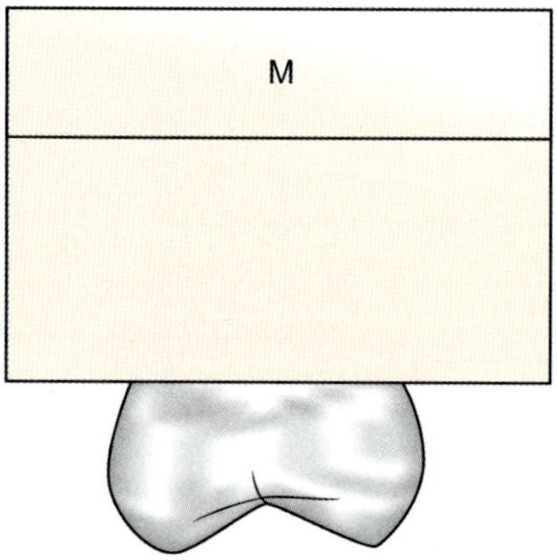

Fig. 5.14K: Step 11—Carve the mesial aspect

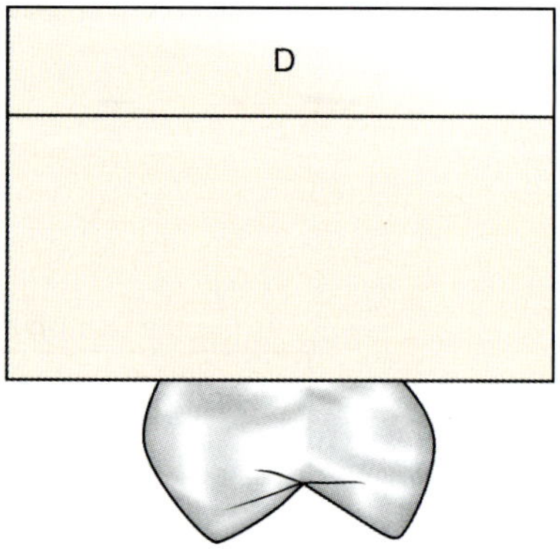

Fig. 5.14L: Step 12—Carve the distal aspect

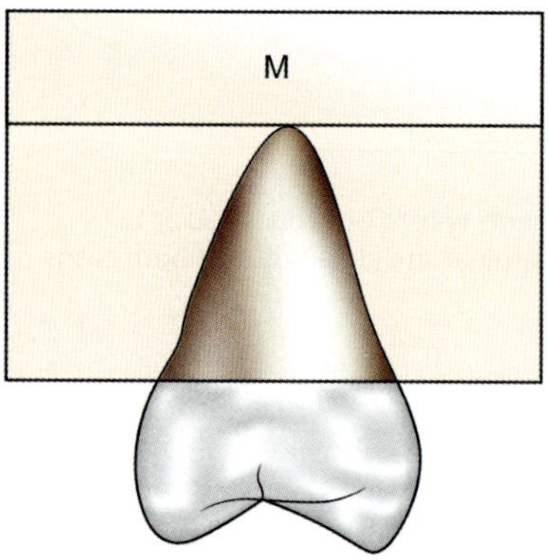

Fig. 5.14M: Step 13—Draw the root outline on the mesial aspect

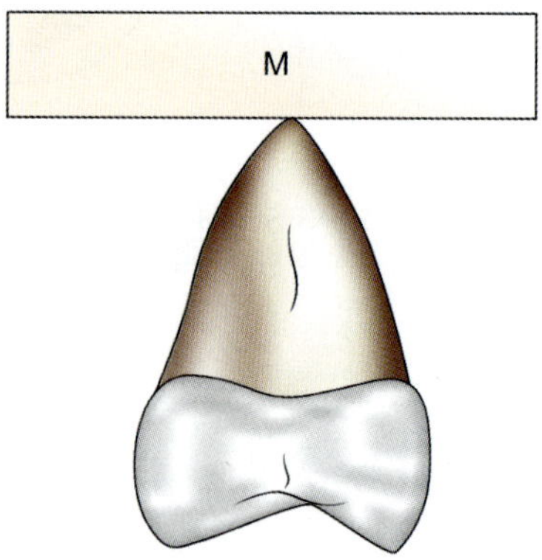

Fig. 5.14N: Step 14—Carve according to the root outline

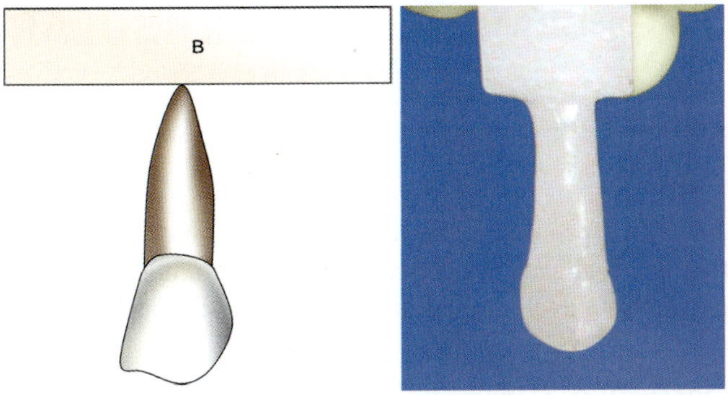

Fig. 5.14O: Carved permanent maxillary second premolar, buccal aspect

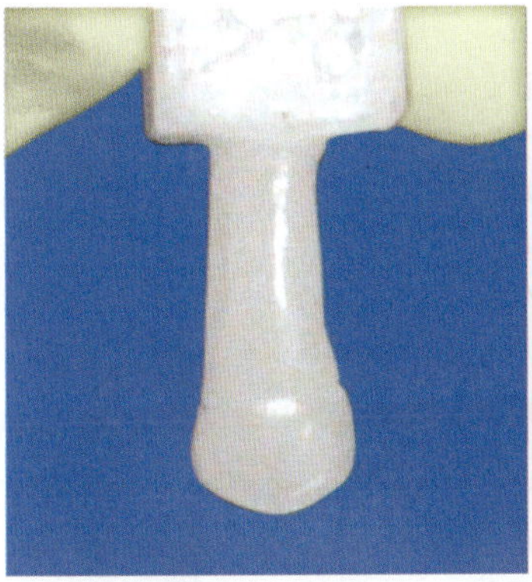

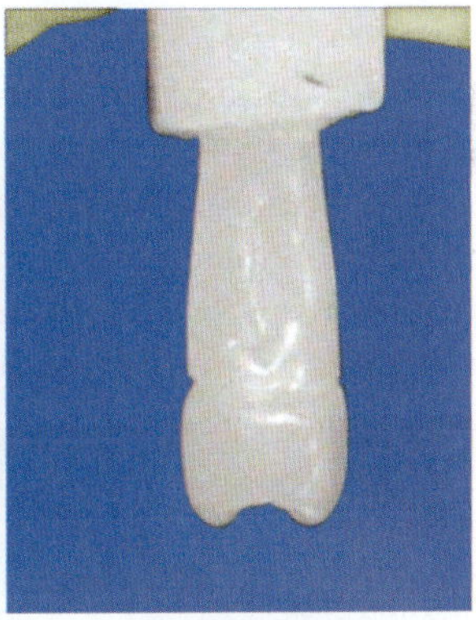

Lingual aspect **Mesial aspect**

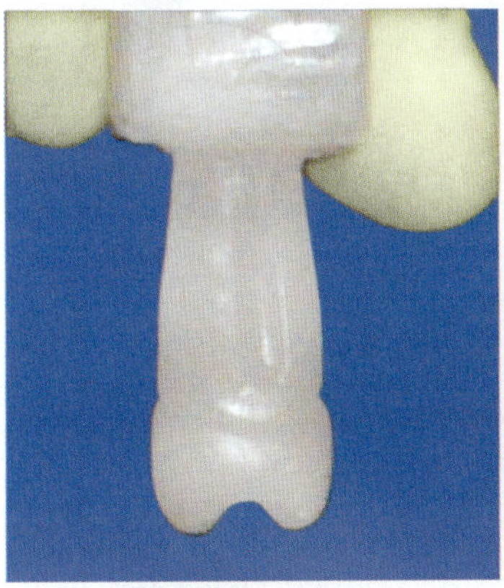

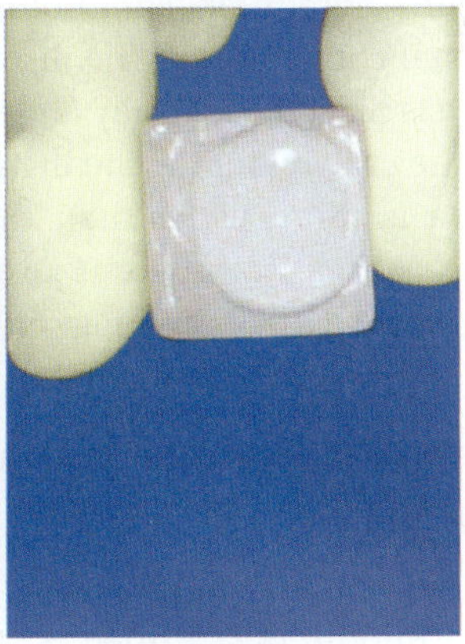

Distal aspect **Occlusal aspect**

Fig. 5.15: Permanent maxillary second premolar

REFERENCES

1. Woelfel JB, Scheid RC. Dental Anatomy. Williams & Wilkins. 1997.
2. Ash, Nelson. Wheelers Dental Anatomy, Physiology & Occlusion. 8th edition. Elsevier. 2003.

THE PERMANENT MANDIBULAR FIRST PREMOLAR

Morphology

The mandibular first premolar develops from four lobes and second premolar develops from five lobes; three buccal and two lingual lobes.[2] They are the succedaneous teeth to deciduous first and second molars.[1,2]

Buccal Aspect[1,2] *(Fig. 5.16)*

The crown is roughly trapezoidal.

Outline

Crown: The cervical third of the mesial outline from the cervical line is slightly concave, from here it joins the mesial contact area which is placed occlusal to half of the crown length. The outline from here joins the mesial slope which is shorter than distal slope and is straight. So the buccal cusp tip is placed mesially.

The cervical third of distal outline from the cervical line is slightly concave from here it is continuous with the distal contact area. The distal contact area is placed occlusally above the half of the crown length. The distal contact area is more wider than the mesial contact area from here it joins the distal slope which is long and concave.

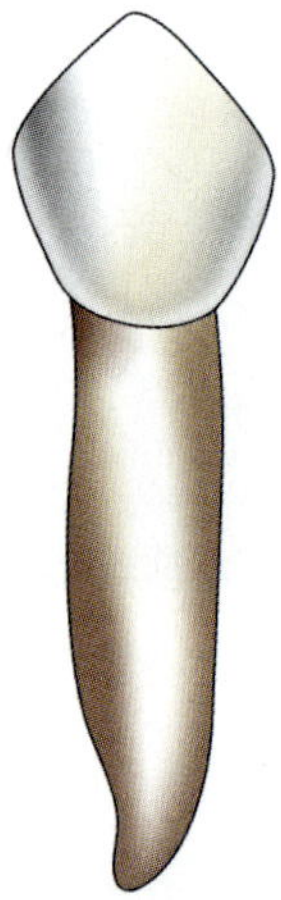

Fig. 5.16: Mandibular right first premolar, buccal aspect

Root: The mesial outline of the root inclines distally. Gradual tapering of the root with more pointed root apex is seen.

Surface

Crown: The middle buccal lobe is well developed giving rise to buccal ridge. Adjacent to the buccal ridge mesially and distally a developmental depression is present. The buccal surface is more convex at the cervical and middle third than the maxillary first premolar.

Root: The root surface is smooth and convex.

Lingual Aspect[1,2] *(Fig. 5.17)*

The crown and the root taper lingually.

Outline

Crown and root outline is similar to buccal aspect.

Surface

Crown: The crown tapers lingually, part of mesial and distal surfaces are seen. The lingual cusp is small or rudimentary. The lingual cusp is more pointed than the buccal cusp tip. Since the buccal cusp inclines lingually in a cervical direction, the occlusal portion is seen from lingual aspect. That is the buccal triangular ridge and occlusal fossae are seen. The very important characteristic feature of this tooth is the presence of mesiolingual developmental groove in the mesiolingual depression.

Root: The root tapers lingually with a lingual ridge. Part of developmental depression from mesial and distal aspect may be seen.

Mesial Aspect[1,2] *(Fig. 5.18)*

Outline

Crown: Buccal outline of the crown—the cervical third and middle third is convex, the occlusal third slopes straight towards the cusp tip. The buccal outline inclines lingually in a cervical direction. The greatest convexity is seen at the middle of the crown. The buccal cusp tip is placed over the center of the root.

The lingual outline from the cervical line is straight at the cervical third; middle third shows convexity that is the lingual cusp outline. The lingual cusp is in line with the lingual border of the root. The length of lingual cusp is about two thirds of crown length.

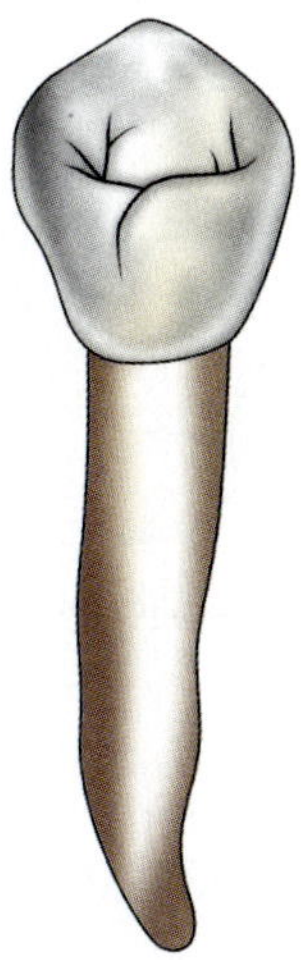

Fig. 5.17: Mandibular right first premolar, lingual aspect

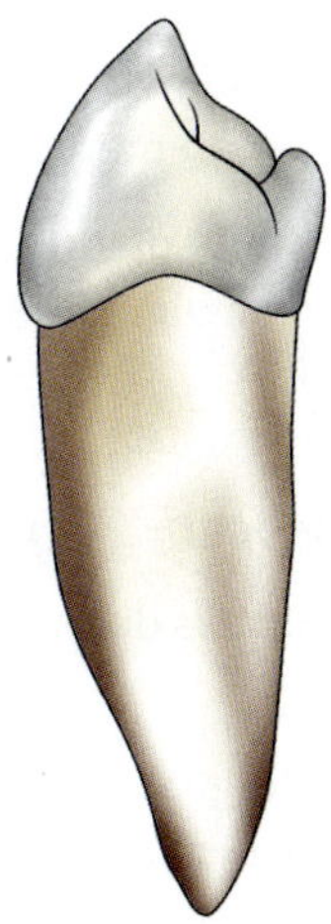

Fig. 5.18: Mandibular right first premolar, mesial aspect

The outline of mesial marginal ridge is parallel to outline of buccal triangular ridge. The curvature of cervical line is regular and curved occlusally and is about 1 mm.

Surface

Crown: The surface of the crown is smooth. The mesial contact area is occlusal to half of the crown length and shows convexity. Below the contact area the surface is flat and smooth. The mesiolingual developmental groove is present at the mesiolingual line angle.

Distal Aspect[1,2] *(Fig. 5.19)*

The outline of the crown and root is almost similar to mesial aspect. The differences from mesial aspect are:

1. The distal marginal ridge is placed at a higher level and is at right angles to the long axis of the crown and root.
2. The marginal ridge is confluent with the lingual cusp ridge and no developmental groove is seen on the distal marginal ridge.
3. Major portion of the distal surface of the crown is smoothly convex.
4. Cervical third of the distal surface shows concavity. The distal contact area is broader and placed at halfway of the crown length.
5. Surface of the root is more convex and a shallow developmental depression is centered on the root.

The curvature of the cervical line distally is irregular and similar to mesial aspect.

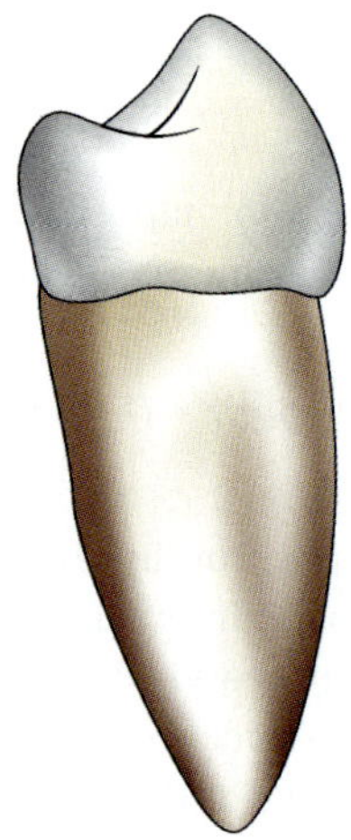

Fig. 5.19: Mandibular right first premolar, distal aspect

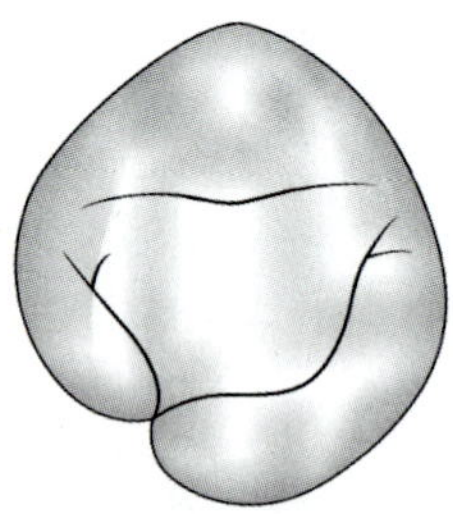

Fig. 5.20: Mandibular right first premolar, occlusal aspect

Occlusal Aspect[1,2] *(Fig. 5.20)*

The outline form is diamond shaped.

Dimensions

- The buccolingual width is greater than the mesiodistal width.
- The buccal cusp makes up the major portion of the occlusal aspect.

Ridges: The mesiobuccal and distobuccal cusp, ridge of buccal cusp, mesiolingual and distolingual cusp ridge of lingual cusp, the mesial and distal marginal ridges are present. The buccal triangular ridge of buccal cusp and lingual triangular ridge of lingual cusp are also present on the occlusal aspect.

Fossa: Mesial fossa is linear in form and distal fossa is circular in form. Mesial fossa is present distal to mesial marginal ridge and distal fossa is present mesial to distal marginal ridge.

Grooves: Mesial and distal developmental grooves are seen. The mesial developmental groove runs buccolingually and extends over the mesiolingual developmental depression to give rise to mesiolingual developmental groove. The distal developmental groove is crescent shaped and has accessory supplemental grooves radiating from it.

Pits: A distal pit is present from which the supplemental grooves are radiating.

Carving technique

Measurements (in mm)

Cervico-occlusal length of crown	-	8.5
Length of root	-	14.0
Mesiodistal diameter of crown	-	7.0
Mesiodistal diameter of crown at cervix	-	5.0
Buccolingual diameter of crown	-	7.5
Buccolingual diameter of crown at cervix	-	6.5
Curvature of cervical line - mesial	-	1.0
Curvature of cervical line - distal	-	0.0

The detailed carving steps can be followed as the permanent maxillary first premolar. The morphological features (Fig. 5.22) should be followed. Steps in carving are represented by diagrammatic illustrations as given below (Figs 5.21A to 5.21O).

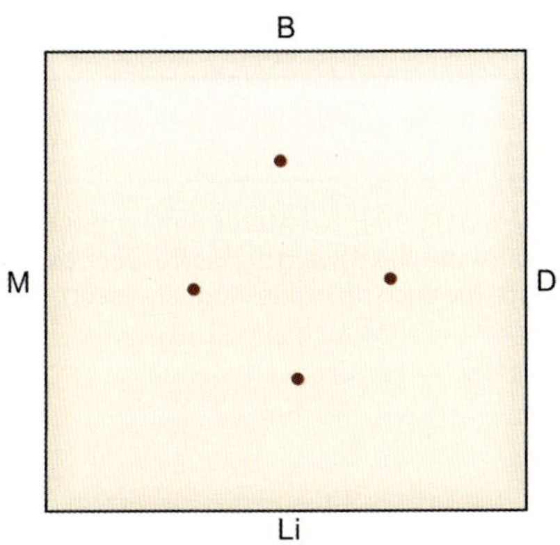

Fig. 5.21A: Step 1—Mark the buccolingual and mesiodistal width

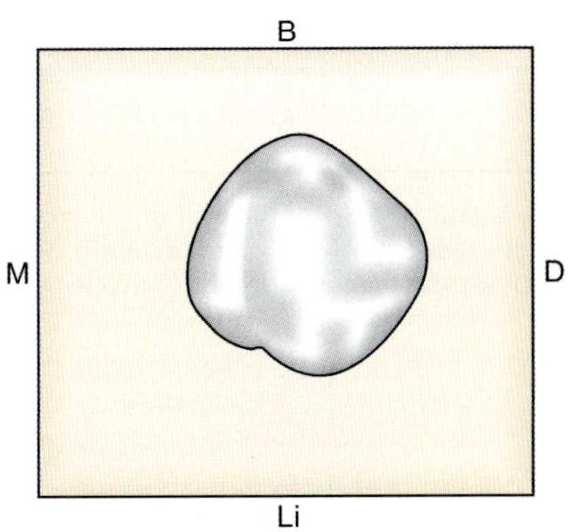

Fig. 5.21B: Step 2—Draw the occlusal outline

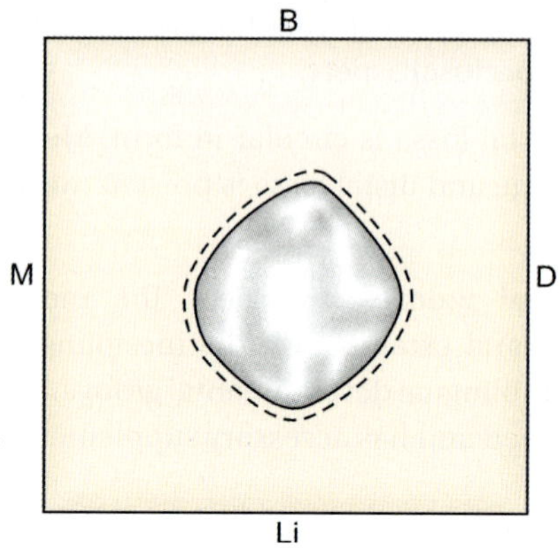

Fig. 5.21C: Step 3—Carve according to the outline leaving about 0.5 mm of wax extra

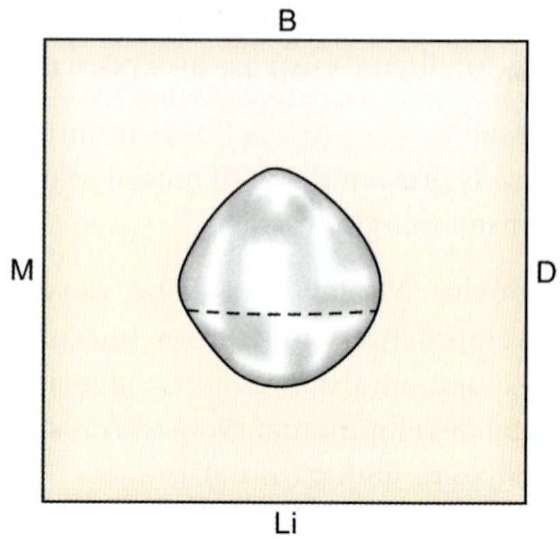

Fig. 5.21D: Step 4—Draw a midline to carve two cusps

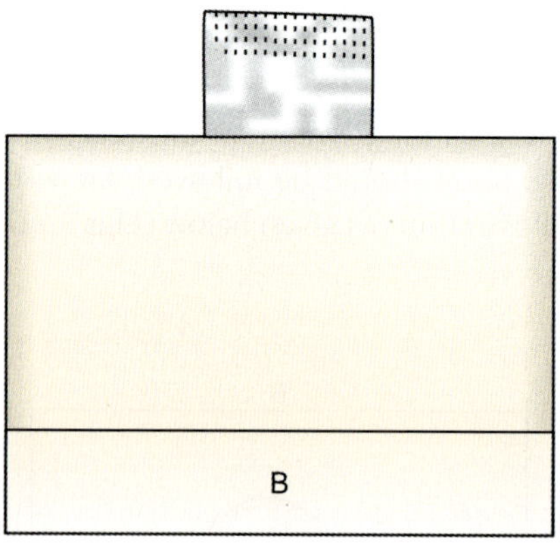

Fig. 5.21E: Step 5—About half of the crown length, reduce the wax toward occlusal aspect, this is to place the cusp tip inside (buccal aspect)

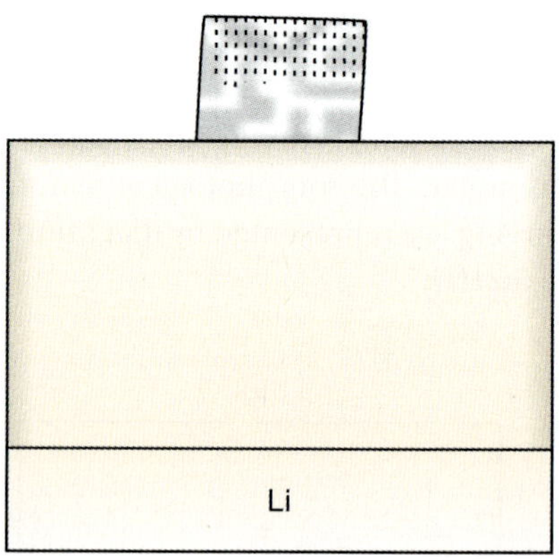

Fig. 5.21F: Step 6—About half of the crown reduce the wax toward occlusal aspect, this is to place the cusp tip inside (lingual aspect)

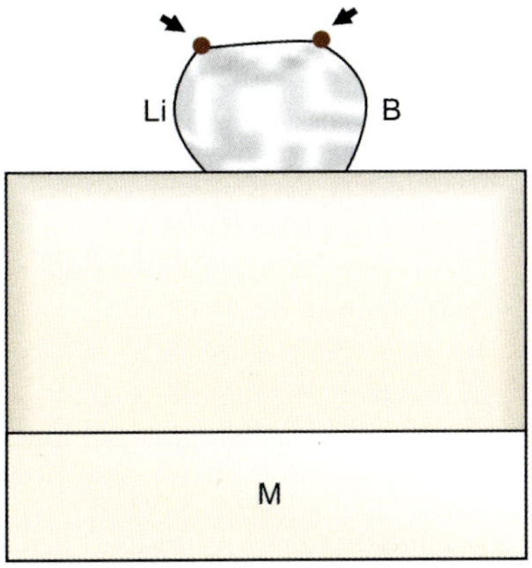

Fig. 5.21G: Step 7—The arrow mark pointing the buccal and lingual cusp tips placed and inside from mesial aspect

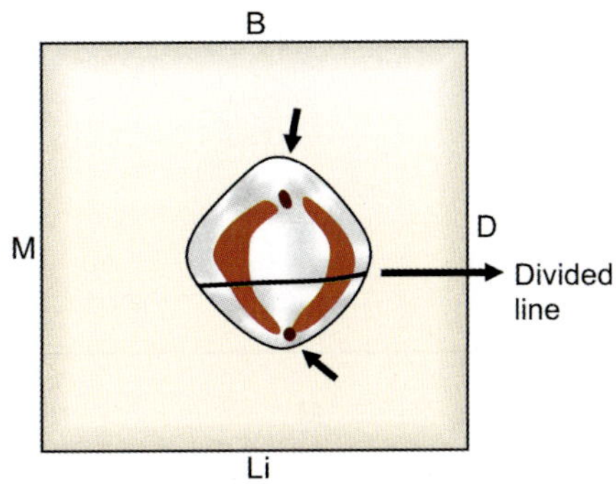

Fig. 5.21H: Step 8—The shaded part represents wax to be reduced so as to carve the buccal lingual triangular ridges, marginal and cusp ridges of both cusps

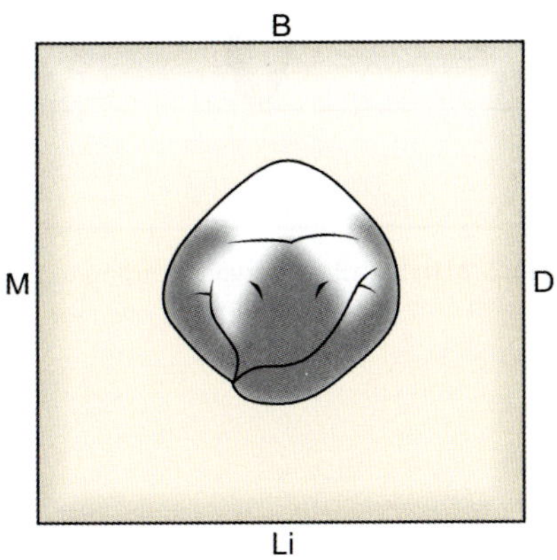

Fig. 5.21I: Step 9—Carve the grooves. The shaded parts are ridges

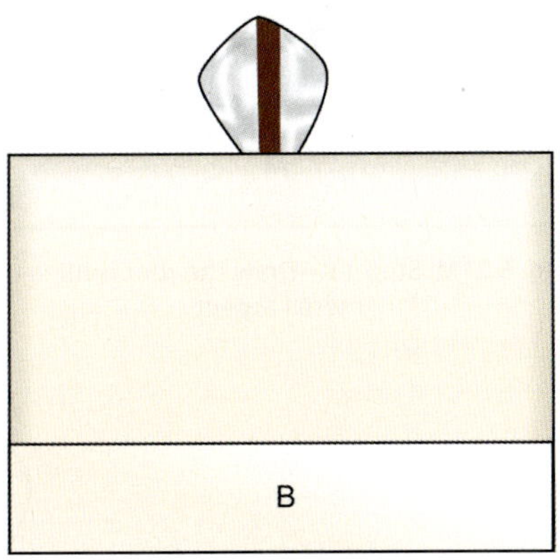

Fig. 5.21J: Step 10—Carve the buccal aspect outline and buccal ridge

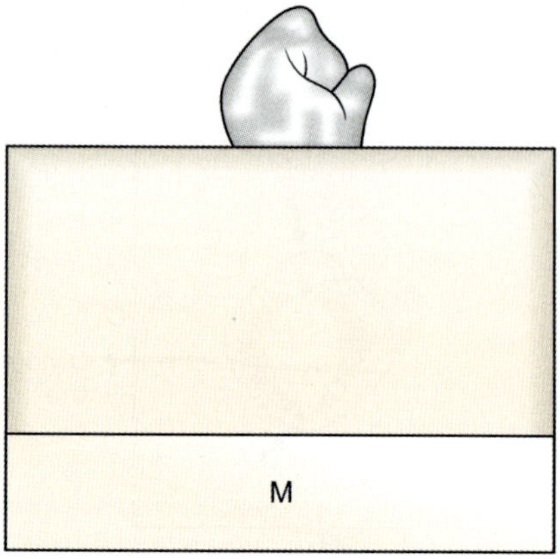

Fig. 5.21K: Step 11—Carve the mesial aspect

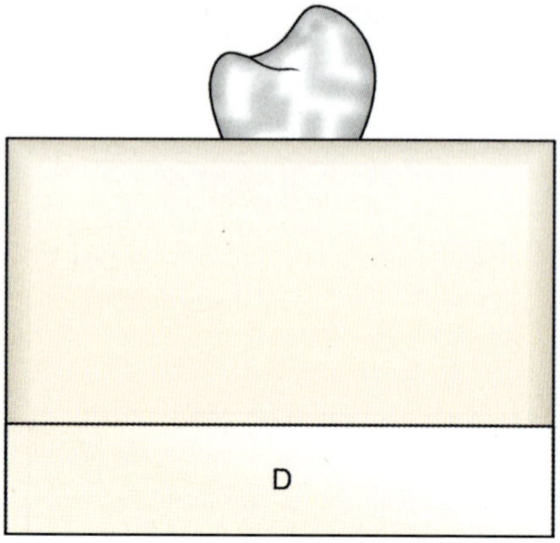

Fig. 5.21L: Step 12—Carve the distal aspect

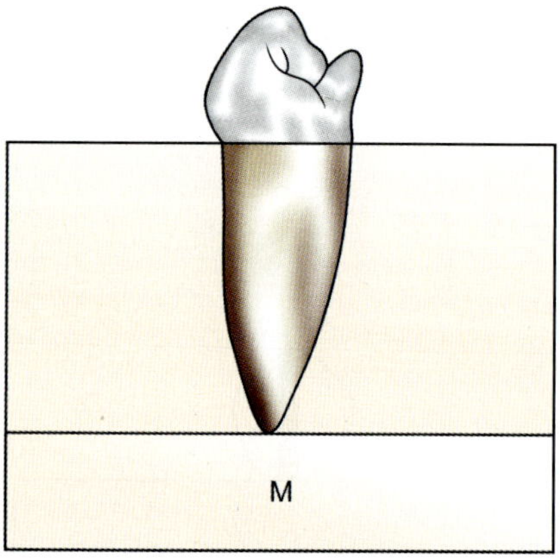

Fig. 5.21M: Step 13—Draw the root outline on mesial aspect

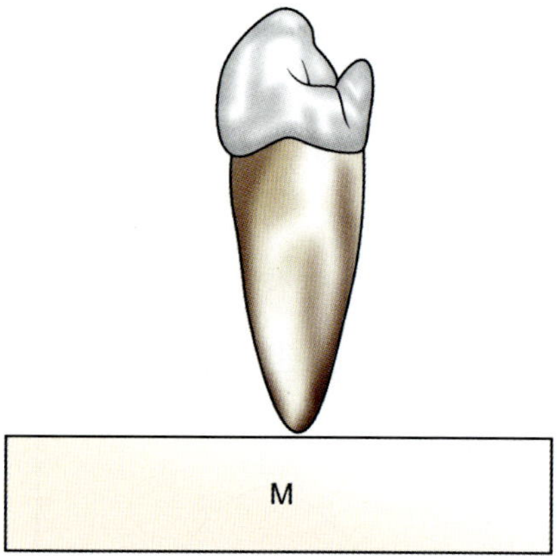

Fig. 5.21N: Step 14—Carve according to the root outline

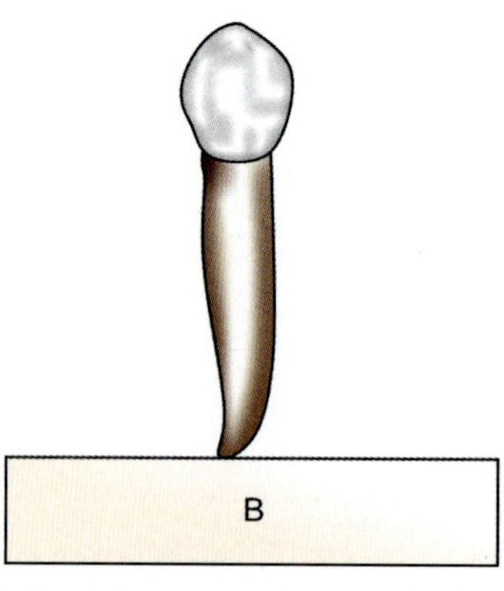

Fig. 5.21O: Carved permanent mandibular first premolar

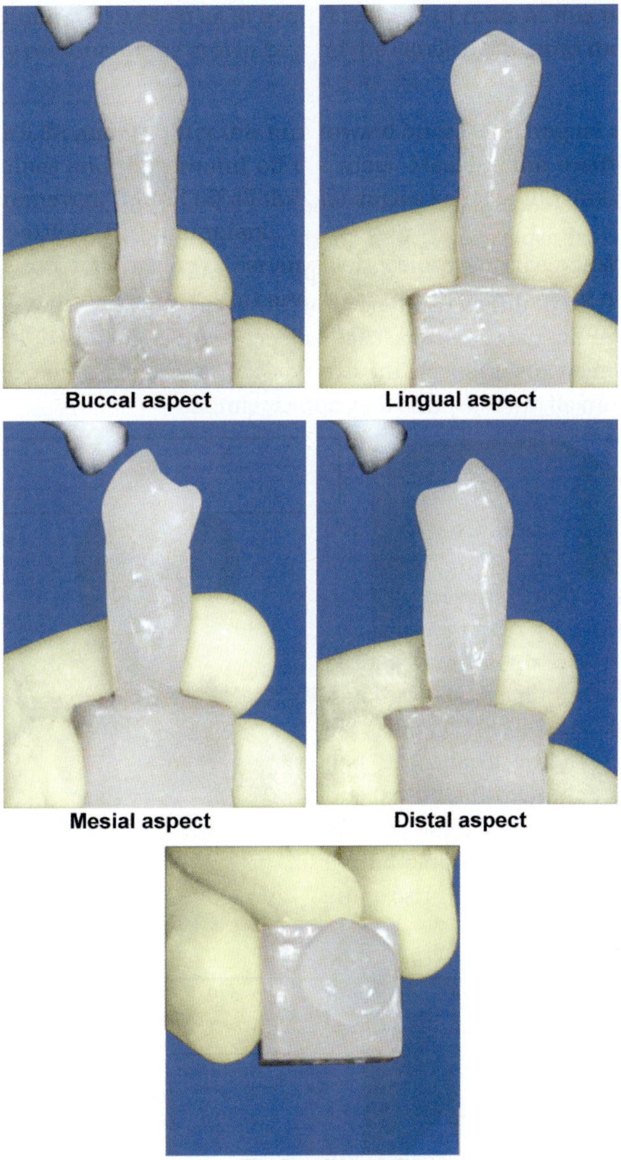

Fig. 5.22: Permanent mandibular first premolar

REFERENCES

1. Woelfel JB, Scheid RC. Dental Anatomy. Williams & Wilkins. 1997.
2. Ash, Nelson. Wheelers Dental Anatomy, Physiology & Occlusion. 8th edition. Elsevier. 2003.

THE PERMANENT MANDIBULAR SECOND PREMOLAR

Morphology

The mandibular second premolar resembles the mandibular first premolar from the buccal aspect only.[2] This tooth is larger and has better development in other aspects. There are two types of mandibular second premolar. **a**. two cusp type **b**. three cusp type.[2] The three cusp type is more common and appears more angular from occlusal aspect. The two cusp type appears more rounded from occlusal aspect. The two types differ mainly from occlusal design otherwise from all other aspects they appear similar.

Buccal Aspect[1,2] (Fig. 5.23)

The buccal cusp is shorter than the mandibular first premolar. The mesial cusp ridge is shorter than the distal cusp ridge. Both the cusp ridges are straight. The buccal cusp tip is less pointed than the mandibular first premolar. The mesial and distal contact areas are broad and placed occlusal to the half of the length of crown. The mesial and distal outline converges at the cervical third of the crown. The middle buccal lobe is well developed giving rise to the buccal ridge.

The root is broader mesiodistally than that of the first premolar. The root apex is more blunt.

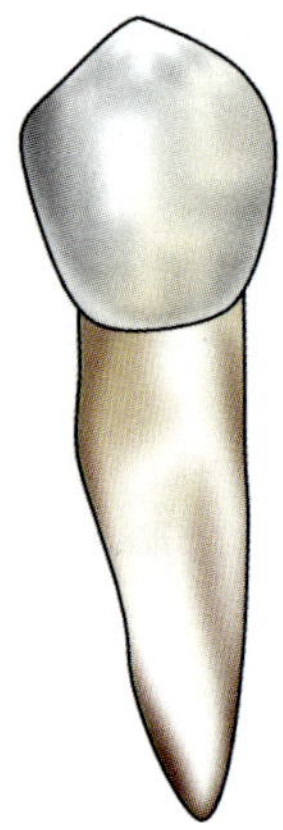

Fig. 5.23: Mandibular right second premolar, buccal aspect

Lingual Aspect[1,2] (Fig. 5.24)

The differences from lingual aspect are:

1. The lingual lobes are well developed giving rise to mesiolingual and distolingual cusp.
2. Less of the occlusal surface seen from lingual aspect.

Two cusp type: The lingual cusp height is equal to buccal cusp.

Outline

Crown: The mesial and distal outline is more curved from cusp tip till the middle third of the crown. The outline converges at the cervical third. The cervical line is irregular.

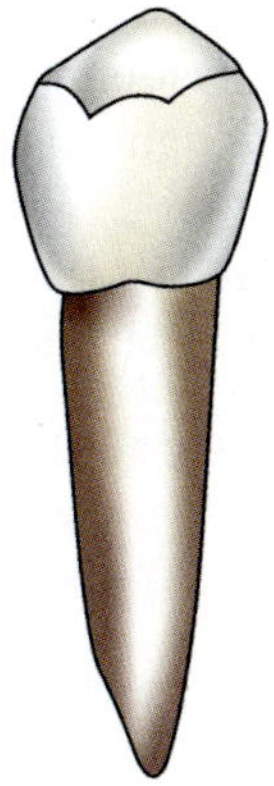

Fig. 5.24: Mandibular right second premolar, lingual aspect

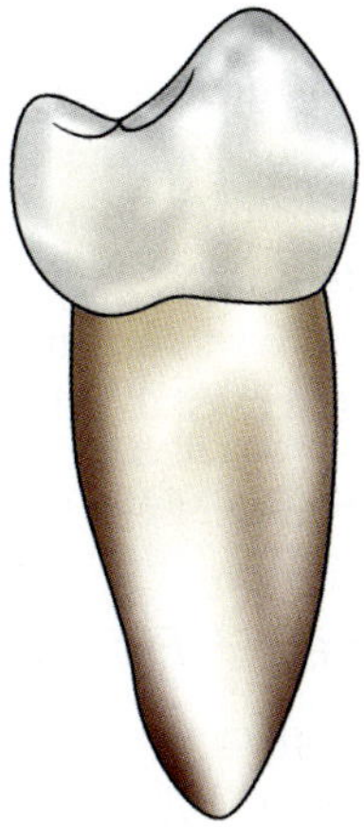

Fig. 5.25: Mandibular right second premolar, mesial aspect

Root: Gradual tapering of the root outline from cervical line till the root apex is seen.

Surface
The surface of the crown is smooth and convex.

Three cusp type
The mesiolingual and distolingual cusp are present. The mesiolingual cusp is larger than the distolingual cusp. The mesiolingual cusp is pointed and it is placed at a higher level than the distolingual cusp tip. The distolingual cusp tip is flat. The height of mesiolingual cusp is almost equal to the buccal cusp.

A lingual groove is seen in between mesiolingual and distolingual cusp, and the groove terminates at the junction of occlusal and middle third of the crown.

The outline of the mesiolingual and distolingual cusp is curved. The single root outline gradually tapers from the cervical line till the root apex. The root apex is blunt.

Mesial Aspect[1,2] (Fig. 5.25)

Outline
Crown: The buccal outline is convex at cervical third and the middle third shows greater convexity. The outline from here shows lingual inclination. The buccal cusp tip is placed at the center of the root. The lingual outline is straight at the cervical third. The middle third and occlusal third is more convex and outwards than the lingual outline of the root. The lingual cusp tip is in line along the lingual outline of the root. Lingual cusp height is about 2 mm shorter than the buccal cusp height. The curvature of cervical line is irregular and is about 1 mm.

Root: The root outline is regular and gradually tapers toward the root apex.

Surface

Crown: Since the mesial marginal ridge is placed at a higher level, less of occlusal surface is seen from mesial aspect. No mesiolingual developmental groove on the crown portion is seen. The mesial marginal ridge is at right angles to the long axis of the tooth.

The maximum convexity is present at occlusal to half of the length of the crown, i.e. the mesial contact area and rest of the surface is flat and smooth.

Root: The surface of the root is slightly convex with a blunt root apex.

Distal Aspect[1,2] (Fig. 5.26)

The distal aspect is similar to mesial aspect except that much of the occlusal surface is seen. This is because the distal marginal ridge is placed at a lower level and also the crown is also tipped distally over the root trunk which is the characteristic of all posterior maxillary and mandibular teeth.

Occlusal Aspect[1,2] (Fig. 5.27)

Two common forms of this tooth is already described, i.e. two cusp type and three cusp type.

Three cusp type: The occlusal shape is squarish to lingual to buccal cusp tip.

Dimensions: The buccolingual width is greater than the mesiodistal width.

Size of the cusps: The buccal cusp is largest followed by mesiolingual then the distolingual cusp.

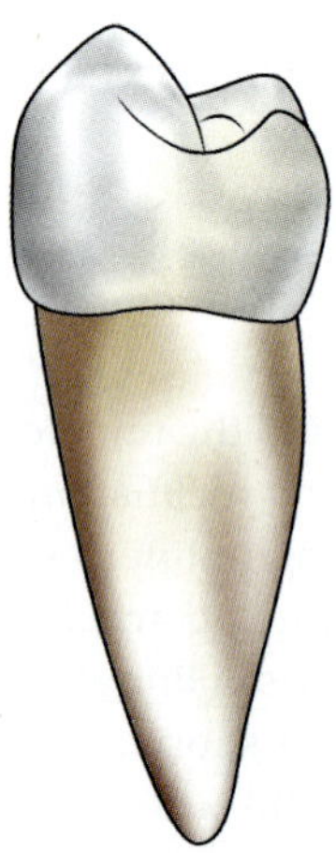

Fig. 5.26: Mandibular right second premolar, distal aspect

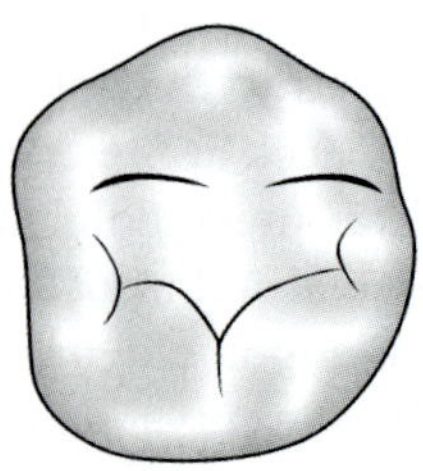

Fig. 5.27: Mandibular right second premolar, occlusal aspect

Ridges: Mesiobuccal and distobuccal cusp ridge of buccal cusp, mesiolingual and distolingual cusp ridges of mesiolingual cusp, mesiolingual and distolingual cusp ridges of distolingual cusp are present. Triangular ridges of buccal cusp, mesiolingual cusp and distolingual cusp are also seen. The buccal triangular ridge being larger among the three.

The mesial marginal ridge and distal marginal ridges are present. The mesial marginal ridge is placed at a higher level.

Grooves and Pit: The mesial developmental groove extends mesially towards mesial marginal ridge from central pit. The distal developmental groove extends distally towards distal marginal ridge from central pit. Both the grooves extend from the central pit mesially and distally, a groove from central pit extends lingually in between the mesiolingual and distolingual cusp termed as lingual groove. This groove terminates at $^1/_3$rd of the crown length on the lingual aspect.

All the three grooves combined together form a typical Y-shaped groove on the occlusal aspect.

Fossa: Mesial and distal triangular fossae are seen adjacent to mesial and distal marginal ridges, respectively.

Two Cusp type

The occlusal form is rounded. The mesiolingual and distolingual line angles are rounded.

Dimensions: The buccolingual width is greater than the mesiodistal width.

Ridges: Mesiobuccal and distobuccal cusp ridges of buccal cusp and mesiolingual and distolingual cusp ridges of lingual cusp are present.

- Buccal and lingual triangular ridges are presen.
- Transverse ridge running from buccal to lingual cusp is seen.
- Mesial marginal ridge and distal marginal ridges are also present.

Grooves: A central developmental groove which is crescent shaped on the occlusal surface travels in a mesiodistal direction and terminates in the mesial and distal fossae, respectively and branches out to give rise to supplemental grooves.

Fossa: A circular mesial and distal fossae harboring supplemental grooves are seen.

Pits: Mesial and distal developmental pits are present where the groove gives supplemental grooves.

Carving technique

[Measurements (in mm)]

Cervico-occlusal length of crown	–	8.0
Length of root	–	14.5
Mesiodistal diameter of crown	–	7.0

Mesiodistal diameter of crown at cervix	–	5.0
Buccolingual diameter of crown	–	8.0
Buccolingual diameter of crown at cervix	–	7.0
Curvature of cervical line - mesial	–	1.0
Curvature of cervical line - distal	–	0.0

The detailed carving steps can be followed as for the permanent maxillary first premolar (Figs 5.28A to 5.28O). Figure 5.29 is a carved mandibular second premolar.

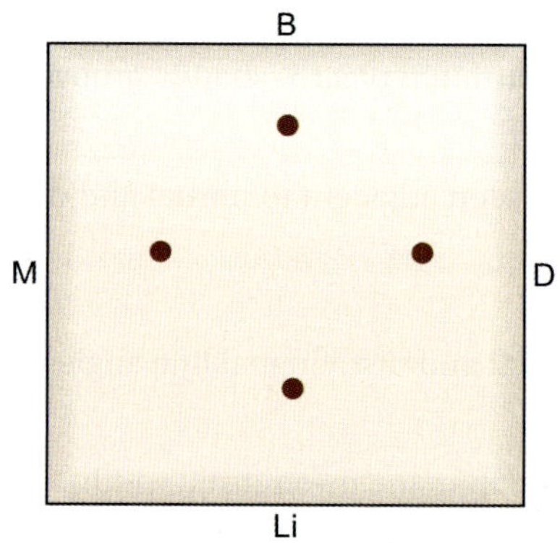

Fig. 5.28A: Step 1—Mark the buccolingual and mesiodistal width

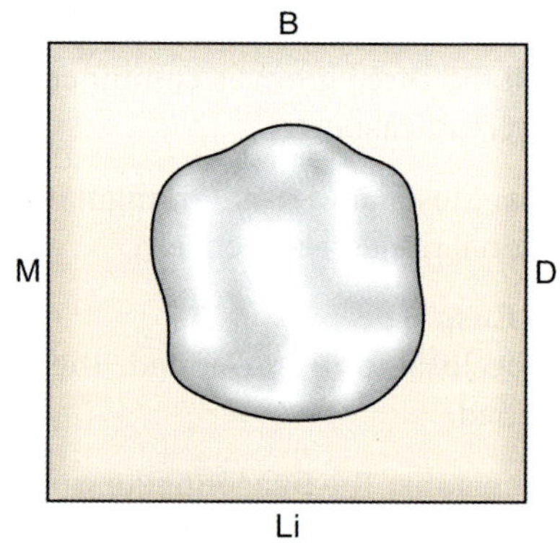

Fig. 5.28B: Step 2—Draw the occlusal outline

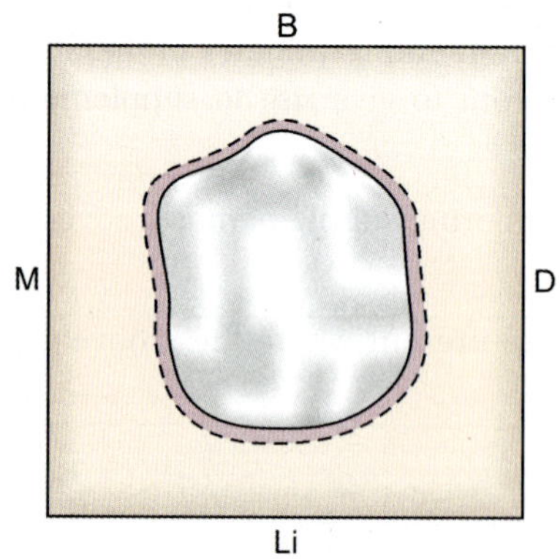

Fig. 5.28C: Step 3—Carve according to the outline leaving about 0.5 mm of wax extra

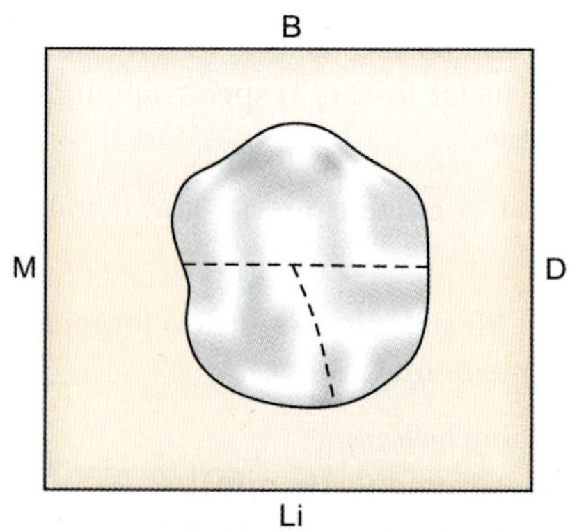

Fig. 5.28D: Step 4—Draw the outline of three cusps on occlusal surface

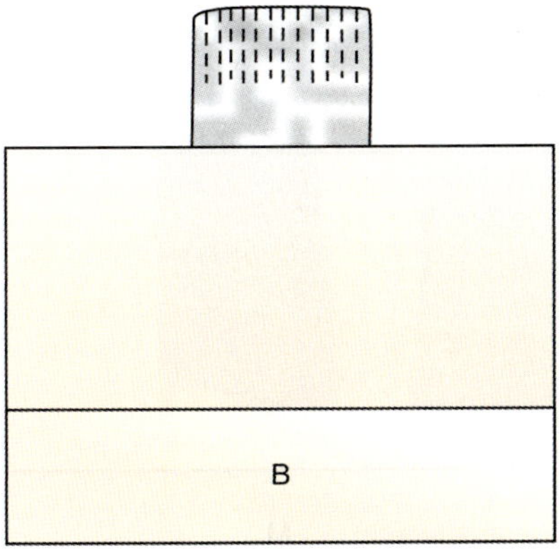

Fig. 5.28E: Step 5—About half of the crown length, reduce the wax toward occlusal aspect this is to place the cusp tip inside (buccal aspect)

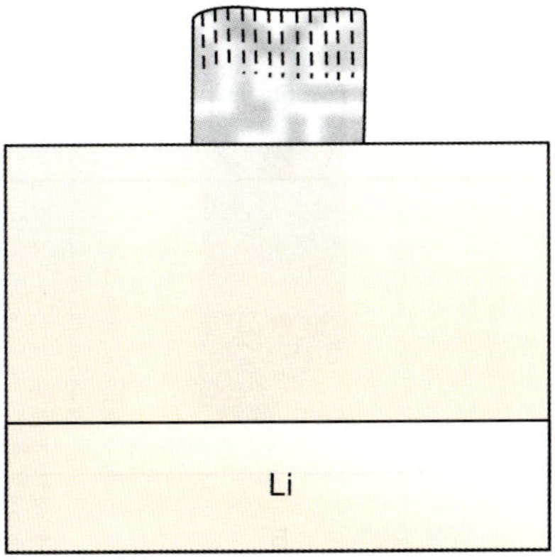

Fig. 5.28F: Step 6—About half of the crown length reduce the wax toward occlusal aspect this is to place the cusp tip inside (lingual aspect)

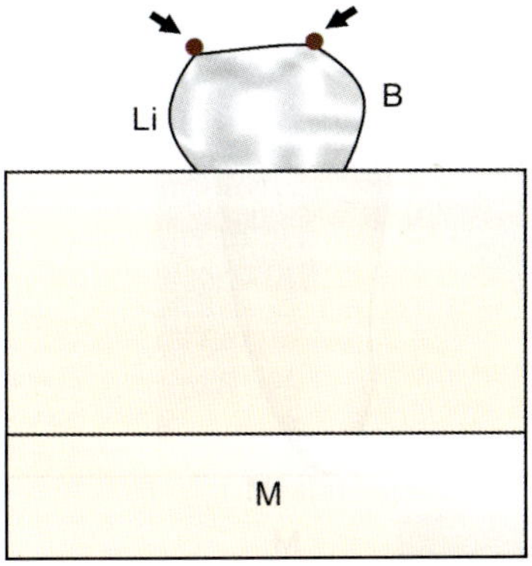

Fig. 5.28G: Step 7—The arrow mark pointing the buccal and lingual cusp tip placed inside from mesial aspect

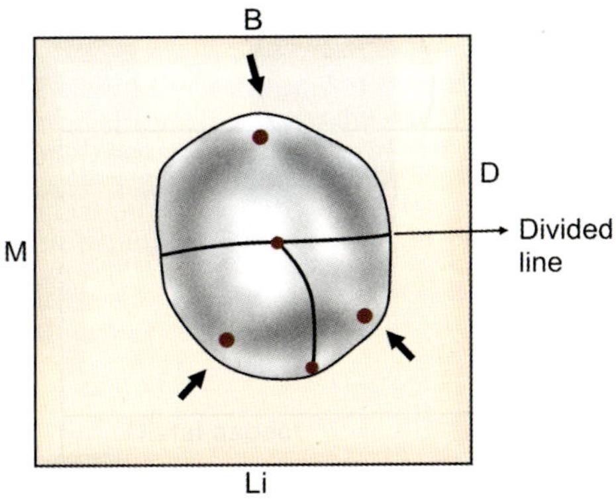

Fig. 5.28H: Step 8—The shaded part represents wax to be reduced so as to carve the buccal and lingual triangular ridges, marginal ridges and cusp ridges of all three cusps

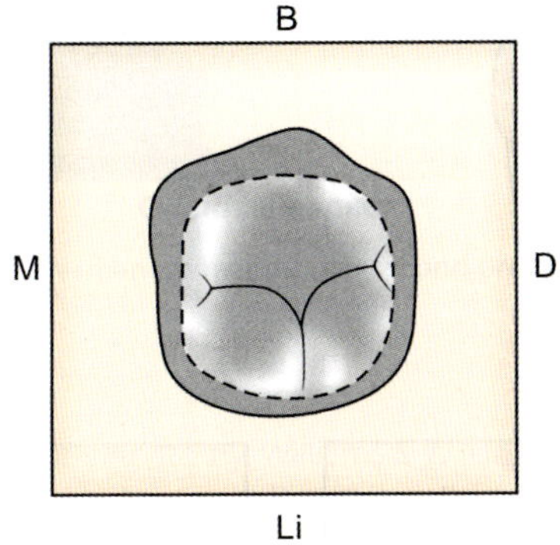

Fig. 5.28I: Step 9—Carve the grooves. The shaded parts are ridges

CHAPTER

6

The Permanent Molars

The human mouth contains upper (maxillary) and lower (mandibular) molars. They are, maxillary first molar, maxillary second molar, maxillary third molar, mandibular first molar, mandibular second molar and mandibular third molar.[1,2]

Molars are the rearmost and most complicated kind of tooth in most mammals. In many mammals they grind food; hence the Latin name *mola*, "millstone".[3]

Molars differ considerably from one species to another, so there are many terms describing them:[3]

- **Tribosphenic:** This kind is found in insectivores and young platypuses (adults have no teeth). Upper molars look like three-pointed mountain ranges; lowers look like two peaks and a third off to the side.
- **Quadrate:** This kind is found in humans and various other species. Four cusps are arranged in a rectangle; there may be a fifth.
- **Bunodont:** The cusps, instead of being sharp peaks, are rounded hills. The entire tooth is covered in enamel, and is most common among omnivores such as the pig, the bear and humans.
- **Hypsodont:** There is a lot of enamel and dentin above the gumline and the top of the pulp. This kind of molar is found in mammals that wear their teeth a lot, such as the horse.
- **Zalambdodont:** The tooth has two ridges that meet at an angle, forming the letter lambda.
- **Dilambdodont:** Like zalambdodont, but there are two lambdas on one tooth.
- **Lophodont:** The tooth has a few ridges perpendicular to the jaw.
- **Selenodont:** The tooth has a crescent-shaped ridge or ridges.
- **Loxodont:** The tooth has several parallel oblique ridges on its surface. The elephant *Loxodonta* is so named for this feature.

THE PERMANENT MAXILLARY FIRST MOLAR

Morphology

These teeth assist mandibular molars in performing mastication and comminution of food.[1,2] They are largest and strongest maxillary teeth by virtue of their bulk and anchorage in the jaws.[2] Maxillary first molar erupts after the eruption of mandibular first molar around the age of 6 years.[2] They erupt distal to the deciduous second molar.

Importance of Permanent First Molar

a. They are present in the center of the fully developed jaw anteroposteriorly. So, they are considered as the "corner stones" of the dental arches.[2]
b. They provide "Key of Occlusion".[2]
c. Because of their proper occlusion they help in "Mastication".[1,2]
d. Since they are the first permanent teeth to erupt in the oral cavity they are more "prone for dental caries".[1,2]

Buccal Aspect[1,2] (Fig. 6.1)

The crown is roughly trapezoidal in shape. The cusps seen from this aspect are the mesiobuccal, distobuccal, mesiolingual and distolingual. The mesiobuccal cusp is larger than the distobuccal cusp. The roots visible are mesiobuccal, distobuccal and lingual root. The lingual root is longer by 1 mm than the buccal roots.

Outline

Crown: The mesial outline of the crown from cervical line is straight sloping down till the mesial contact area. The mesial contact area is placed at the junction of occlusal and middle third. The distal outline of the crown is more curved from cervical line till the distolingual cusp tip. The distal contact area is present at the middle of middle third. The curvature of cervical line is irregular, the convexity is facing towards the root apex.

The mesial and distal slope of mesiobuccal cusp meet at obtuse angle, i.e. the cusp tip is rounded. The mesial and distal slope of distobuccal cusp meets acute angle, i.e. the cusp tip is more pointed.

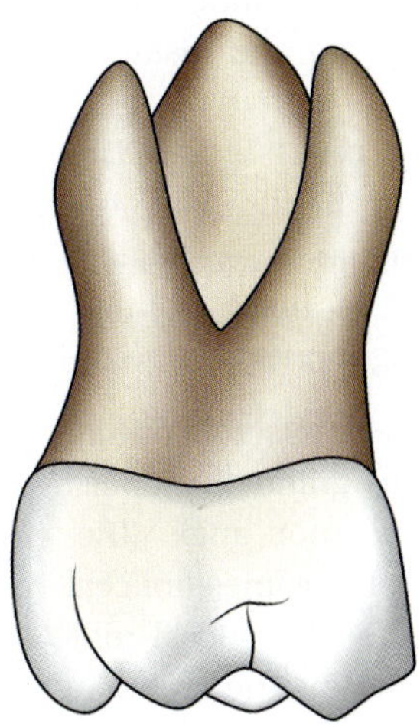

Fig. 6.1: Permanent maxillary right first molar, buccal aspect

Root: The cervical third of mesiobuccal and distobuccal root is concave. From the middle third the outline curves outward showing convexities on both the buccal roots.

The greatest convexity is seen at the middle of the length of bifurcation. The mesial root inclines distally and the distal root is straight. The buccal root apices are pointed.

Surface

Crown: A buccal developmental groove is present at the middle of width from mesiobuccal outline and the distolingual outline. This groove terminates at the half of the crown length. Immediately above the terminus of buccal groove, an enamel dip is present. The rest of crown surface from buccal aspect is smooth and convex.

Root: The cervical third of the root is flat and the remaining root surface is smooth and convex. The root trunk length is about 4 mm on buccal aspect.

Lingual Aspect[1,2] (Fig. 6.2)

The cusps seen from lingual aspect are mesiolingual cusp, fifth cusp and distolingual cusp. The roots visible are the lingual root, mesiobuccal root and the distobuccal root.

Outline

Crown: The mesial outline is straight sloping downward and outward till it joins the distal slope of mesiolingual cusp. The angle formed by the mesial outline and distal slope of mesiolingual cusp is very sharp (90°). The distal outline is more curved from cervical line and is continuous with the slopes of the cusp and with the lingual developmental groove. Because of this curving of this outline, it looks like a semicircle. The mesiolingual cusp tip is rounded (Obtuse angle of the mesial and distal slope of this cusp).

The cervical line is irregular. The outline of the fifth cusp is seen at the mesiolingual line angle. The fifth cusp tip is more pointed than the mesiolingual cusp tip.

Root: The lingual root outline is conical in shape, gradually tapering toward the blunt root apex. The complete outline of the mesiobuccal root and half of the distobuccal root outline is seen including the root apex from this aspect.

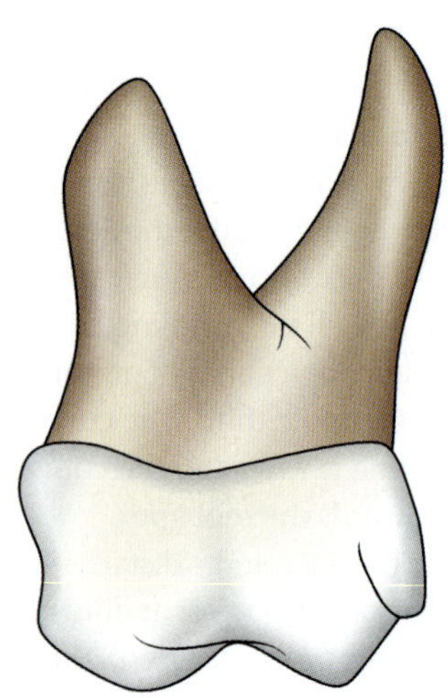

Fig. 6.2: Permanent maxillary right first molar, lingual aspect

Surface

Crown: The cusp of Carabelli (fifth cusp) is present about 2 mm cervical to the mesiolingual cusp tip. The distolingual cusp surface is more convex compared to the mesiolingual cusp surface. The lingual development terminates at about half of the crown length. The mesiolingual cusp is about $^3/_5$th of the mesiodistal width of the crown and this is the largest cusp among the other cusps.

Root: The surface of the root is smooth and convex.

Mesial Aspect[1,2] (Fig. 6.3)

The cusps and roots seen from mesial aspect are the mesiobuccal, mesiolingual and fifth cusp (Cusp of Carabelli), roots are mesiobuccal and lingual root.

At the cervical third the buccal outline from the cervical line is convex, middle third is slightly concave and occlusal third is slightly convex. This outline progresses downward and inward compared to the root outline.

The lingual outline is convex throughout the fifth cusp outline, from here the outline dips inward suddenly. The mesiolingual cusp is on a line with the long axis of the lingual root.

The cervical line is irregular that shows curvature of about 1 mm on mesial aspect.

Root: The buccal outline of the root extends upward and outward from the crown with a slightly pointed root apex sloping down toward the bifurcation. The lingual outline of the root inclines buccally and it is banana shaped. The lingual root is longer than the mesiobuccal root.

Surface

Crown and Root: The mesial marginal ridge is irregular and is placed about 2 mm from the mesiolingual cusp tip. Just above the mesial marginal ridge the mesial contact area is present, i.e. at the junction of middle and occlusal third. Cervical to this contact area the crown surface is flat or slightly concave, this concavity crosses the cervical line, extends till the bifurcation of root and also a developmental depression is present within this concavity.

The buccal root surface is broad and flat. The lingual surface of the root is smooth and convex. The length of root trunk is about 3 mm.

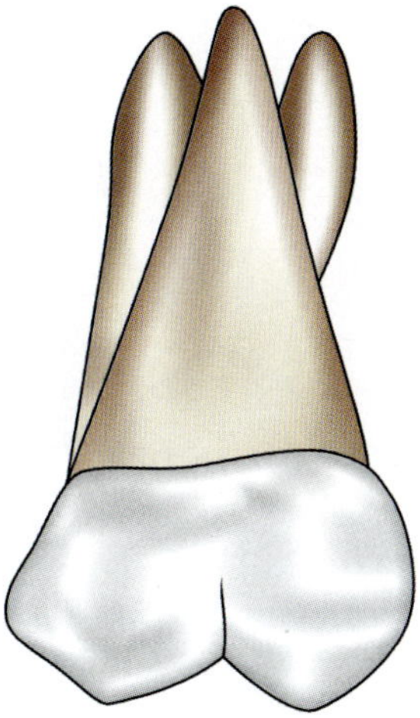

Fig. 6.3: Permanent maxillary right first molar, mesial aspect

Distal Aspect[1,2] (Fig. 6.4)

The outline of the crown and root is almost similar to mesial aspect except for the following differences. The differences are:

1. Because the crown tapers distally, part of the buccal surface is seen.
2. The distal marginal ridge is irregular and is placed more cervically, i.e. about 3 mm from the cusp tips. Because of this the triangular ridges on the occlusal surface is visible.
3. The cervical line curvature is 0 mm.
4. The distal surface is more convex.
5. Only the cervical third of root is concave.
6. Since the distobuccal root is smaller than the mesiobuccal root, part of the mesiobuccal root is visible.
7. The distobuccal root outline is straight from cervical line till the root apex and then slopes downward till the bifurcation.
8. The lingual root is concave at the bifurcation.
9. The length of root trunk is about 5 mm on distal aspect.

Occlusal Aspect[1,2] (Fig. 6.5)

The shape of the occlusal aspect is rhomboidal. The cusps seen from occlusal aspect are mesiolingual, mesiobuccal, distobuccal, distolingual and fifth cusp (cusp of Carabelli).

Dimensions: The buccolingual width is greater than the mesiodistal width. The mesiolingual cusp is the largest, followed by mesiobuccal, distolingual, distobuccal cusp and fifth cusp.

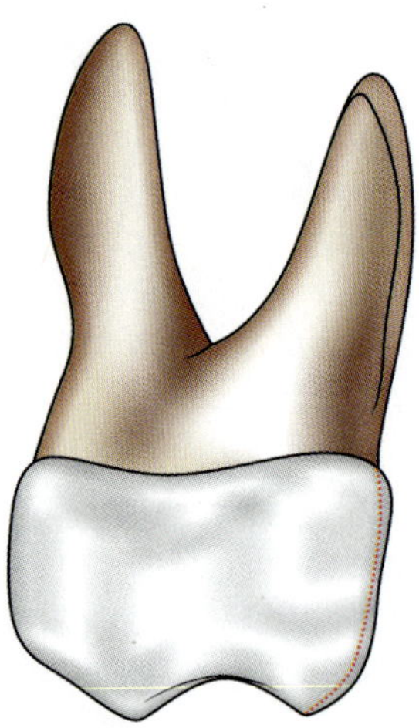

Fig. 6.4: Permanent maxillary right first molar, distal aspect

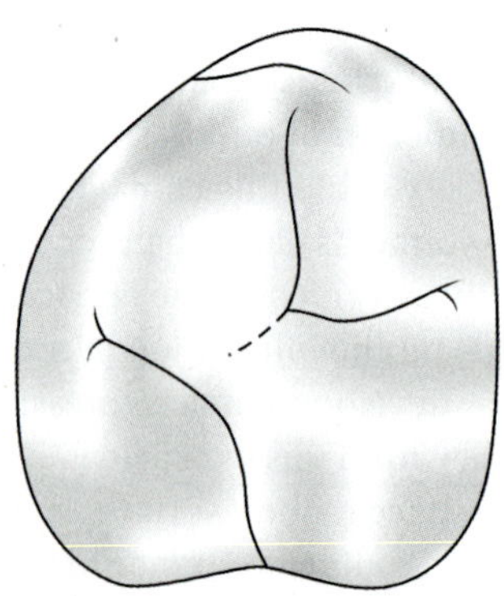

Fig. 6.5: Permanent maxillary right first molar, occlusal aspect

Developmentally, only three cusps are major cusps, i.e. mesiolingual, mesiobuccal, distobuccal cusp which are the primary cusps. The other cusps, distolingual and fifth cusp are secondary cusps. Cope Osborn hypothesis put forward the "Maxillary molar primary cusp triangle" theory. During human tooth development only three major cusps are formed that is why even the roots are three, i.e. the mesiobuccal, distobuccal cusp and lingual root. This is explained by, i.e. the fifth cusp is absent in second and third molar and the distolingual cusp is reduced in size in second molar and it disappears in third molar.

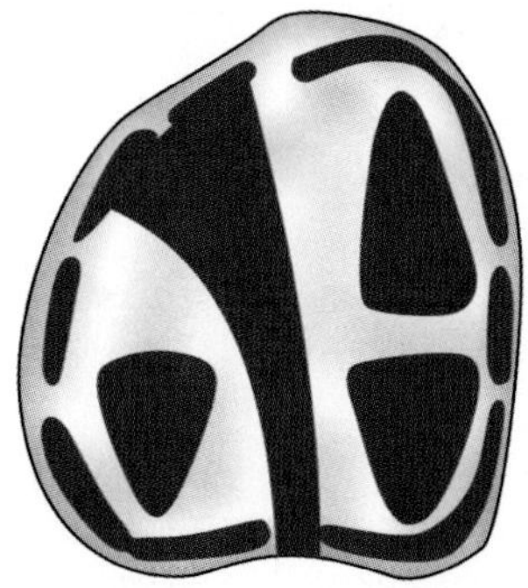

Fig. 6.5A: Ridges (shaded parts)

Ridges: Mesial and distal cusp ridges of all the five cusps are present. The mesial and distal marginal ridges, the buccal triangular ridge of mesiobuccal cusp, the lingual triangular ridges of mesiolingual, distolingual and fifth cusp are seen. The oblique ridge is present obliquely on the occlusal surface formed by the union of triangular ridge of distobuccal cusp and distal ridge of mesiolingual cusp (Fig. 6.5A).

Fossa:

Two major fossae:
1. Central fossa
2. Distal fossa

Two minor fossae:
1. Mesial triangular fossa
2. Distal triangular fossa

Central fossa is triangular in form and is present mesial to oblique ridge. Distal fossa is linear in form and seen distal to oblique ridge.

Mesial triangular fossa is present distal to mesial marginal ridge.

Distal triangular fossa is present mesial to distal marginal ridge (Fig. 6.5B).

Sulcus: Central sulcus extends buccally and mesially from the central fossa.

Grooves: The Central developmental groove is present within the central sulcus and extends buccally giving rise to buccal developmental groove which terminates on the buccal aspect (refer buccal aspect). Then the groove extends mesially giving rise to mesial developmental groove and branches within the mesial triangular fossa. When this central groove crosses over the oblique ridge it is called as transverse groove of the oblique ridge (Fig. 6.5C).

The distal groove begins at the center of distal fossa extends distally and lingually giving rise to lingual developmental groove which terminates on lingual aspect (refer lingual aspect). When the groove extend distally it gives branches

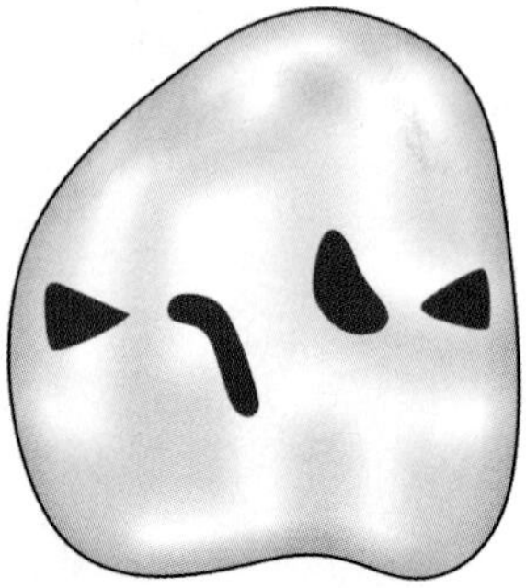

Fig. 6.5B: Fossae (shaded part)

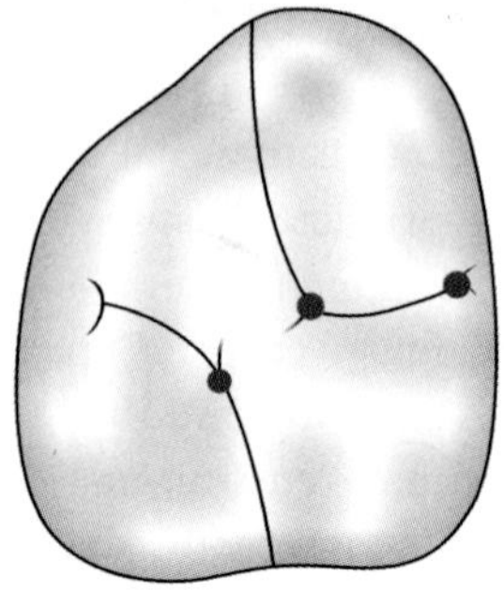

Fig. 6.5C: Grooves, pits (dots)

and lies within the distal triangular fossa (Fig. 6.5C). A groove from the distal groove extends over the oblique ridge is termed as distal oblique groove.

Pits: Wherever the groove gives supplemental branches the pits are found. The pits seen are central pit and distal pit (Fig. 6.5C).

Carving Technique

Measurements (in mm)

Cervico-occlusal length of crown	–	7.5
Length of root	–	b-12, li-13
Mesiodistal diameter of crown	–	10
Mesiodistal diameter of crown at cervix	–	8.0
Buccolingual diameter of crown	–	11.0
Buccolingual diameter of crown at cervix	–	10.0
Curvature of cervical line - mesial	–	1.0
Curvature of cervical line - distal	–	0.0

To carve molar teeth, first carve the crown and then the root. Figure 6.7 is a carved maxillary first molar. Carve the occlusal aspect first and then the other aspects.

Step 1: Smoothen the wax block. Mark the butt end to retain as base for carving. Mark the aspects, i.e. **B** for buccal aspect, **L** for lingual aspect, **M** for mesial aspect and **D** for distal aspect.

Step 2: Mark the length of crown and root on all the four aspects.

Step 3 (Fig. 6.6A): To carve the occlusal aspect, first mark the buccolingual width (11 mm) and mesiodistal width (10 mm) of crown, on the other end of the butt end (base) of the wax block.

Step 4 (Fig. 6.6B): Draw the occlusal outline

Step 5 (Fig. 6.6C): After drawing the occlusal outline, carve according to this outline upto the length of crown which is marked on the wax block, leaving about 0.5 mm extra wax than the outline.

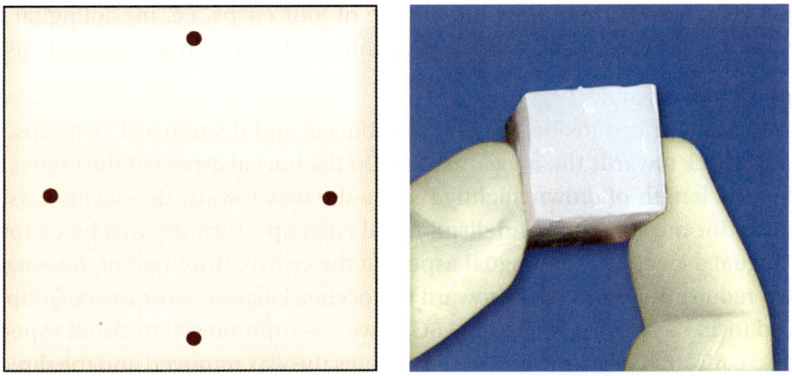

Fig. 6.6A: Step 3

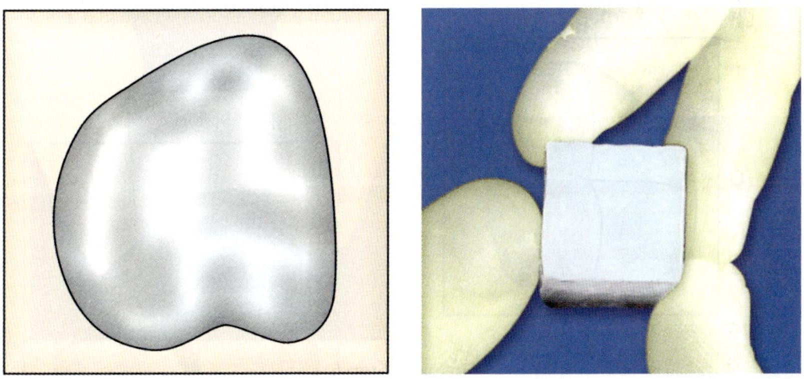

Fig. 6.6B: Step 4

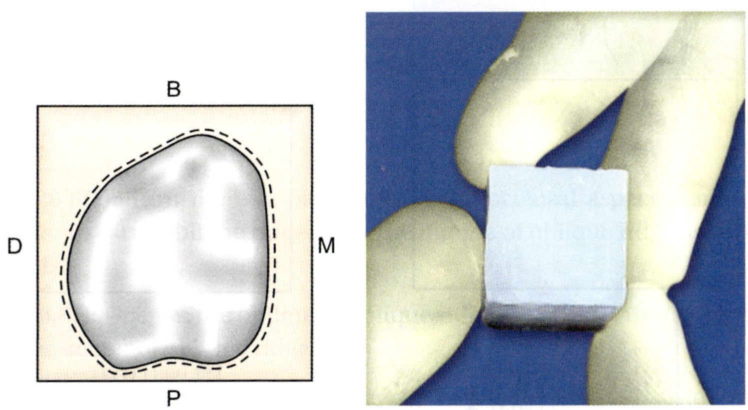

Fig. 6.6C: Step 5, the dotted line represents the extra wax retained apart from the outline (left), picture to show carving done according to the outline (right)

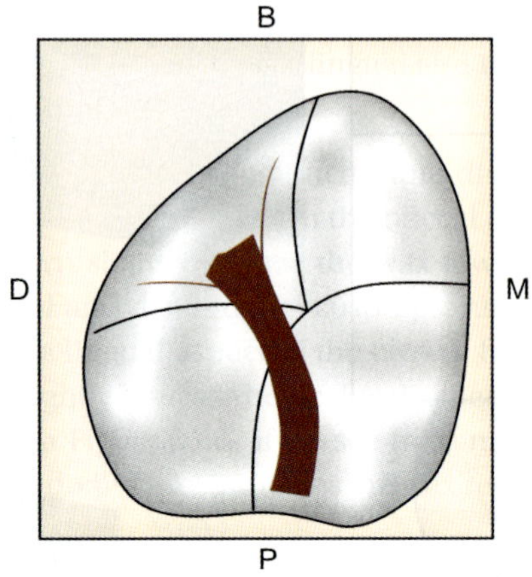

Fig. 6.6I: Step 9 (The shaded part of oblique ridge represents the gradual reduction of wax toward the center of oblique ridge)

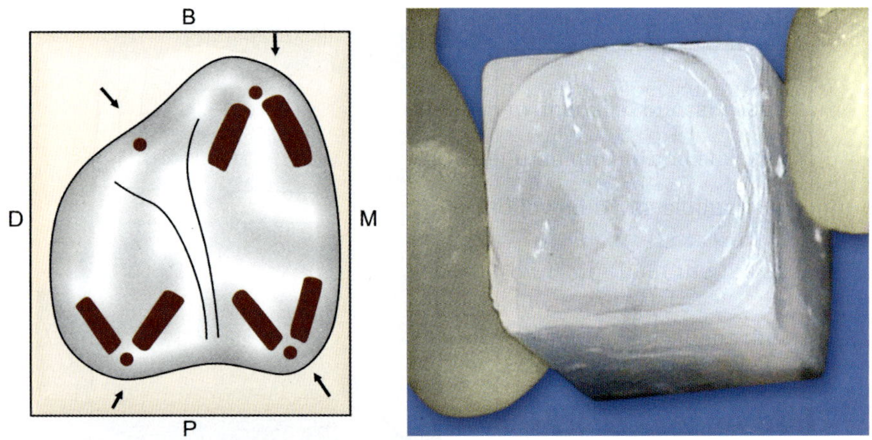

Fig. 6.6J: Step 10—The shaded part in the diagram represents wax to be reduced, arrow mark points the cusp tips. Photograph (right) showing the ridges

Once this is done, automatically the cusp ridges of mesiobuccal (mesial and buccal cusp ridges), mesiolingual cusp (mesial and lingual cusp ridge), the mesial marginal ridge and distal marginal ridge and the triangular ridges of mesiobuccal, distolingual and mesiolingual cusp is obtained (the unshaded portion of the Figure 6.6J, represents all the above ridges).

Reduce the distal marginal ridge level about 3 mm from distal cusp tips and mesial marginal ridge by 2 mm from mesial cusp tips. Now carve the cusp tips, i.e. mesiobuccal and mesiolingual cusp tips round, distobuccal cusp tip more pointed and distolingual more rounded.

Step 11 (Fig. 6.6K): Carve the fifth cusp. To carve this turn wax block towards mesial aspect. About 2 mm from mesiolingual cusp tip draw a groove mesiolingually for some distance and then deepen this groove. After this from the groove reduce the wax towards cusp tip till the fifth cusp is prominently seen. Then the fifth cusp tip appears more pointed.

Step 12 (Fig. 6.6L): Carve a triangular shaped concavity mesial to oblique ridge and a linear shaped concavity distal to oblique ridge for central fossa and distal fossa, respectively. Carve a triangular shaped concavity near the marginal ridges for mesial and distal triangular fossae.

Step 13 (Fig. 6.6M): Carve the central developmental groove deeper starting from the central fossa, extend it mesially for mesial developmental groove along with supplemental grooves. Then extend buccally for buccal developmental groove and also extend over the oblique ridge for transverse groove.

From the distal fossa extend the groove distally with supplemental grooves for distal developmental groove and lingually for lingual developmental groove.

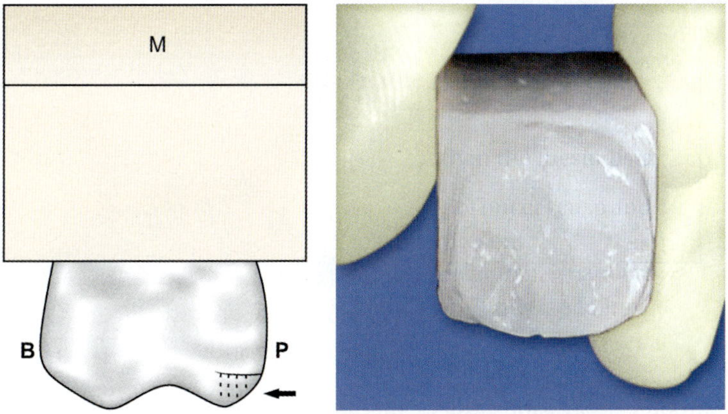

Fig. 6.6K: Step 11—Arrow mark points the groove and the dotted lines represents direction of wax reduced (Photograph showing all the above-mentioned ridges)

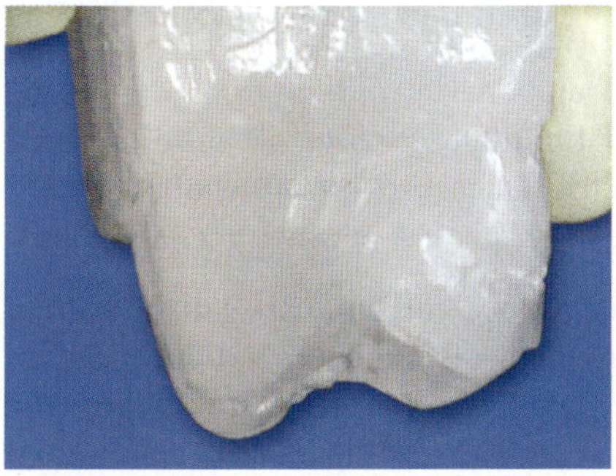

Fig. 6.6K: The groove drawn to carve fifth cusp

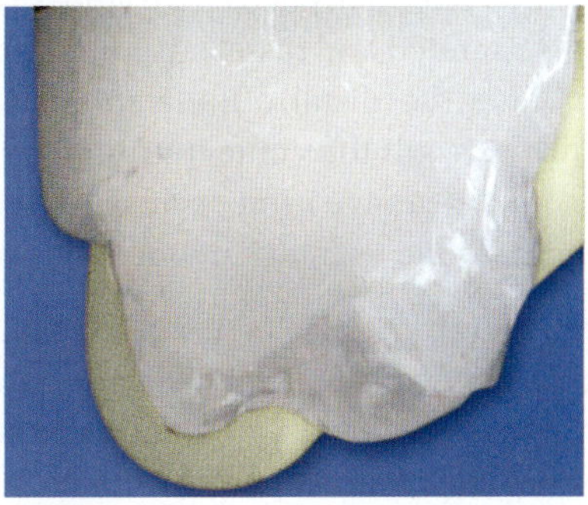

Fig. 6.6K: The groove is deepened

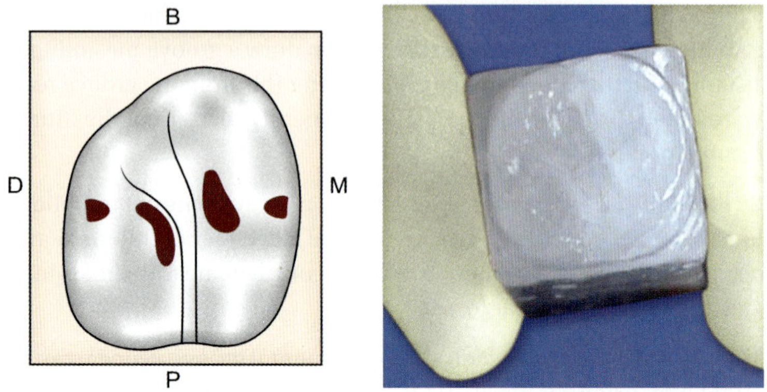

Fig. 6.6L: Step 12—The shaded parts are fossae, the unshaded outline is oblique ridge in the diagram. The photograph on the right shows fossae

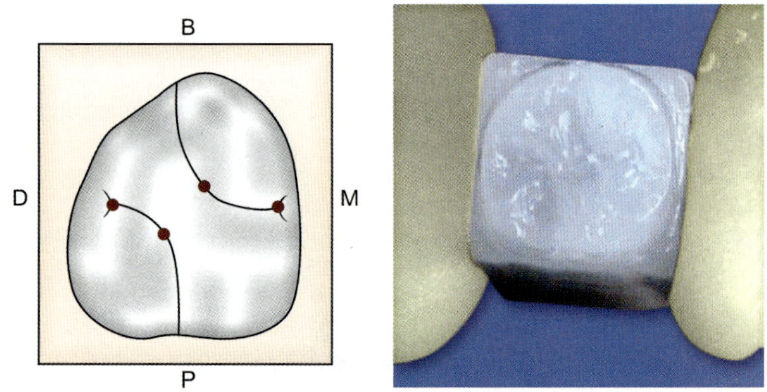

Fig. 6.6M: Step 13—Grooves, pits (dots)

Carve pinpoint depressions where the groove branches mesially, distally and centrally for mesial, distal and central pits, respectively.

Step 14 (Fig. 6.6N): Once the occlusal aspect is carved, turn the wax block towards buccal aspect, carve slopes of both buccal cusps. The mesiobuccal cusp tip is rounded and distal cusp tip is pointed.

Carve the distal outline more curved and mesial outline straight sloping downward till the contact area (junction of middle and occlusal third). Extend the buccal groove from occlusal aspect on the buccal aspect till half of the crown length. At the terminus of buccal groove, carve a shallow concavity (enamel dip).

Step 15 (Fig. 6.6O): Turn toward the mesial aspect, carve the buccal outline, i.e. at the cervical third convexity, middle third concavity and occlusal third slightly convex. Carve the lingual outline, the fifth cusp is completely convex. Carve the mesial and distal slopes for both mesiobuccal and mesiolingual cusps. Both cusp tips should be rounded, flatten the middle and cervical third of mesial aspect.

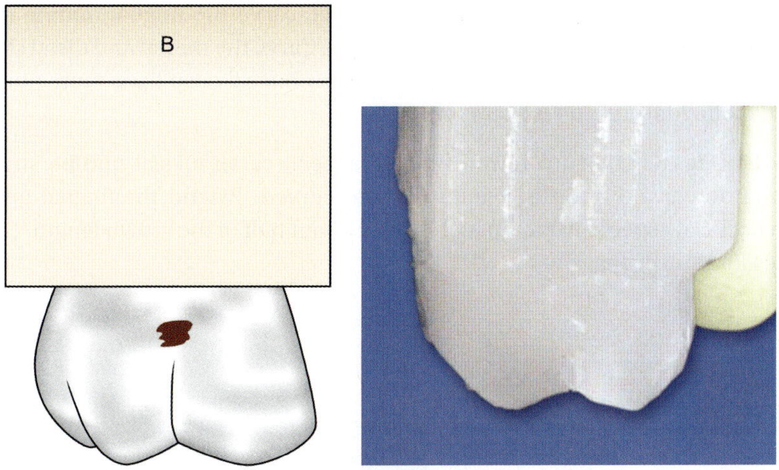

Fig. 6.6N: Step 14

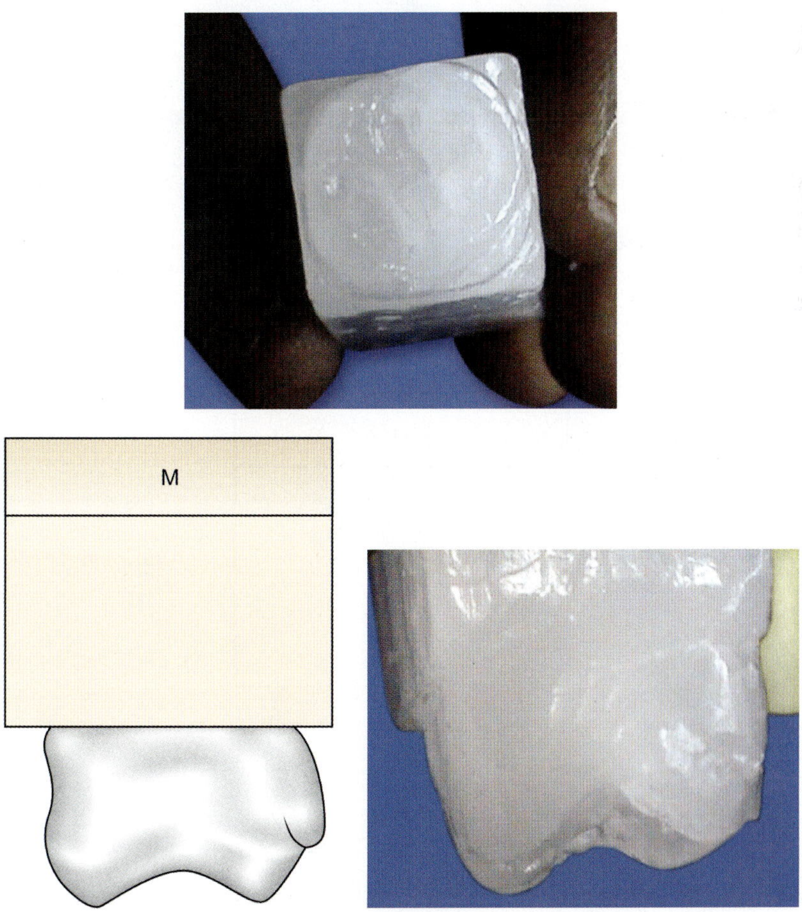

Fig. 6.6O: Step 15 (Photograph showing fifth cusp from occlusal aspect)

Step 16 (Fig. 6.6P): Turn toward distal aspect, carve the lingual outline more convex, buccal outline similar to mesial aspect. Carve the mesial and distal slopes for distobuccal and distolingual cusps. The distobuccal cusp tip is more pointed and distolingual cusp tip is more rounded.

Step 17 (Fig. 6.6Q): Turn toward lingual aspect, carve mesial outline straight sloping downward and distal outline more curved. Extend the lingual groove from occlusal aspect toward lingual surface about half of the crown length. Carve slopes for both cusps.

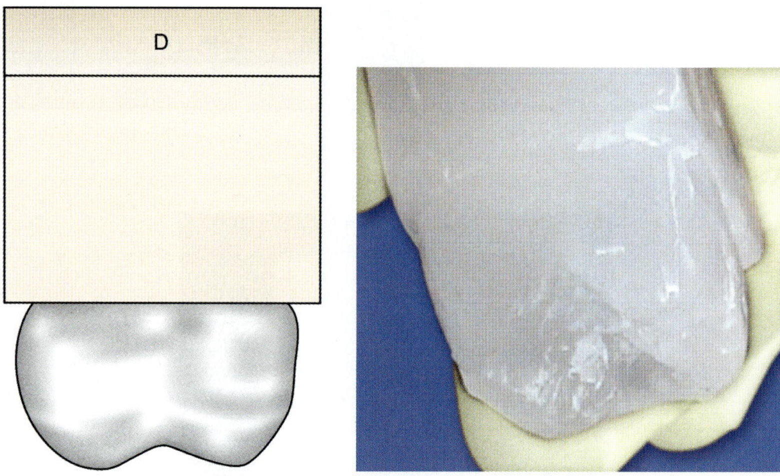

Fig. 6.6P: Step 16

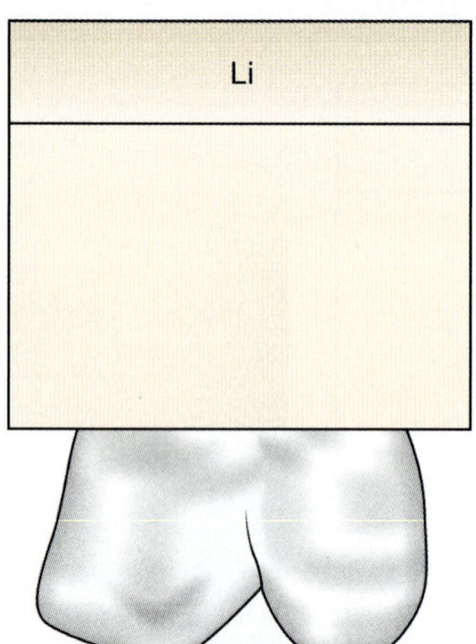

Fig. 6.6Q: Step 17

Step 18 (Figs 6.6R and S): Once the crown is completed, carve the roots: first draw the mesiobuccal and distobuccal root outline. Then start bifurcating the roots. Remove the wax only about half of the wax block width buccolingually; this is very important because wax is needed for lingual root, i.e. bifurcate only half of the wax block width.

Step 19 (Figs 6.6T and U): Turn toward the mesial aspect. Draw the mesiobuccal and lingual outline of the root. Then start bifurcating completely, i.e. the carver should pass through the distal aspect. Now the roots are trifurcated.

Step 20 (Figs 6.6V and W): Turn toward the lingual aspect, draw the lingual outline of root, carve according to the outline and round off the root.

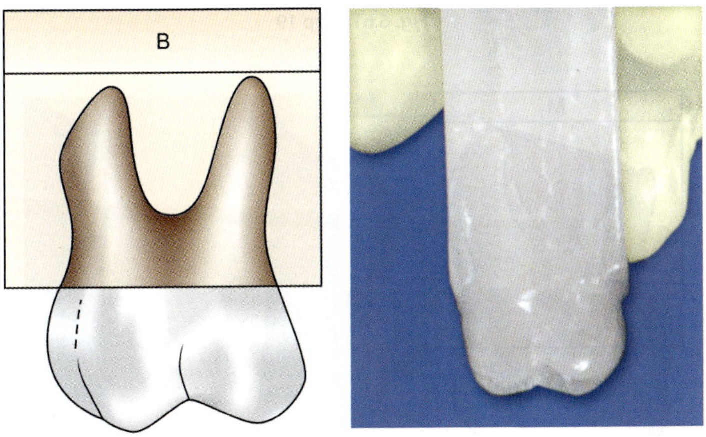

Fig. 6.6R: Step 17

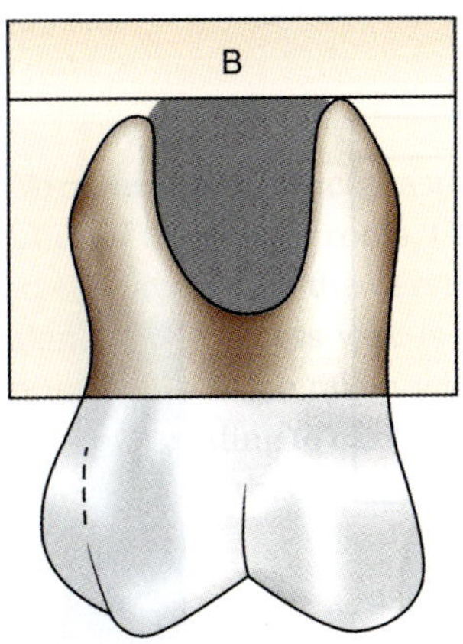

Fig. 6.6S: Step 17—Shaded part represents the reduction of wax for bifurcation but not completely

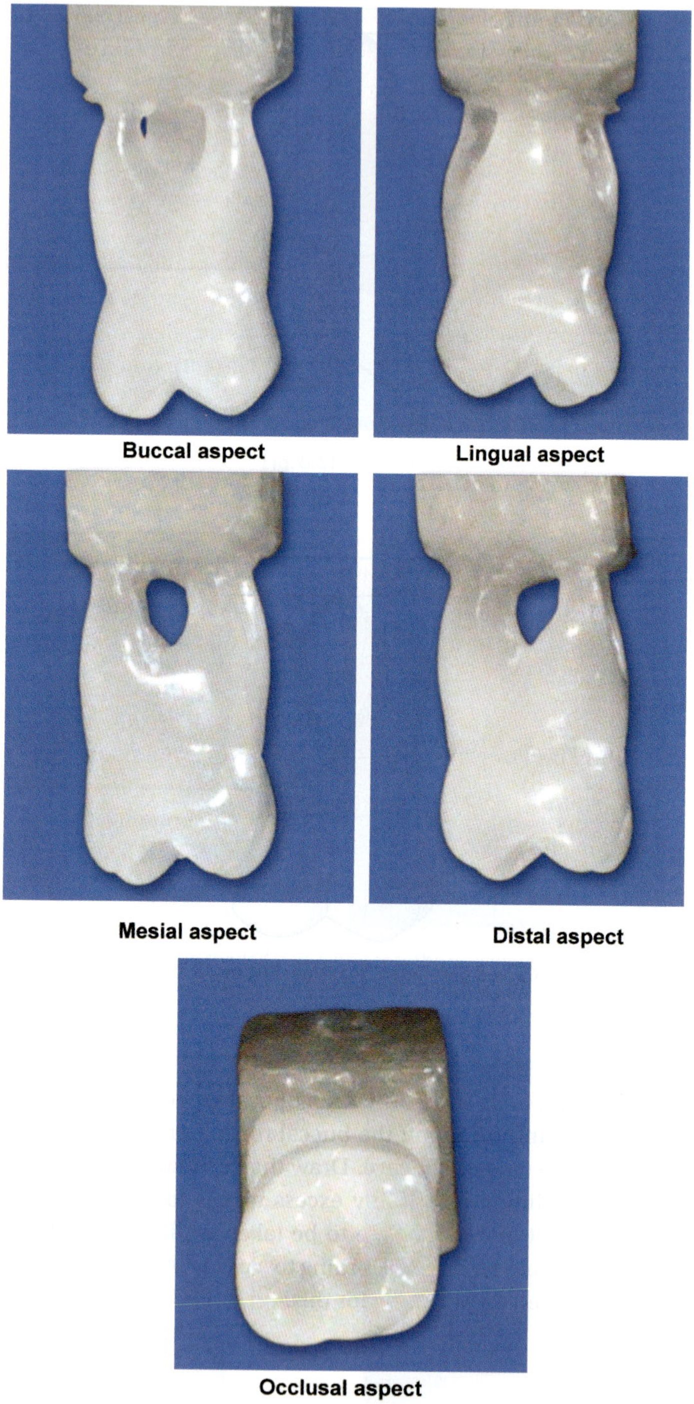

Fig. 6.7: Permanent maxillary first molar

REFERENCES

1. Woelfel JB, Scheid RC. Dental Anatomy. Williams & Wilkins. 1997.
2. Ash, Nelson. Wheelers Dental Anatomy, Physiology & Occlusion. 8th edition. Elsevier. 2003.
3. Stokstad E. Tooth Theory Revises History of Mammals. Science. 2001;291(5501):26. doi: 10.1126/science.10.1126/SCIENCE.291.5501.26.PMID 11191993. http://www.sciencemag.org/cgi/content/full/291/5501/26?ck=nck.
4. www.wikepedia.com.

THE PERMANENT MAXILLARY SECOND MOLAR

Morphology

The maxillary second molar supplements the first molar in function.[2] Direct comparison is made with the maxillary first molar.

Buccal Aspect[1,2] (Fig. 6.8)

The crown length is reduced and also the mesiodistal width is reduced. The distobuccal cusp is smaller. Even the distal marginal ridge is seen from this aspect.

Lingual Aspect[1,2] (Fig. 6.9)

The differences from buccal aspect are:

1. The distolingual cusp is smaller.
- 2. The distobuccal cusp is seen from palatal aspect.
- 3. Fifth cusp is absent.

   The apex of lingual root is in line with the distolingual cusp tip.

Mesial Aspect[1,2] (Fig. 6.10)

The buccolingual width is similar to first molar. The buccal and lingual outline is curved compared to the first molar. The root outlines are similar to first molar. The difference is that the distance between the roots is reduced.

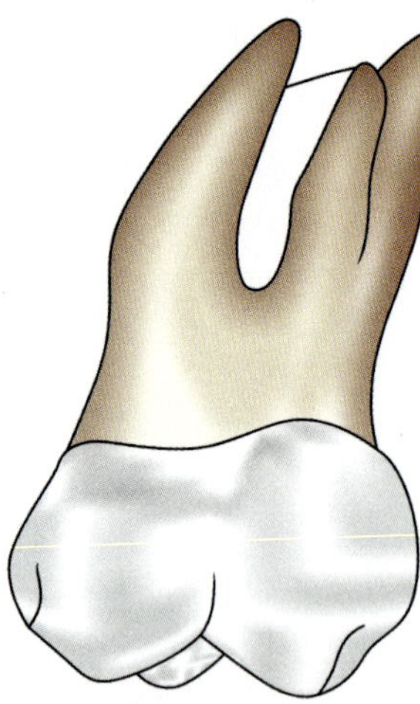

Fig. 6.8: Permanent maxillary left second molar, buccal aspect

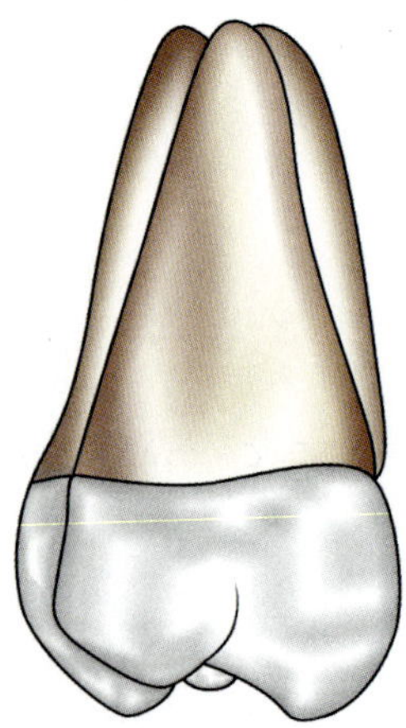

Fig. 6.9: Permanent maxillary left second molar, lingual aspect

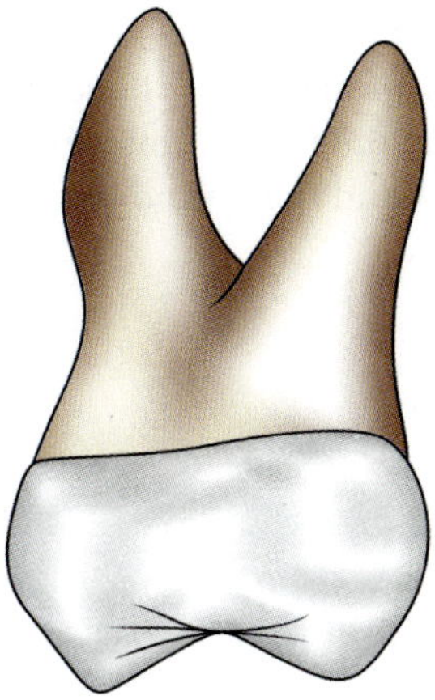

Fig. 6.10: Permanent maxillary left second molar, mesial aspect

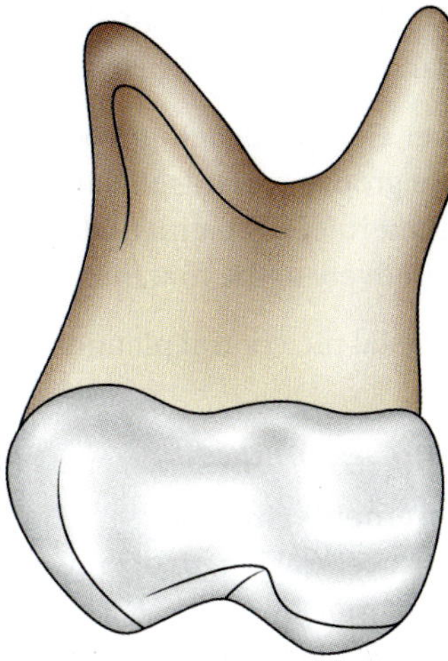

Fig. 6.11: Permanent maxillary left second molar, distal aspect

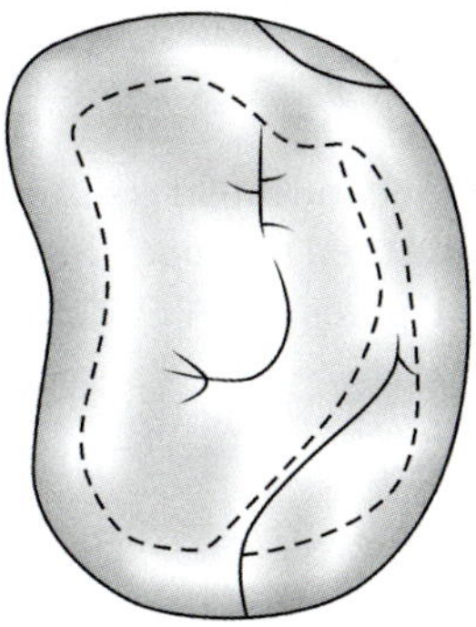

Fig. 6.12: Permanent maxillary left second molar, occlusal aspect

Distal Aspect[1,2] (Fig. 6.11)

Since the distobuccal cusp is smaller than the maxillary first molar, the mesiobuccal cusp is seen from distal aspect. The apex of the lingual root is in line with the distolingual cusp.

Occlusal Aspect[1,2] (Fig. 6.12)

The shape of occlusal outline is rhomboidal. The line angles are more rounded compared to the first molar.

Dimensions: The buccolingual width is greater than the mesiodistal width. The mesiolingual cusp is the largest cusp. The distobuccal and distolingual cusp is smaller compared to first molar.

Ridges: The cusp ridges of all four cusps, the mesial and distal marginal ridges, the triangular ridges of all the 3 cusps and the oblique ridge is present.

Groove: Central developmental groove extends mesially and buccally. Distal oblique groove extends distally and lingually. The difference from first molar is that numerous supplemental grooves are present and these grooves are deeper comparatively to the first molar.

Pits: Mesial pit, central pit and distal pits are present.

Carving Technique

Measurements (in mm)

Cervico-occlusal length of crown	-	7.0
Length of root	-	b-11, li-12
Mesiodistal diameter of crown	-	9.0
Mesiodistal diameter of crown at cervix	-	7.0
Buccolingual diameter of crown	-	11.0
Buccolingual diameter of crown at c ervix	-	10.0
Curvature of cervical line - mesial	-	1.0
Curvature of cervical line - distal	-	0.0

The technique of carving for second molar is similar to permanent maxillary first molar. First carve the crown and then the root. The technique is diagrammatically illustrated as shown below in Figures 6.13A to 6.13V.

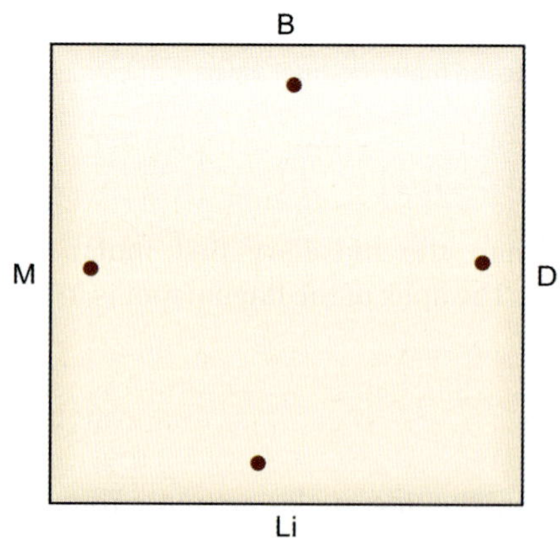

Fig. 6.13A: Step 1—Mark the buccolingual and mesiodistal width

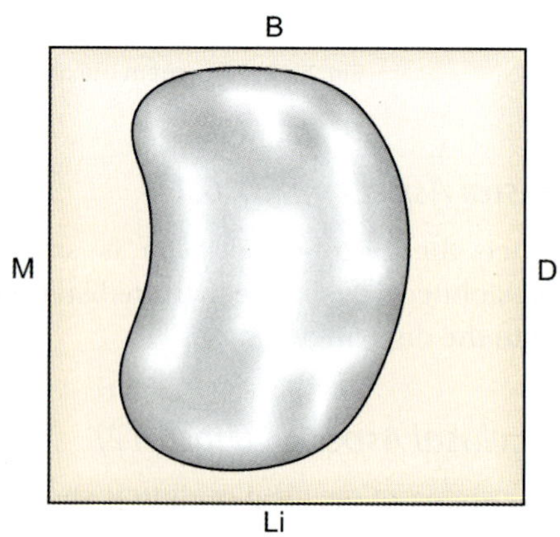

Fig. 6.13B: Step 2—Draw the occlusal outline

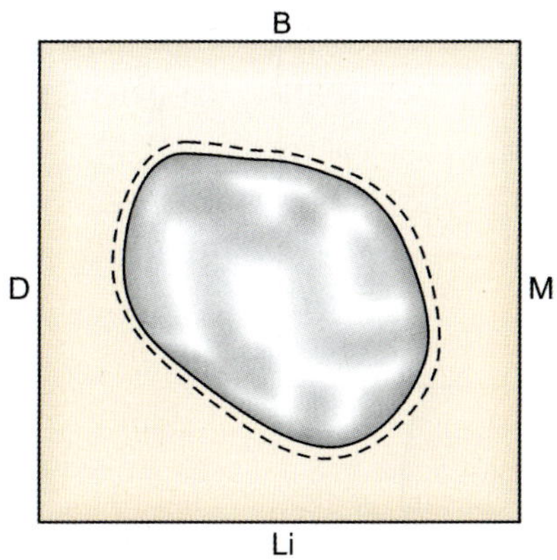

Fig. 6.13C: Step 3—Carve according to the outline, leaving 0.5 mm wax extra

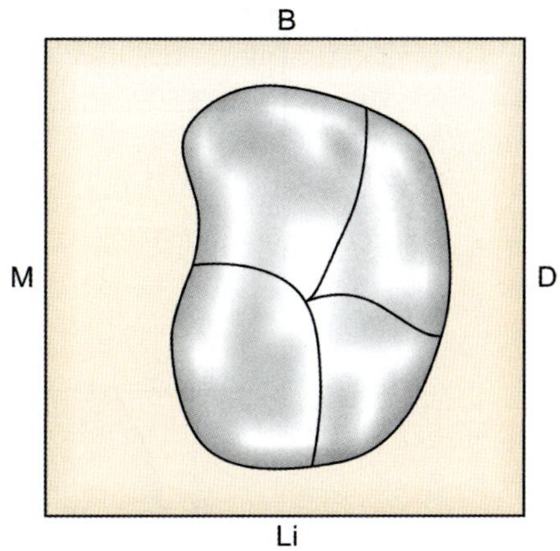

Fig. 6.13D: Step 4—Draw the outline of four cusps based on the size of the cusps

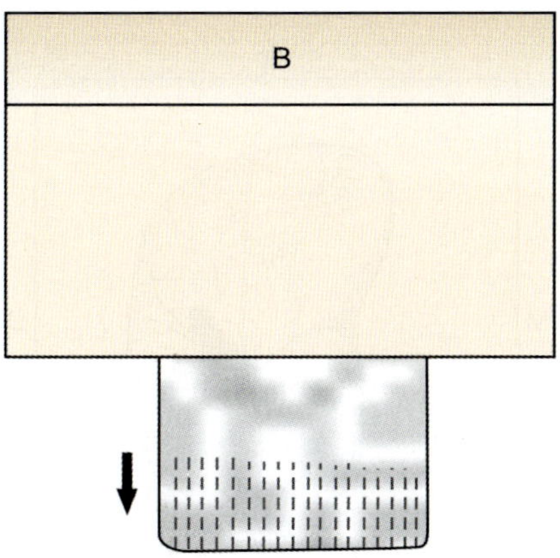

Fig. 6.13E: Step 5—Place the buccal cusp tip inside. For this remove wax from half of the buccal aspect of the crown occlusally. The dotted line represents wax reduced and direction to be removed

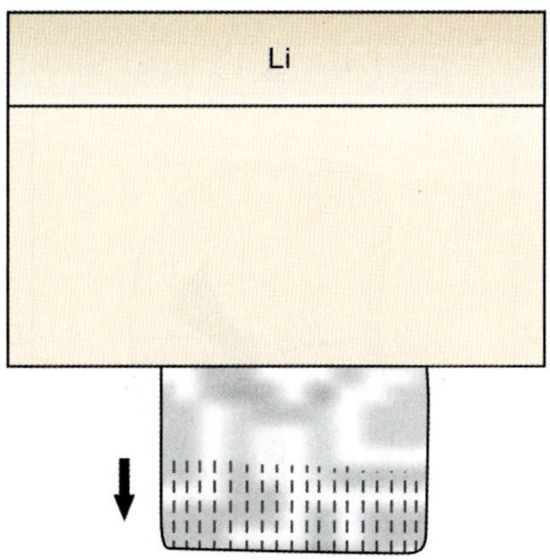

Fig. 6.13F: Step 6—Place the lingual cusp tip inside. For this remove wax from half of the lingual aspect of the crown occlusally. The dotted line represents wax reduced and direction to be removed

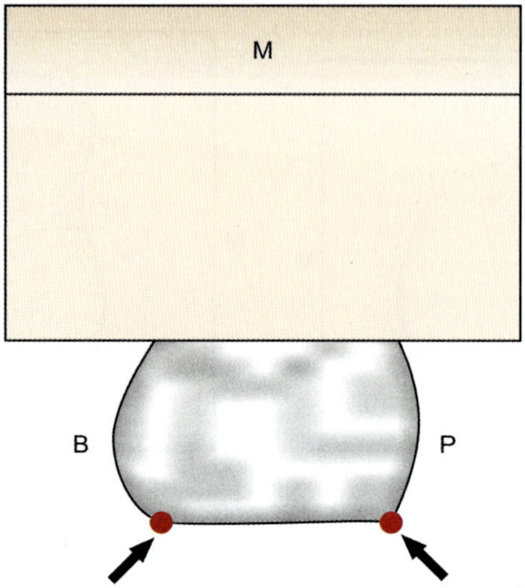

Fig. 6.13G: Step 7—The cusp tips are placed inside. The arrow mark is pointing at the cusp tips

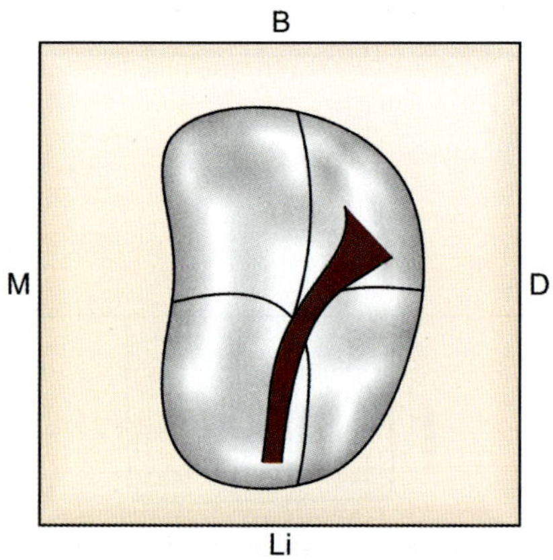

Fig. 6.13H: Step 8—Draw the outline of oblique ridge

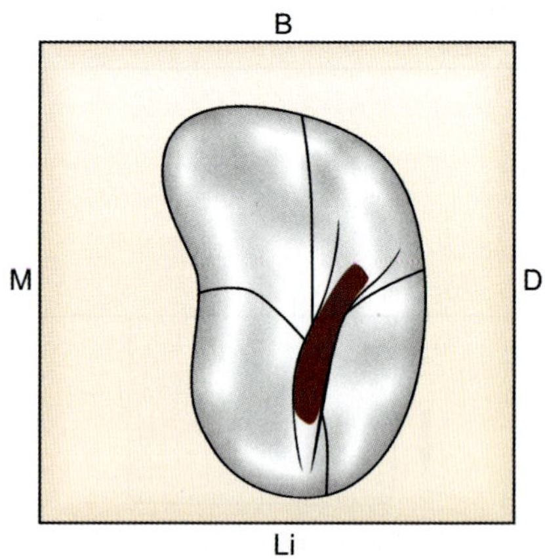

Fig. 6.13I: Step 9—Deepen the outline and depress at the center of oblique ridge

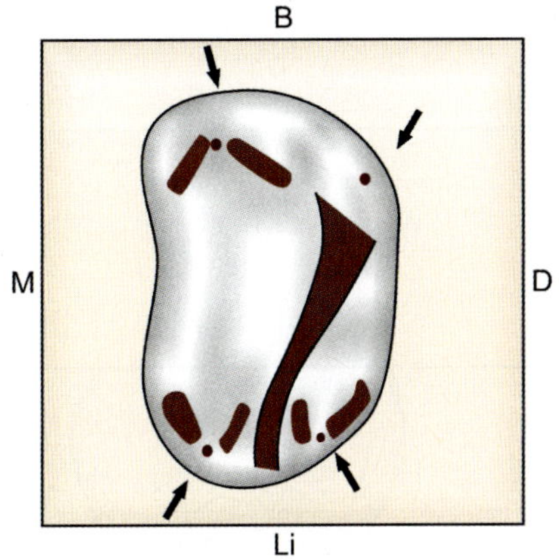

Fig. 6.13J: Step 10—Carve the triangular ridges, cusp ridges and marginal ridges. The shaded part represents the wax to be reduced. The arrow mark represents cusp tips

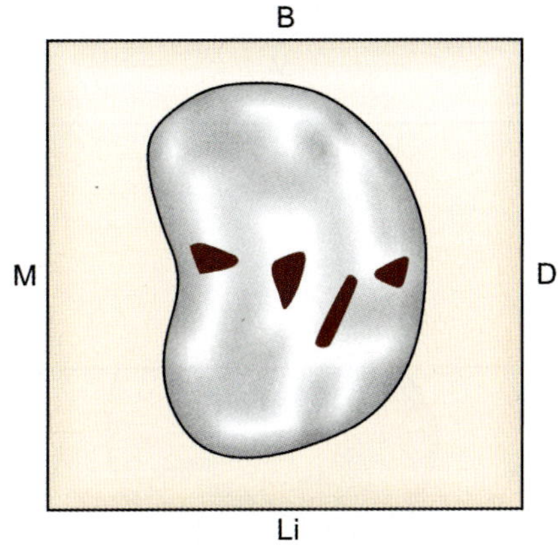

Fig. 6.13K: Step 11—Carve the central fossa, distal fossa, mesial triangular fossa and distal triangular fossa (shaded part)

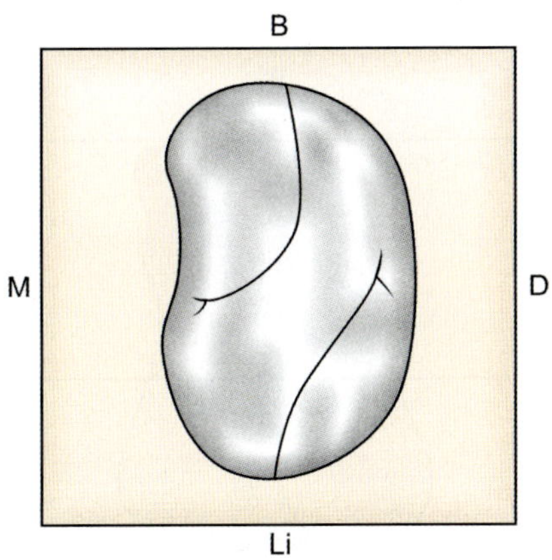

Fig. 6.13L: Step 12—Carve the central developmental groove, buccal groove, distal groove, lingual groove, transverse groove, distal oblique groove and numerous supplemental grooves

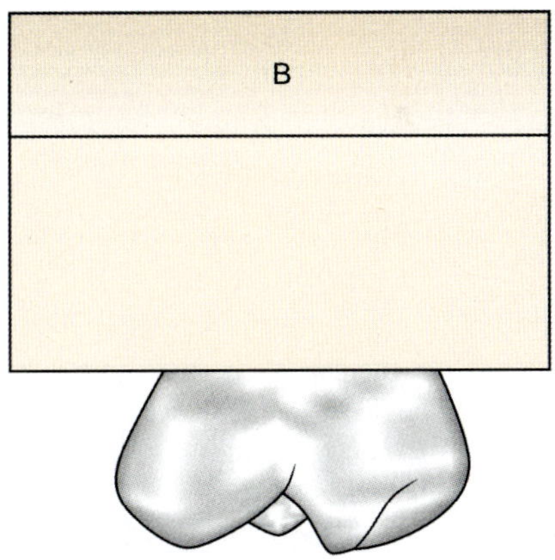

Fig. 6.13M: Step 13—Turn toward buccal aspect to carve the outlines of buccal aspect. Extend the buccal groove from central developmental groove. Carve the cusp tips

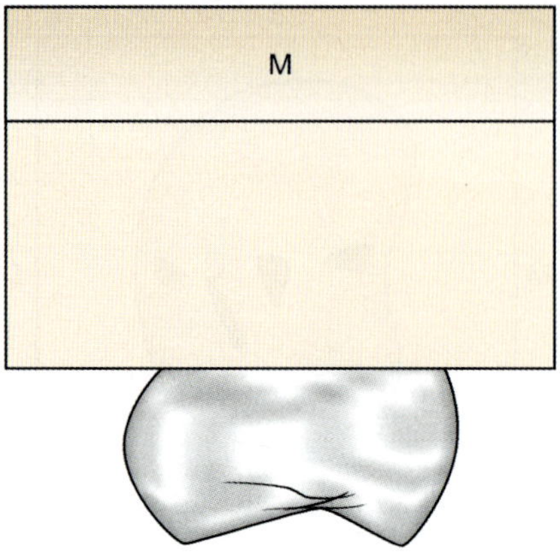

Fig. 6.13N: Step 14—Turn toward mesial aspect, carve the buccal and lingual outline of the crown. Carve the cusp tips

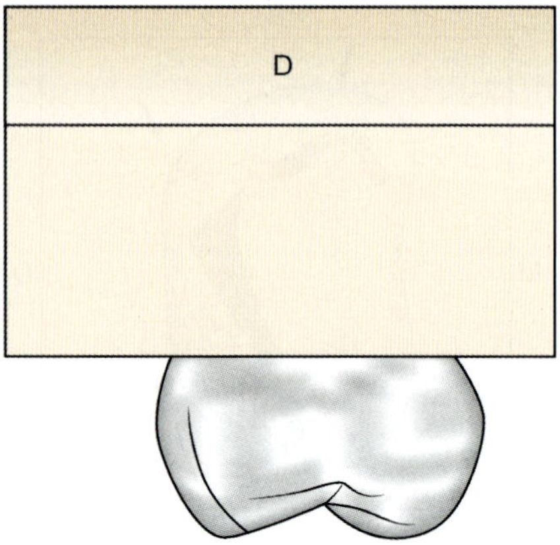

Fig. 6.13O: Step 15—Similarly carve the distal aspect of the crown

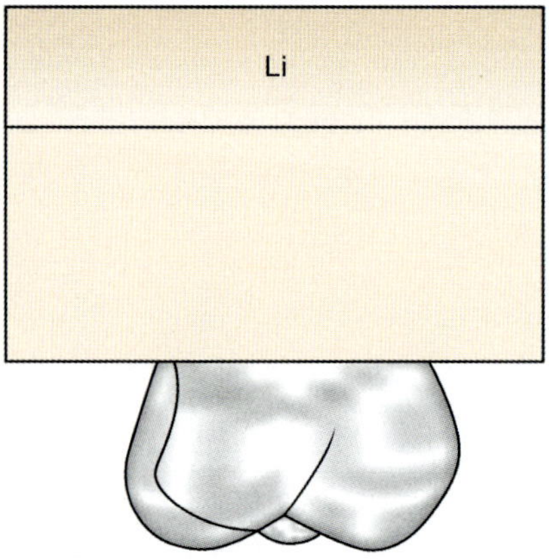

Fig. 6.13P: Step 16—Turn toward lingual aspect, carve the mesial and distal outline of the crown. Carve the cusp tips also

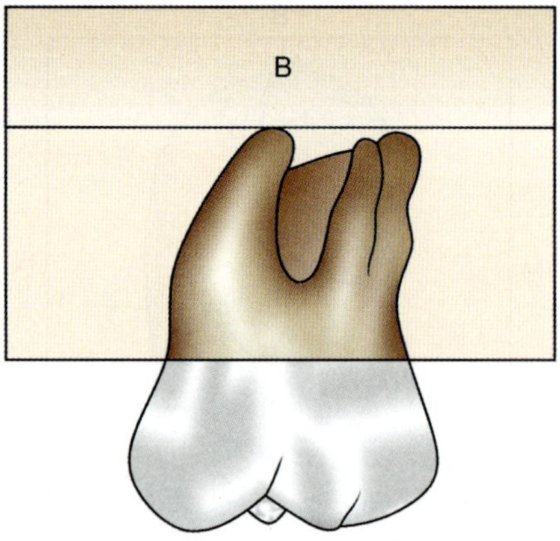

Fig. 6.13Q: Step 17—Draw the root outline on the buccal aspect

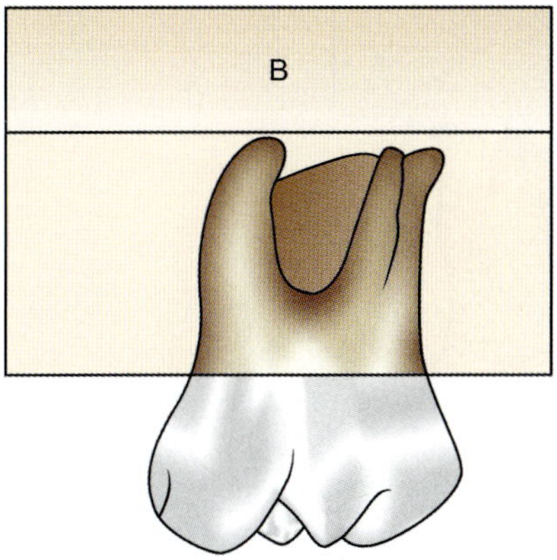

Fig. 6.13R: Step 18—Remove the wax for bifurcation. The shaded part represents the reduction of wax for bifurcation but not completely

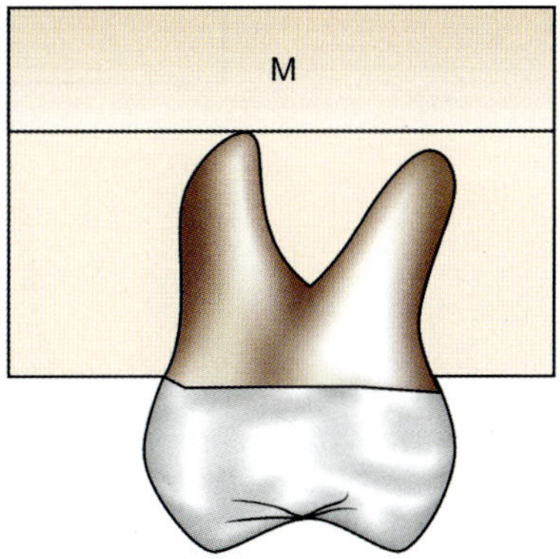

Fig. 6.13S: Step 19—Turn toward mesial aspect. Draw the mesiobuccal and lingual outline of the root. Carve according to the mesial outline of the root

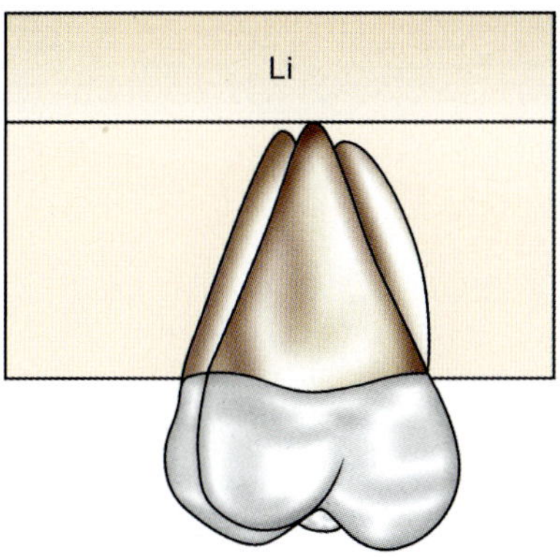

Fig. 6.13T: Step 20—Draw the lingual outline

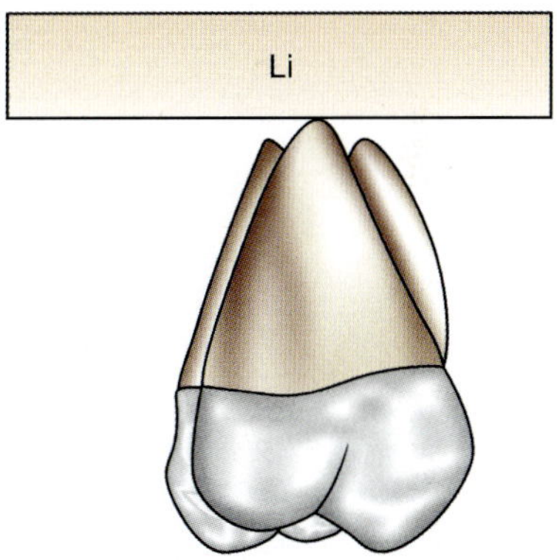

Fig. 6.13U: Step 21—Carve according to the outline

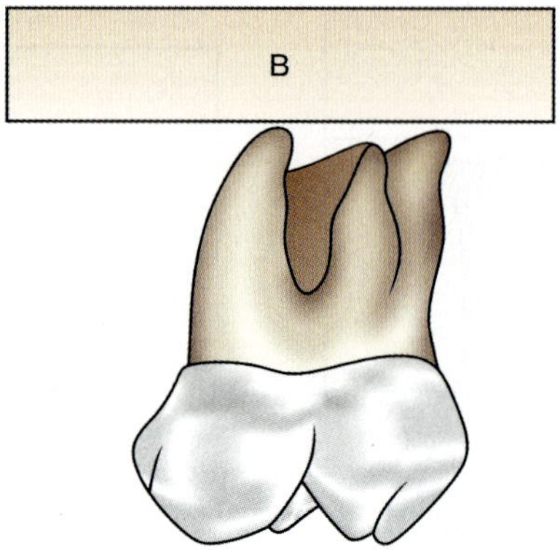

Fig. 6.14V: Carved permanent maxillary second molar

REFERENCES

1. Woelfel JB, Scheid RC. Dental Anatomy. Williams & Wilkins. 1997.
2. Ash, Nelson. Wheelers Dental Anatomy, Physiology & Occlusion. 8th edition. Elsevier. 2003.

THE PERMANENT MAXILLARY THIRD MOLAR

The third molar can vary in size, contour and relative position to the other teeth.[2] The well developed third molar often bears resemblance to the maxillary second molar.[2] The third molar supplements the second molar in function.[1,2] The crown of third molar is smaller and the roots are short, with the inclination toward fusion.[1,2]

Morphology

Buccal Aspect[1,2] (Fig. 6.14)

The crown is shorter cervico occlusally and narrower mesiodistally than that of the second molar. The roots are usually fused, shorter and function as one large root. The fused roots end in a taper at the apex. The root apex is inclined distally.

Lingual Aspect[1,2] (Fig. 6.15)

Only one large lingual cusp is seen from lingual aspect. So no lingual groove is evident. Sometimes a poorly developed distolingual cusp with a developmental groove is seen from lingual aspect.

Mesial Aspect[1,2] (Fig. 6.16)

Apart from the differences in measurement, the main feature is the taper towards the fused roots and a bifurcation usually towards the apical third. The root

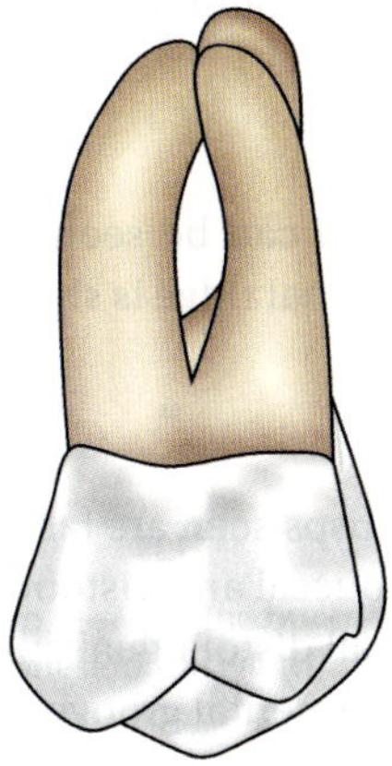

Fig. 6.14: Permanent maxillary left third molar, buccal aspect

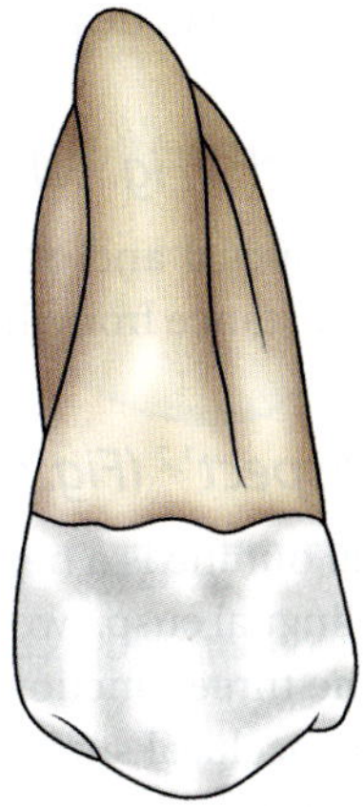

Fig. 6.15: Permanent maxillary left third molar, lingual aspect

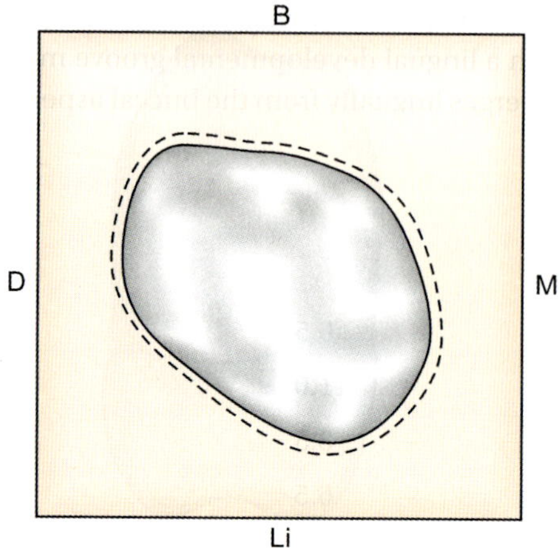

Fig. 6.19C: Step 3—Carve according to the outline leaving 0.5 mm wax extra

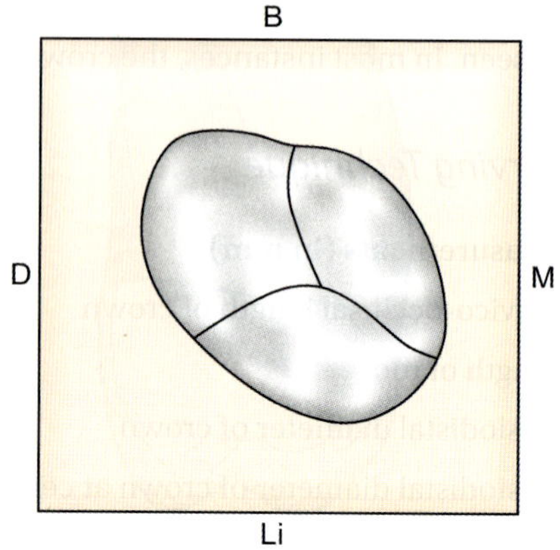

Fig. 6.19D: Step 4—Draw the outline of four cusps based on the size of the cusps

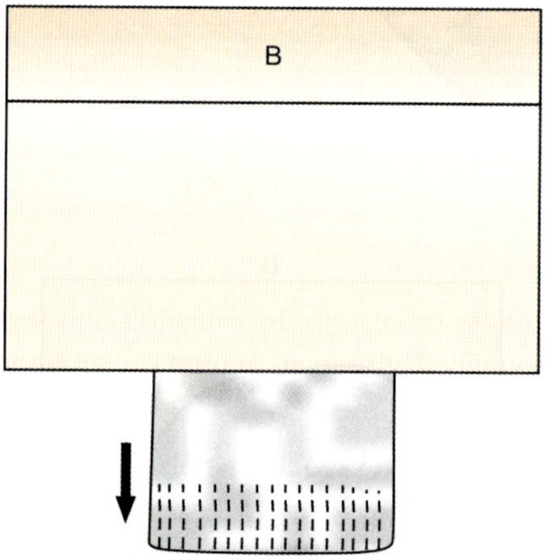

Fig. 6.19E: Step 5—Place the buccal cusp tip inside. For this remove wax from half of the buccal aspect of the crown occlusally. The dotted line represents wax reduced and direction to be removed

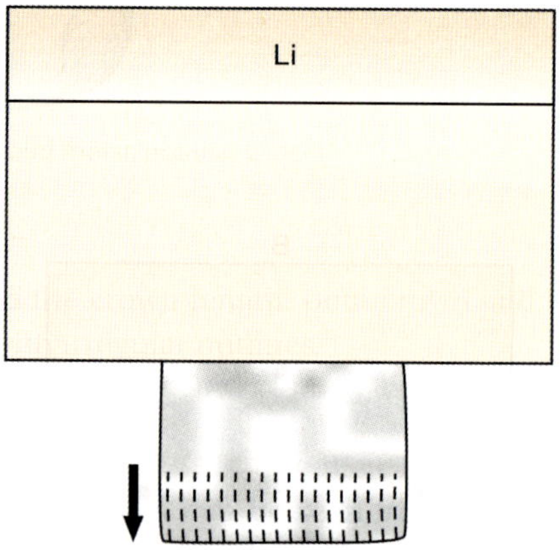

Fig. 6.19F: Step 6—Place the lingual cusp tip inside. For this remove wax from half of the lingual aspect of the crown occlusally. The dotted line represents wax reduced and direction to be removed

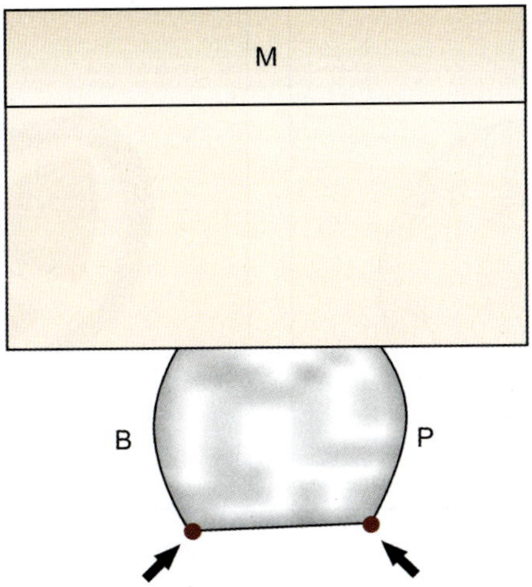

Fig. 6.19G: Step 7—The cusp tips are placed inside. The arrow mark is pointing at the cusp tips

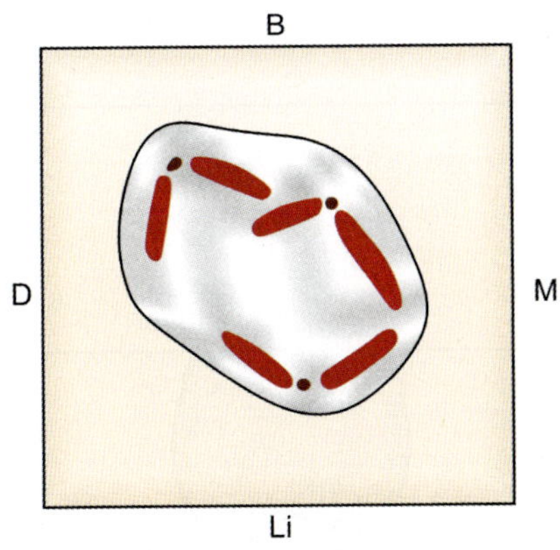

Fig. 6.19H: Step 9—Carve the triangular ridges, cusp ridges and marginal ridges. The shaded part represents the wax to be reduced

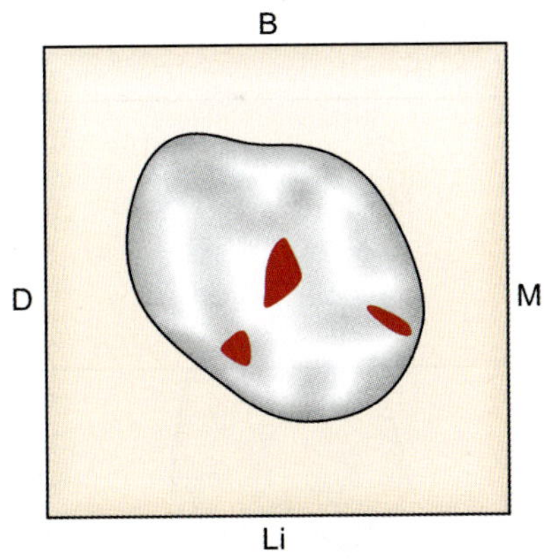

Fig. 6.19I: Step 10—Carve the central fossa, mesial triangular fossa and distal triangular fossa

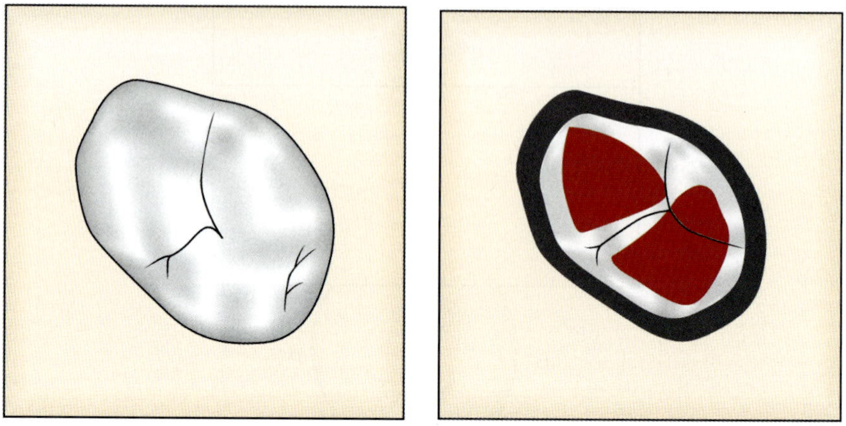

Fig. 6.19J: Step 11—Carve the central developmental groove, buccal groove, distal groove, and numerous supplemental grooves (The shaded part of the figure represents cusp ridges, marginal ridges and triangular ridges)

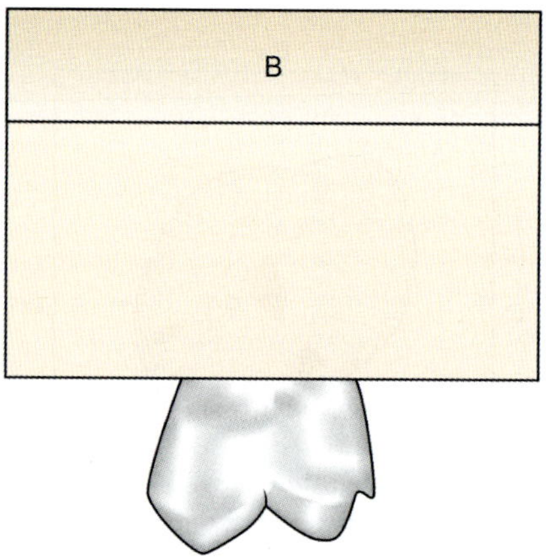

Fig. 6.19K: Step 12—Turn toward buccal aspect and carve the outlines of buccal aspect. Extend the buccal groove from central developmental groove. Carve the cusp tips

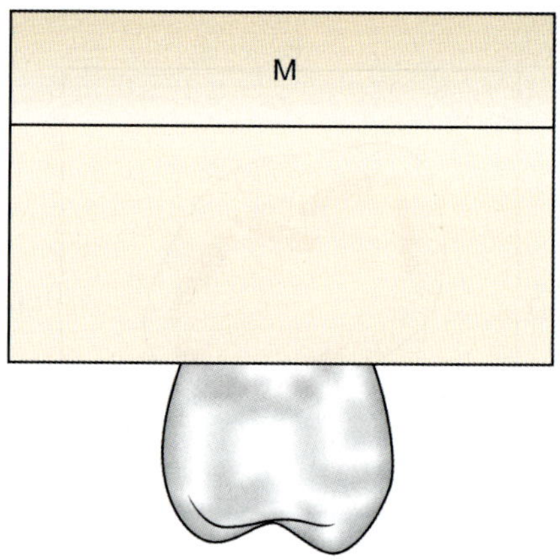

Fig. 6.19L: Step 13—Turn toward mesial aspect, carve the buccal and lingual outline of the crown. Carve the cusp tips also

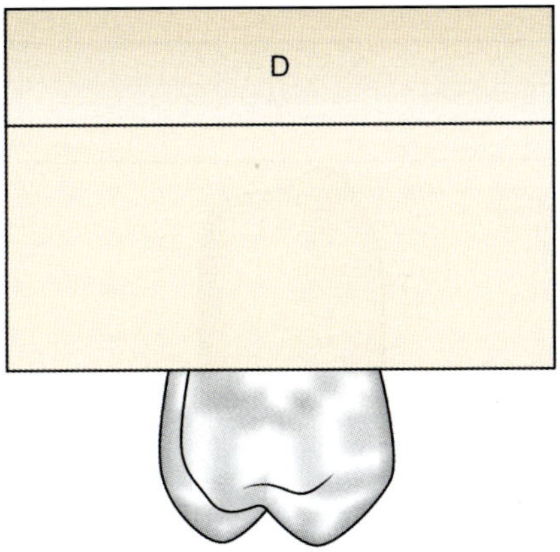

Fig. 6.19M: Step 14—Similarly carve the distal aspect of the crown

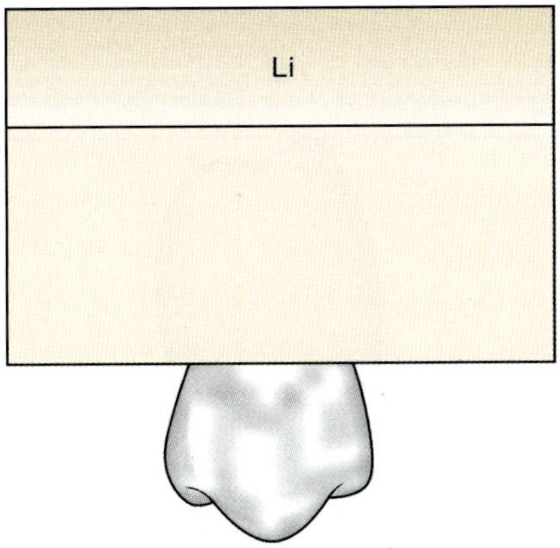

Fig. 6.19N: Step 15—Turn toward lingual aspect, carve the crown outlines

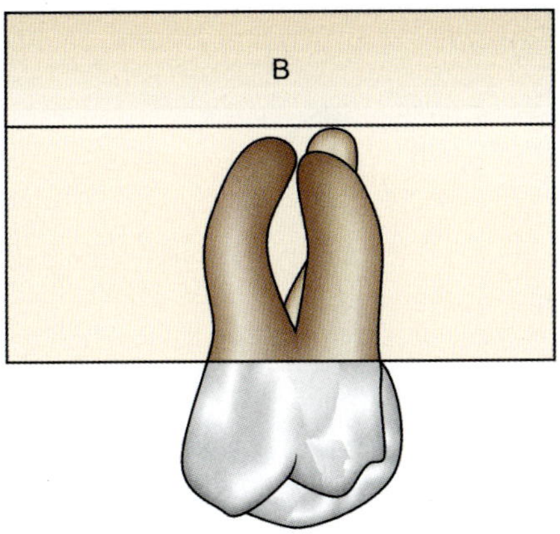

Fig. 6.19O: Step 16—Turn the carving toward buccal aspect, draw the buccal outline of the roots

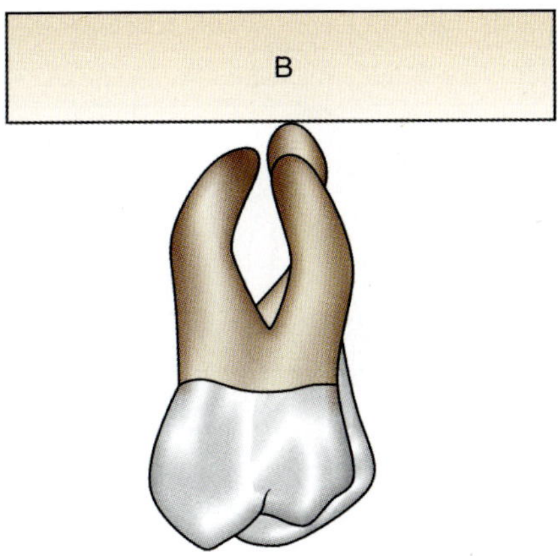

Fig. 6.19P: Step 17—Carve according to the outline

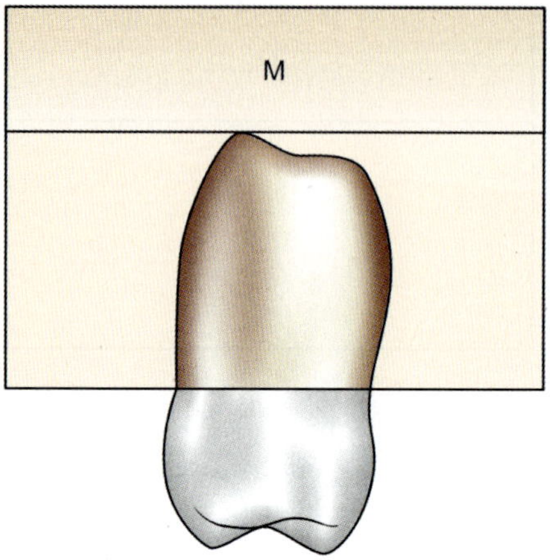

Fig. 6.19Q: Step 18—Turn toward mesial aspect. Draw the mesiobuccal and lingual outline of the root

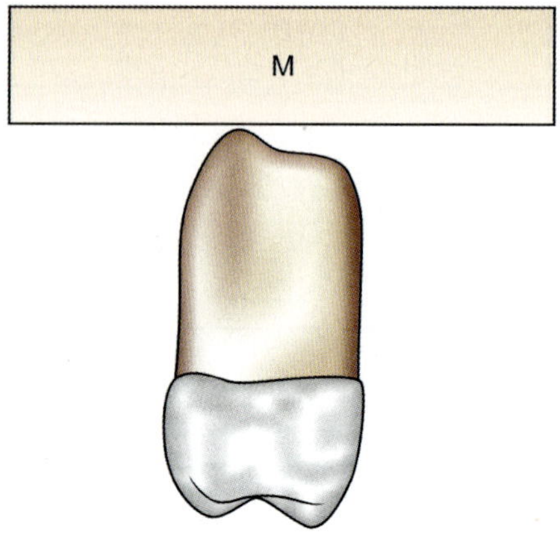

Fig. 6.19R: Step 19—Carve according to the root outline

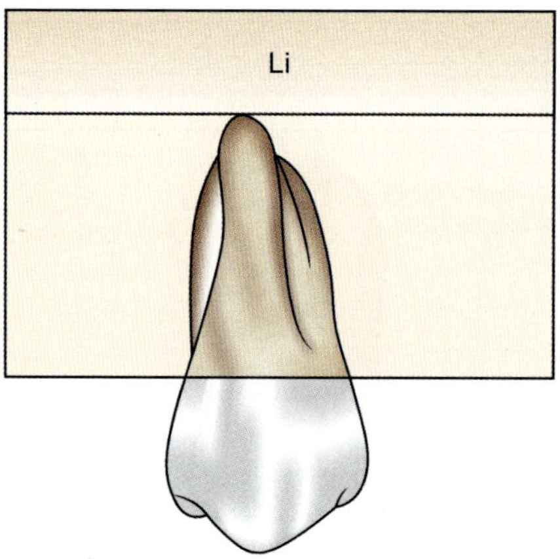

Fig. 6.19S: Step 20—Draw the lingual outline

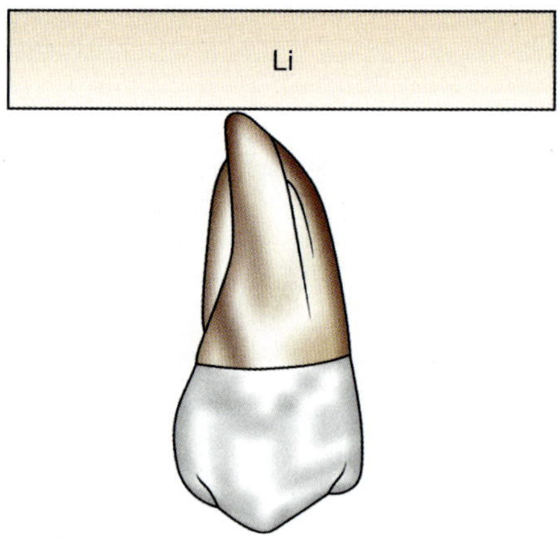

Fig. 6.19T: Step 21—Carve according to the outline

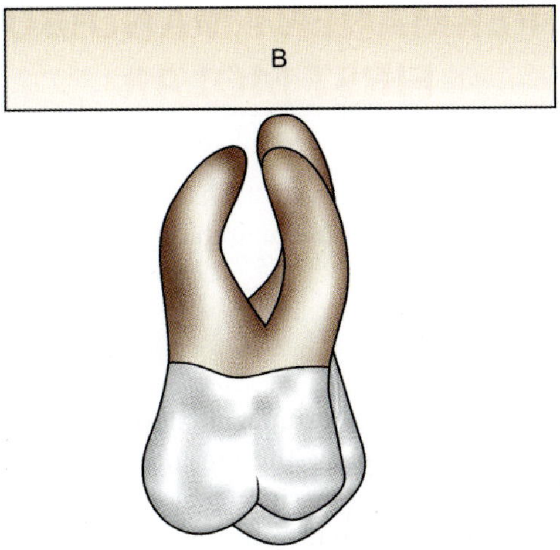

Fig. 6.19U: Step 22—Carved permanent maxillary third molar

REFERENCES

1. Woelfel JB, Scheid RC. Dental Anatomy. Williams & Wilkins. 1997.
2. Ash, Nelson. Wheelers Dental Anatomy, Physiology & Occlusion. 8th edition. Elsevier. 2003.

THE PERMANENT MANDIBULAR FIRST MOLAR

Morphology

This is the largest tooth in the mandibular arch.[2]

Buccal Aspect[1,2] (Fig. 6.20)

Outline

Crown: The crown outline is roughly trapezoidal from buccal aspect. All the five cusps are visible from buccal aspect. The mesiobuccal cusp, distobuccal cusp, part of distal cusp and cusp tips of mesiolingual and distolingual cusp are seen. The mesiobuccal cusp is larger than distobuccal cusp and distal cusp is smallest of all five cusps.

The mesial outline at the cervical third is concave, the middle third and occlusal third is convex. The distal outline is straight from cervical line till the cusp tip. The distal cusp tip is pointed whereas the mesiobuccal and distobuccal cusp tips are flat. The mesiolingual and distolingual cusp tips are more pointed and placed at a higher level than the buccal cusp tips.

The cervical line is regular and shows convexity apically toward the root bifurcation. The mesial contact area is at middle third of the crown. The distal contact area is at center of distal cusp. The crown converges cervically.

Root: Mesial and distal roots are present. The mesial root outline at the cervical third curves mesially to the middle third of the root; from middle third it curves distally to the tapered root apex, which is located directly below the mesiobuccal cusp. The crest of curvature of the root mesially is mesial to the crown cervix. The distal outline of mesial root is concave from bifurcation to the root apex.

The distal root is inclined in a distal direction and is less curved than the mesial root. At the apical third the root may show curvature and the distal root is more pointed than the mesial root apex.

Both the roots are wider mesiodistally from buccal area than they are lingually seen.

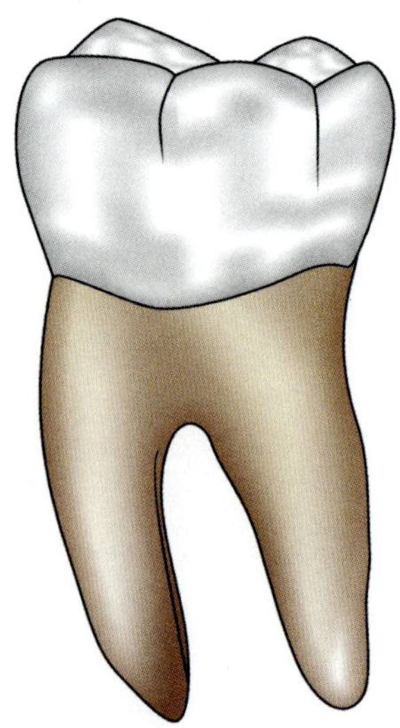

Fig. 6.20: Permanent mandibular left first molar, buccal aspect

Surface

Crown: Two developmental grooves, i.e. mesiobuccal developmental groove and distobuccal developmental groove appear on the buccal crown portion. The mesiobuccal developmental groove acts a line of demarcation between the mesiobuccal lobe and the distobuccal lobe. The distobuccal groove separates the distobuccal lobe from the distal lobe. The mesiobuccal groove is shorter and terminates at middle of the crown length whereas the distobuccal groove is longer and terminates at the junction of middle third and cervical third of the crown.

The surface of the buccal cusps is flat. The distal cusp shows slight convexity. The cervical third of the crown shows convexity and is termed as cervical ridge. In between the cervical ridge and the terminus of the groove, a developmental depression is noticeable.

The surface of the root is smooth and convex; developmental depressions are seen at the cervical third of the roots. On both mesial and distal side of the roots, the depression is more deeper toward the lingual aspect. This natural development provides a better anchorage for the mandibular first molar preventing rotation.

A shallow developmental depression is seen on the root trunk. The level of root bifurcation is located approximately 3 mm below the cervical line.

Lingual Aspect[1,2] (Fig. 6.21)

From this aspect three cusps are seen—mesiolingual, distolingual and part of distal cusp. The mesiolingual cusp is the widest and its cusp tip is placed at a higher level.

Outline

Crown: The mesial outline from cervical line is convex till the mesiolingual cusp ridge, from here the outline slopes toward the pointed cusp tip. Both the mesiolingual and distolingual cusp ridges form obtuse angles at the cusp tips of approximately 100°. The mesial contact area is placed higher than the distal contact area. The mesiolingual cusp tip is placed slightly at a higher level. The distal outline of the crown is straight immediately above the cervical line to a point below the distal contact area. The junction of the distolingual cusp ridge of the distolingual cusp with distal marginal ridge is abrupt. The cervical line is irregular and tends to point sharply toward the root bifurcation and immediately above it.

Root: Lingually the root length appears 1mm longer than the buccal aspect. The length of root trunk is about 4 mm on the lingual aspect. The roots converge lingually and the outlines are similar to roots of buccal aspect.

Surface

Crown: The lingual developmental groove serves as a line of demarcation between the lingual cusps for about occlusal third of the crown. The surface of the crown lingually is smooth and spheroidal on each of the lingual lobes. Toward the lingual groove the surface is concave and the cervical third of crown is flat.

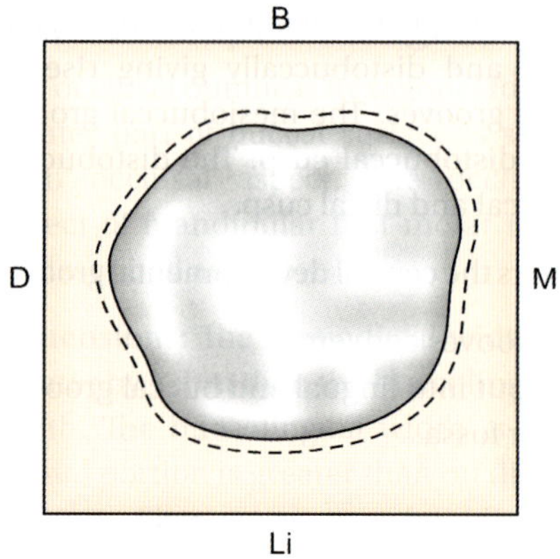

Fig. 6.25C: Step 3—Carve according to the outline leaving 0.5 mm wax extra

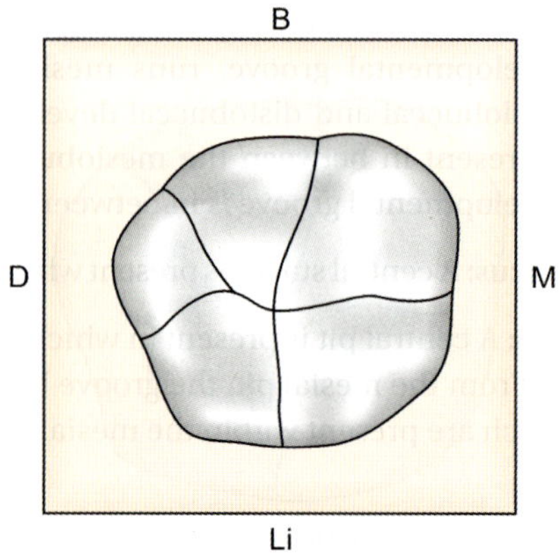

Fig. 6.25D: Step 4—Draw the outline of five cusps based on the size of the cusps

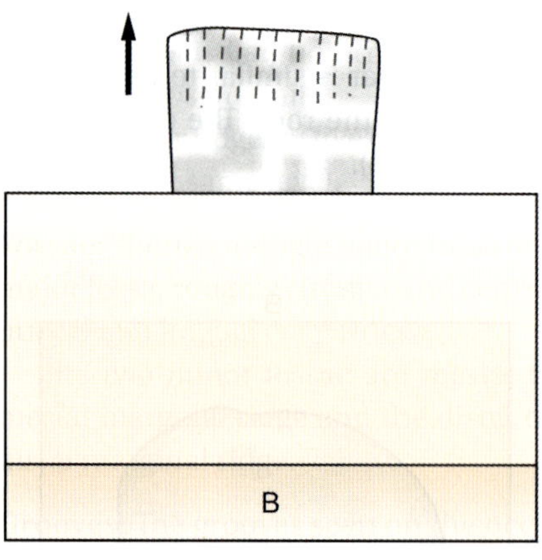

Fig. 6.25E: Step 5—Place the buccal cusp tip inside. For this, remove wax from half of the buccal aspect of the crown occlusally. The dotted line represents wax reduced and direction to be removed

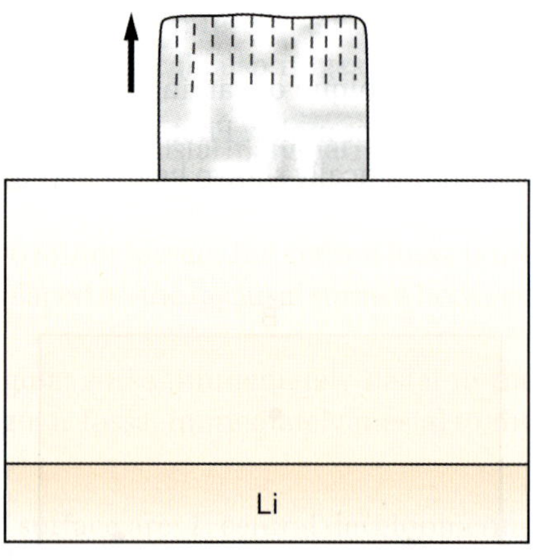

Fig. 6.25F: Step 6—Place the lingual cusp tip inside. For this, remove wax from half of the lingual aspect of the crown occlusally. The dotted line represents wax reduced and direction to be removed

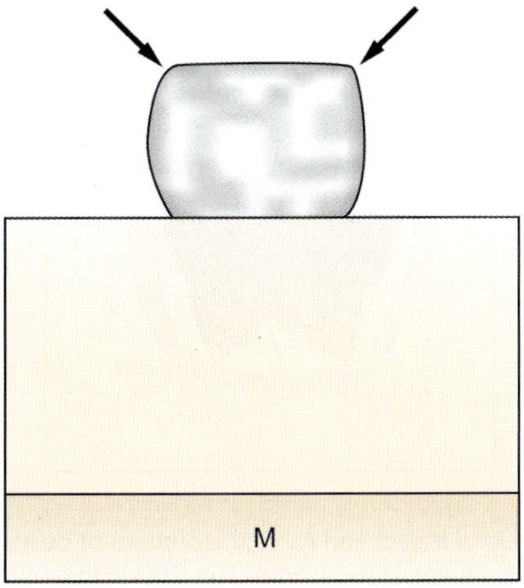

Fig. 6.25G: Step 7—The cusp tips are placed inside. Arrow mark pointing the cusp tips

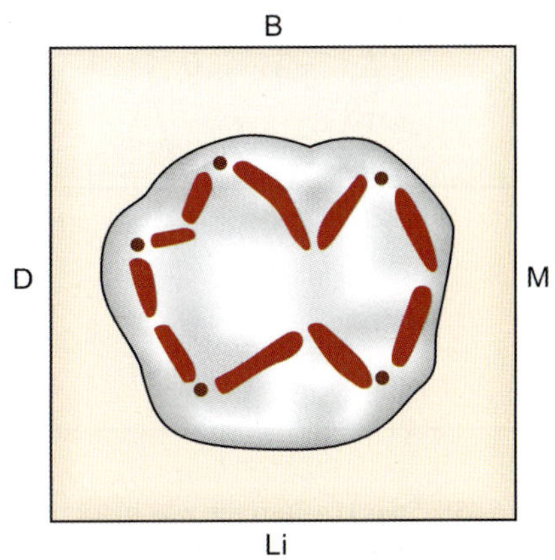

Fig. 6.25H: Step 8—Carve the triangular ridges, cusp ridges and marginal ridges. The shaded part represents the wax to be reduced

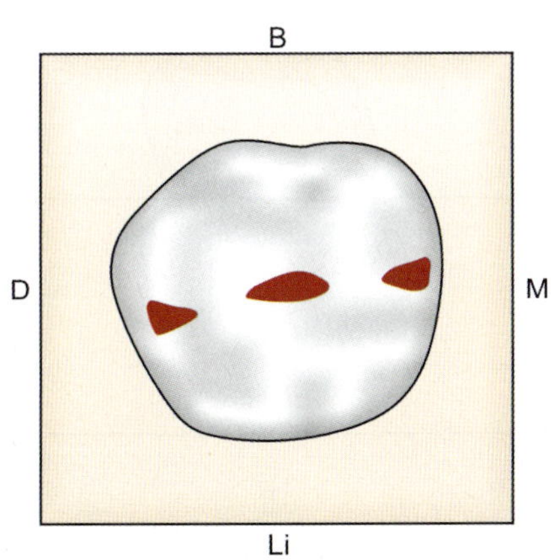

Fig. 6.25I: Step 9—Carve the central fossa, mesial triangular fossa and distal triangular fossa

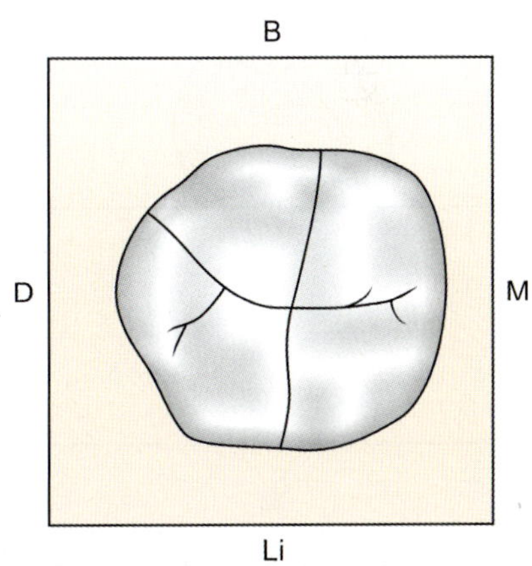

Fig. 6.25J: Step 10—Carve the central developmental groove, mesiobuccal developmental groove, distobuccal developmental groove, lingual developmental groove, mesial and distal development grooves

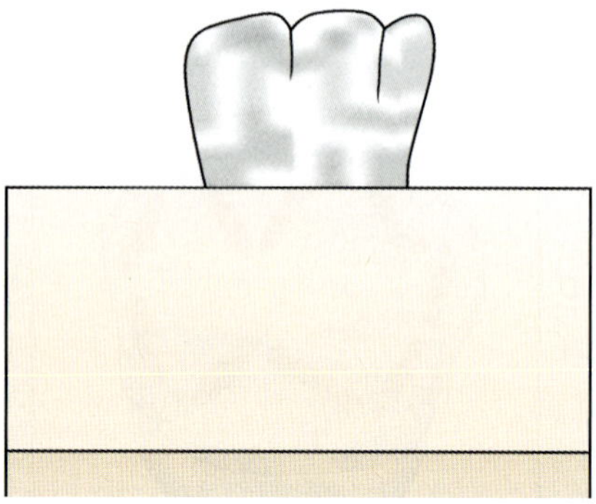

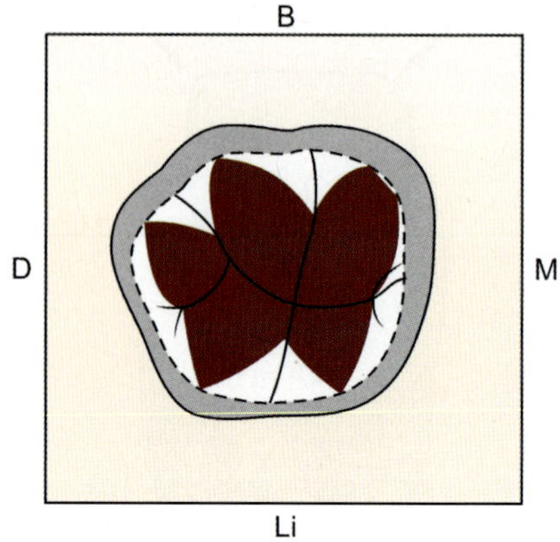

Fig. 6.25K: Step 11—Turn the wax block towards buccal aspect and carve the outlines of buccal aspect. Extend the mesiobuccal and distobuccal developmental groove from central developmental groove. Carve the cusp tips (The shaded part in the figure show cusp ridges, marginal ridges and triangular ridges)

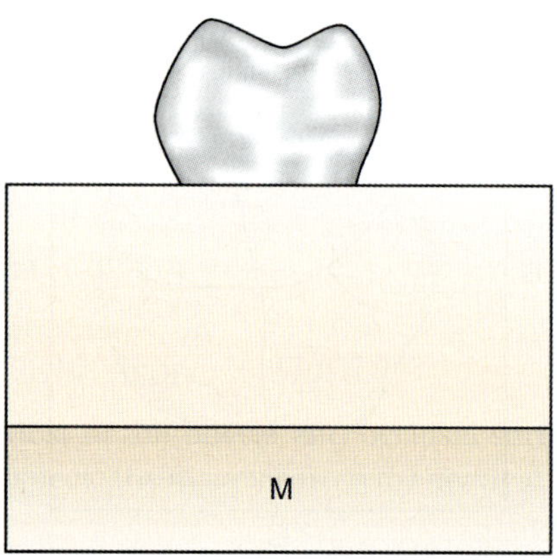

Fig. 6.25L: Step 12—Turn towards mesial aspect, carve the buccal and lingual outline of the crown. Carve the cusp tips also

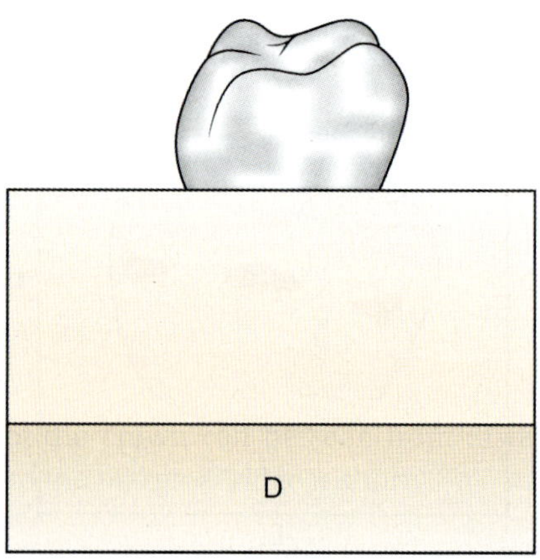

Fig. 6.25M: Step 13—Similarly carve the distal aspect of the crown

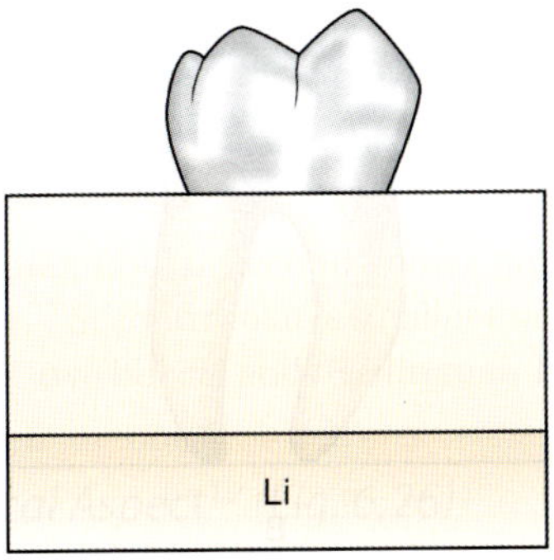

Fig. 6.25N: Step 14—Turn towards lingual aspect, carve the crown outlines

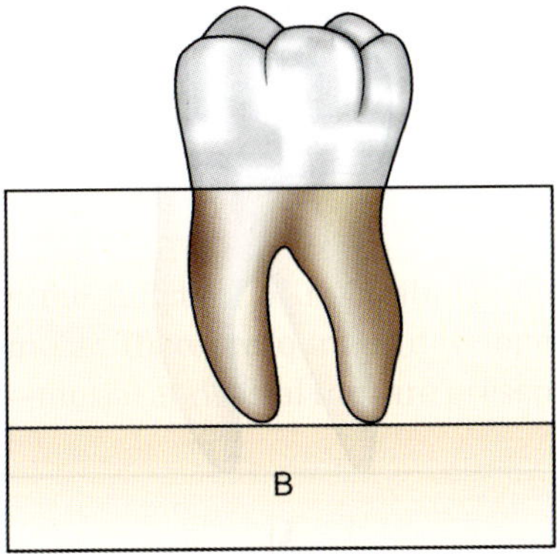

Fig. 6.25O: Step 15—Turn the carving toward buccal aspect, draw the buccal outline of the roots

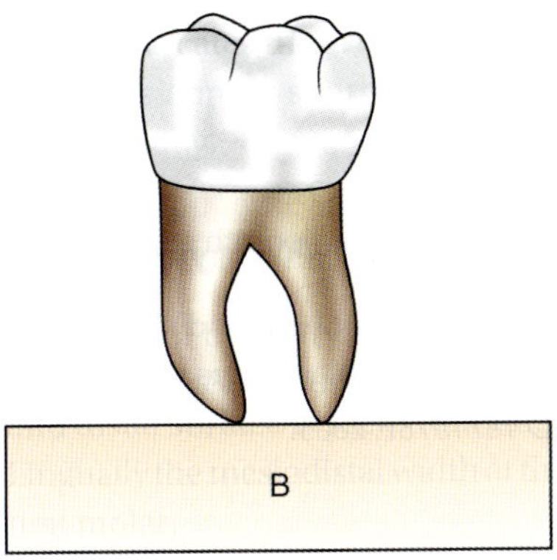

Fig. 6.25P: Step 16—Remove the wax for bifurcation

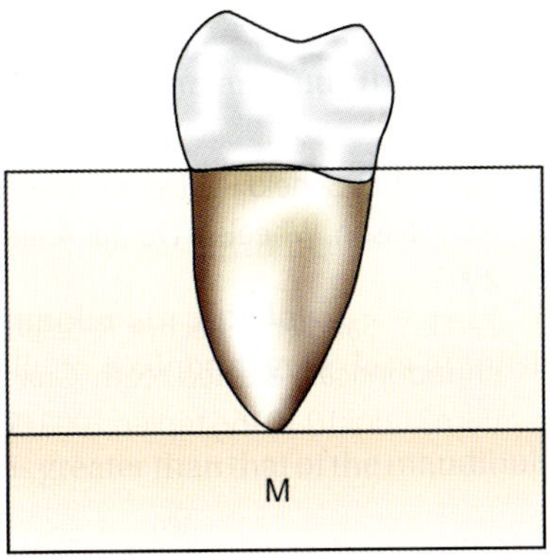

Fig. 6.25Q: Step 17—Turn toward mesial aspect. Draw the outline of the root

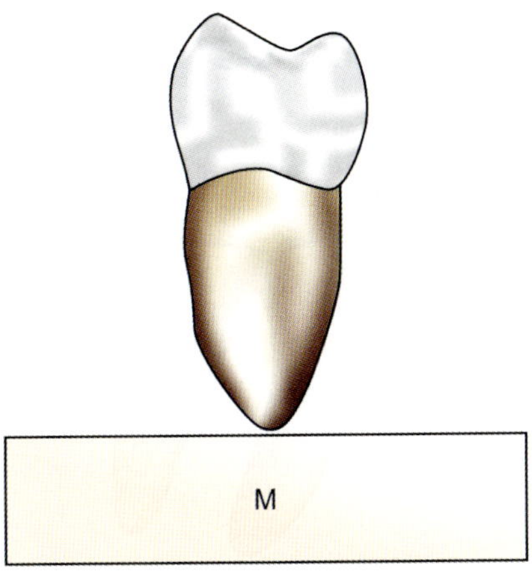

Fig. 6.25R: Step 18—Carve according to the outline

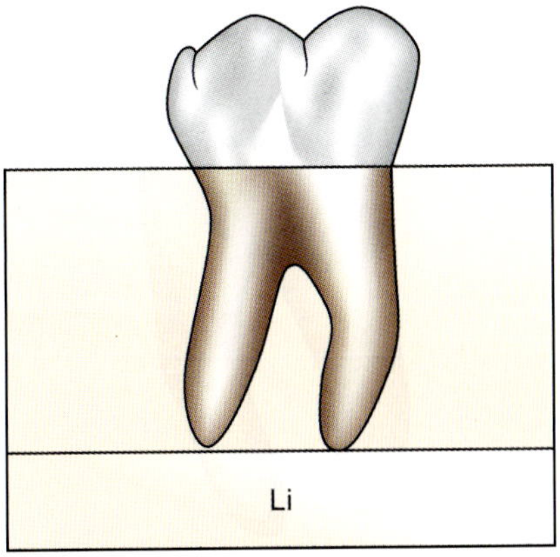

Fig. 6.25S: Step 19—Draw the lingual outline

Mesial Aspect[1,2] (Fig. 6.28)

The buccolingual width is less than that of first molar. The occlusal surface may be more constricted buccolingually. The cervical line is straight and regular. The mesial root apex is pointed and buccal part of distal root is seen.

Distal Aspect[1,2] (Fig. 6.29)

The distal aspect is similar to first molar except for the absence of a distal cusp and distobuccal groove. The contact area is exactly at the center of the crown.

Occlusal Aspect[1,2] (Fig. 6.30)

Variations are seen from occlusal aspect compared with first molar. These variations serve as mark of identity. The occlusal form is rectangular. The distal outline shows more curvature than the mesial outline. The cusp ridge of distobuccal cusp lies buccal to the cusp ridge of the mesiobuccal cusp.

Dimension: The mesiodistal width is slightly greater than the buccolingual width. Four cusps can be viewed from occlusal aspect, i.e. mesiobuccal, distobuccal, mesiolingual and distolingual cusps.

Ridges: Mesial and distal marginal ridges are present. Triangular ridges of all four cusps and cusp ridges of all four cusps are seen.

Grooves: A central developmental groove runs mesially and distally. Buccal developmental groove and lingual developmental groove run buccally and lingually from central developmental groove. Numerous supplemental grooves radiating

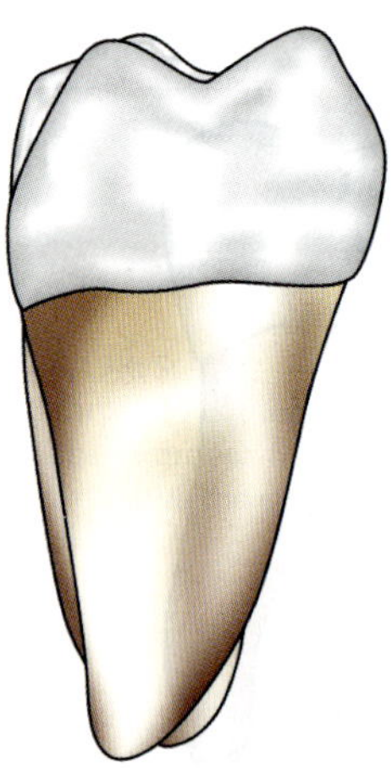

Fig. 6.28: Permanent mandibular right second molar, mesial aspect

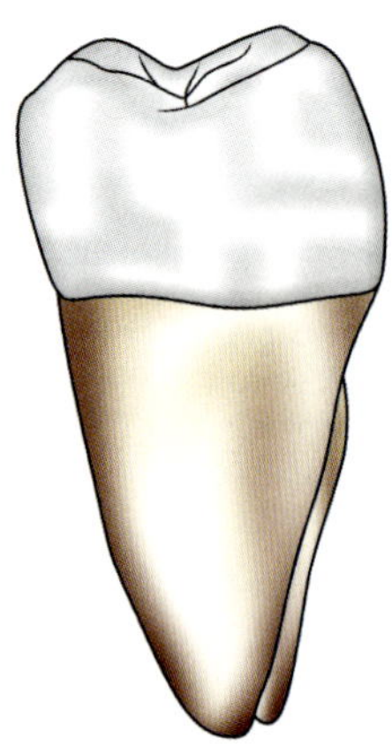

Fig. 6.29: Permanent mandibular right second molar, distal aspect

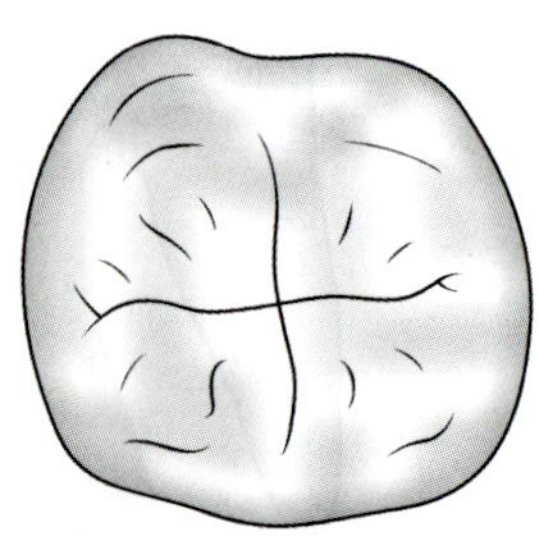

Fig. 6.30: Permanent mandibular right second molar, occlusal aspect

from central developmental grooves are found. All the grooves on mandibular second molar is deeper compared with first molar.

Sulcus: A central sulcus harboring the central developmental groove is seen.

Pit: Central pit, mesial and distal pit are seen.

Carving technique

Measurements (in mm)

Cervico-occlusal length of crown	–	7.0
Length of root	–	13.0
Mesiodistal diameter of crown	–	10.5
Mesiodistal diameter of crown at cervix	–	8.0
Biccolingual diameter of crown	–	10.0
Biccolingual diameter of crown at cervix	–	9.0
Curvature of cervical line - mesial	–	1.0
Curvature of cervical line - distal	–	0.0

The technique of carving for second molar is similar to permanent maxillary first molar. First carve the crown and then the root. The technique is diagrammatically illustrated in Figures 6.31A to 6.31U.

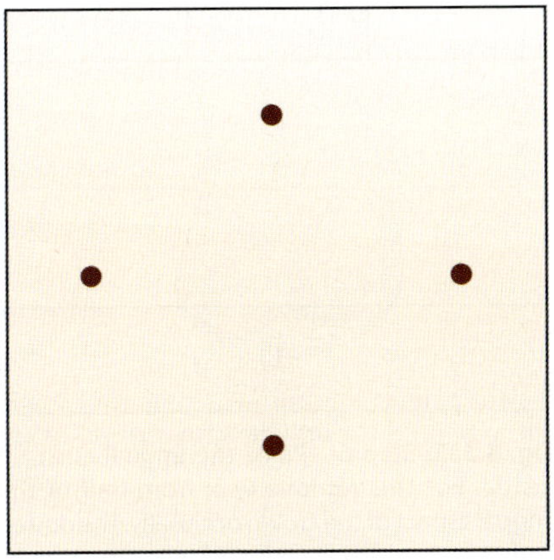

Fig. 6.31A: Step 1—Mark the buccolingual and mesiodistal width

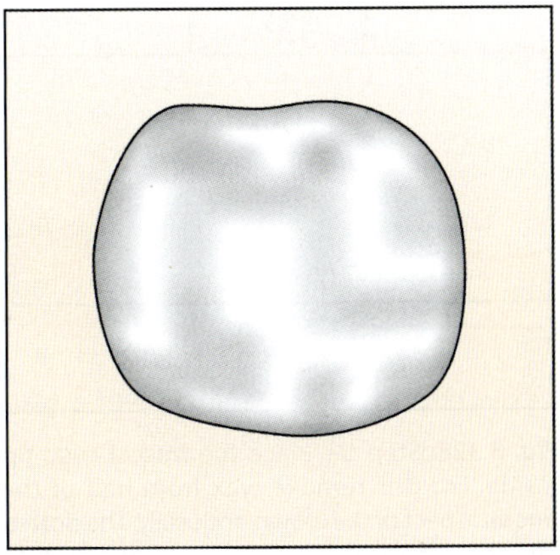

Fig. 6.32B: Step 2—Draw the occlusal outline

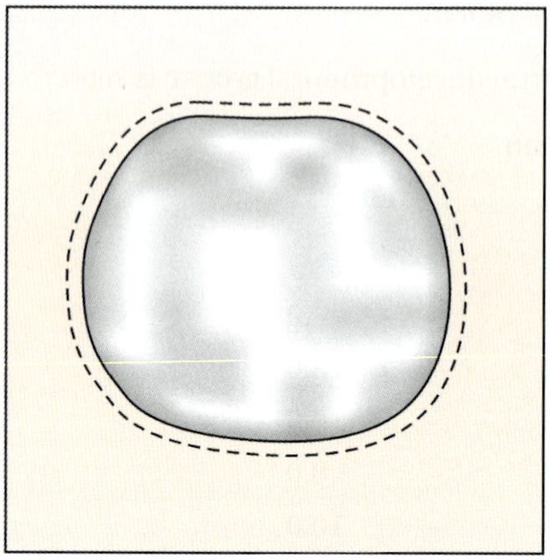

Fig. 6.31C: Step 3—Carve according to the outline leaving 0.5 mm wax extra

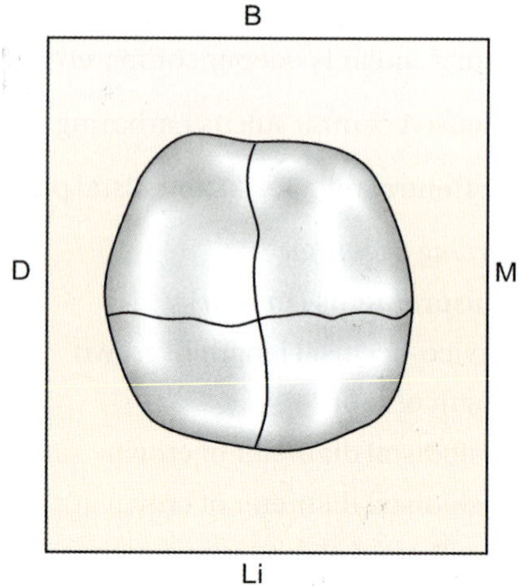

Fig. 6.31D: Step 4—Draw the outline of four cusps based on the size of the cusps

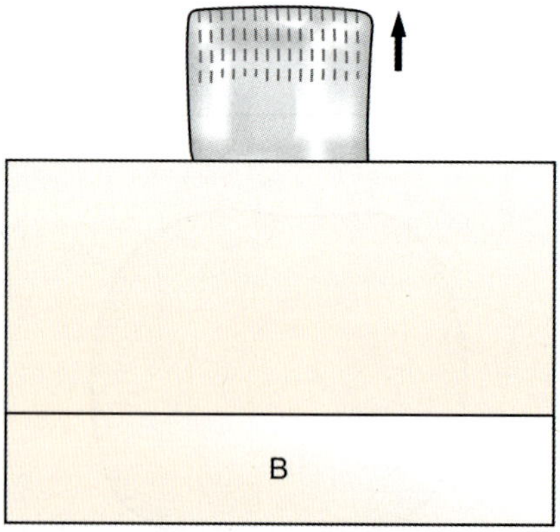

Fig. 6.32E: Step 5—Place the buccal cusp tip inside. For this remove wax from half of the buccal aspect of the crown occlusally. The dotted line represents wax reduced and direction to be removed

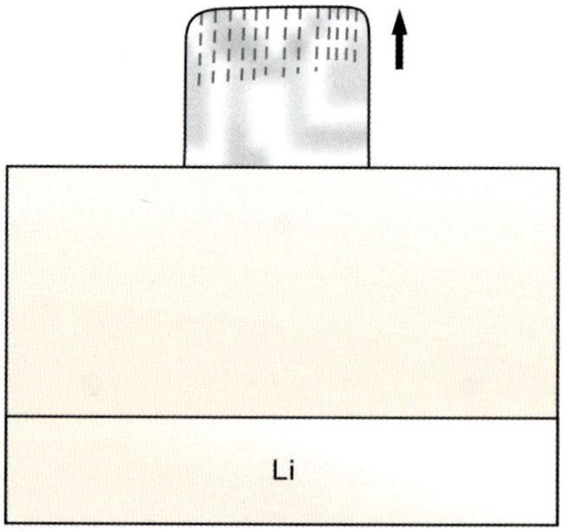

Fig. 6.32F: Step 6—Place the lingual cusp tip inside. For this remove wax from half of the lingual aspect of the crown occlusally. The dotted line represents wax reduced and direction to be removed

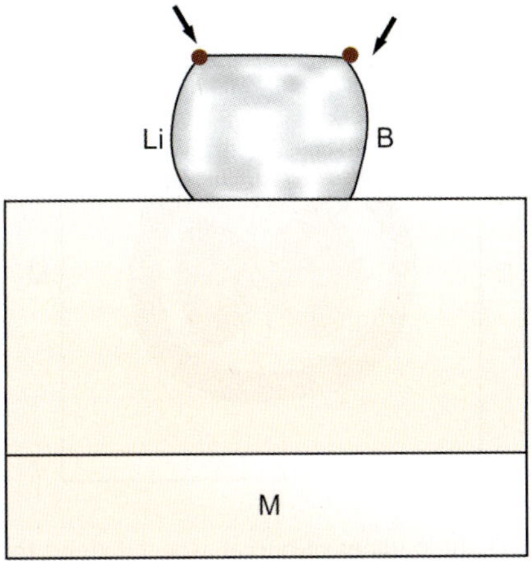

Fig. 6.31G: Step 7—The cusp tips are placed inside. The arrow mark are pointing at the cusp tips

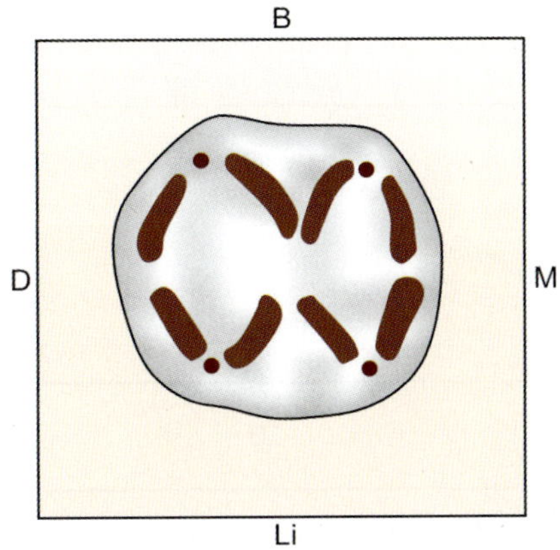

Fig. 6.32H: Step 8—Carve the triangular ridges, cusp ridges and marginal ridges. The shaded part represents the wax to be reduced

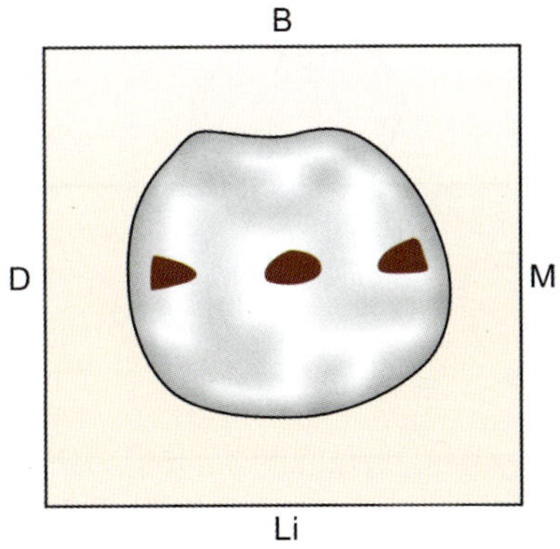

Fig. 6.31I: Step 9—Carve the central fossa, mesial triangular fossa and distal triangular fossa

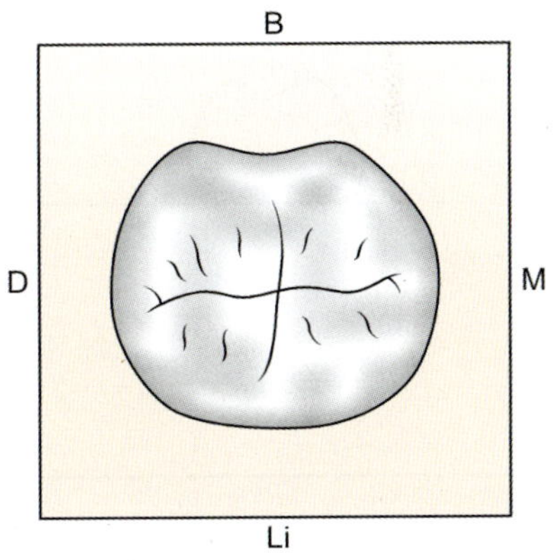

Fig. 6.31J: Step 10—Carve the central developmental groove, buccal develop mental groove, lingual developmental groove, and numerous supplemental grooves

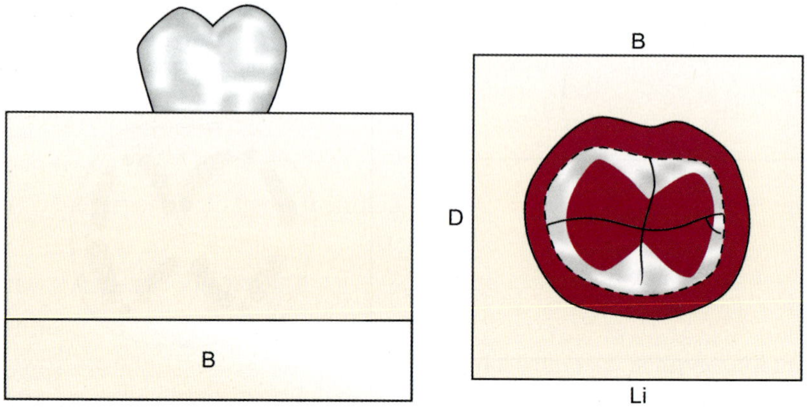

Fig. 6.31K: Step 11—Turn toward buccal aspect carve the outlines of buccal aspect. Extend the buccal groove from central developmental groove. Carve the cusp tips. (The shaded part in the figure represent cusp ridges, marginal ridges and triangular ridges)

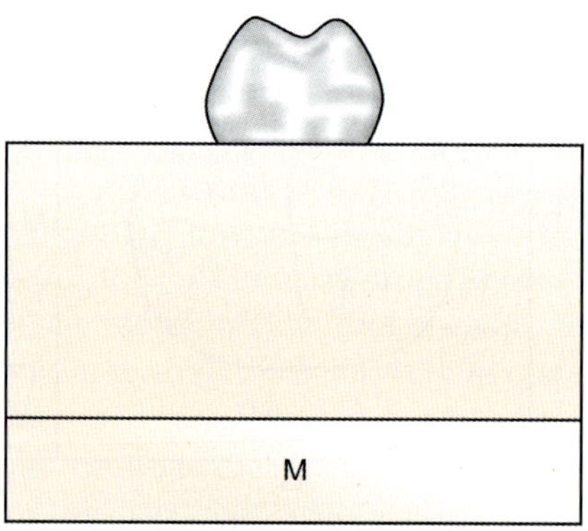

Fig. 6.31L: Step 12—Turn toward mesial aspect, carve the buccal and lingual outline of the crown. Carve the cusp tips also

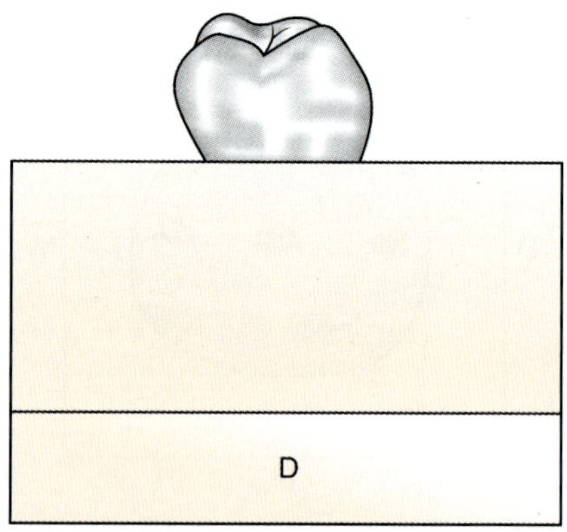

Fig. 6.31M: Step 13—Similarly carve the distal aspect of the crown

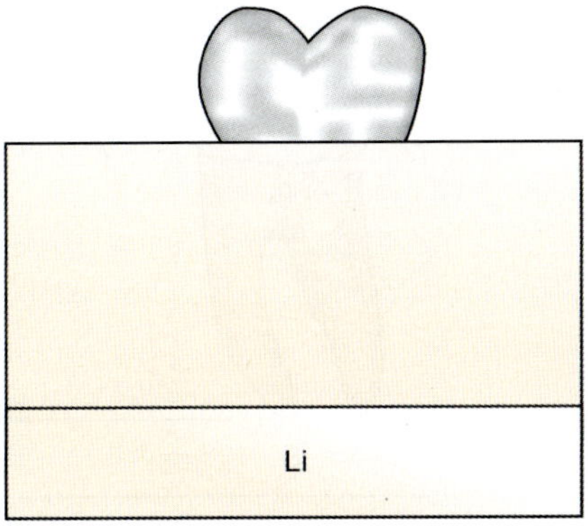

Fig. 6.31N: Step 14—Turn toward lingual aspect, carve the crown outlines

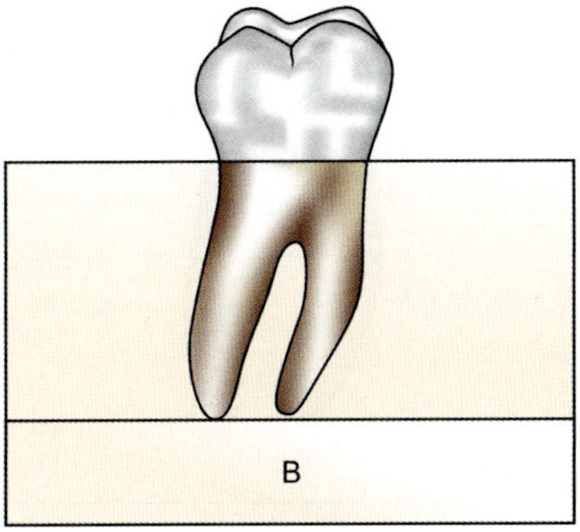

Fig. 6.31O: Step 15—Draw the buccal outline of the roots

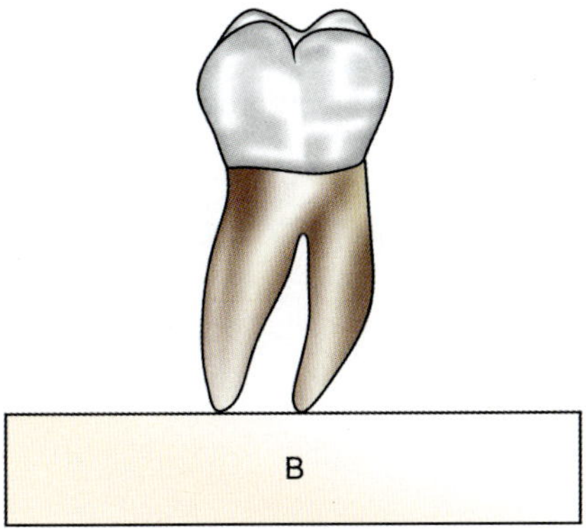

Fig. 6.31P: Step 16—Remove the wax for bifurcation

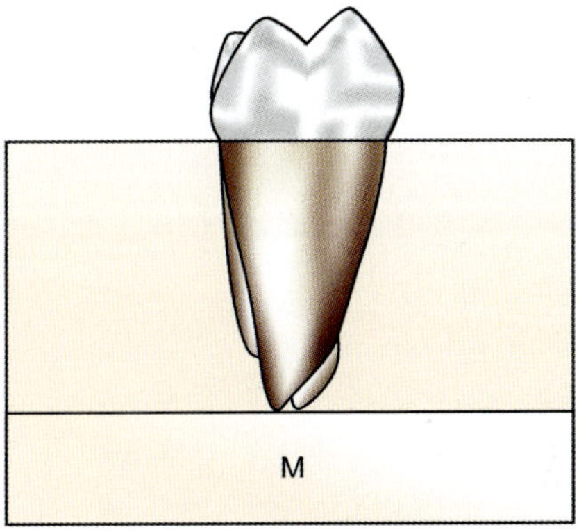

Fig. 6.31Q: Step 17—Turn toward mesial aspect. Draw the root outline

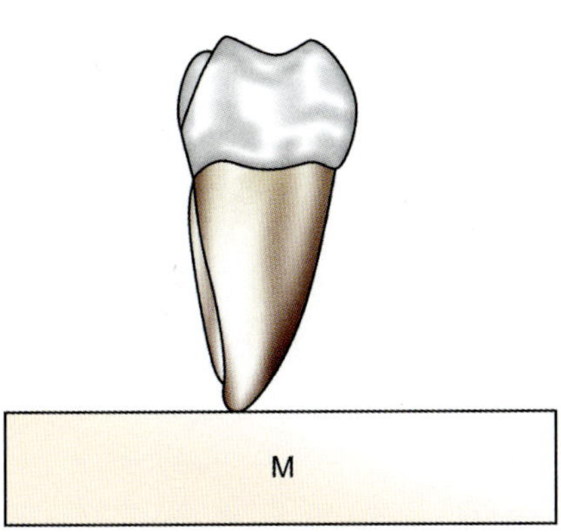

Fig. 6.31R: Step 18—Carve according to the root outline

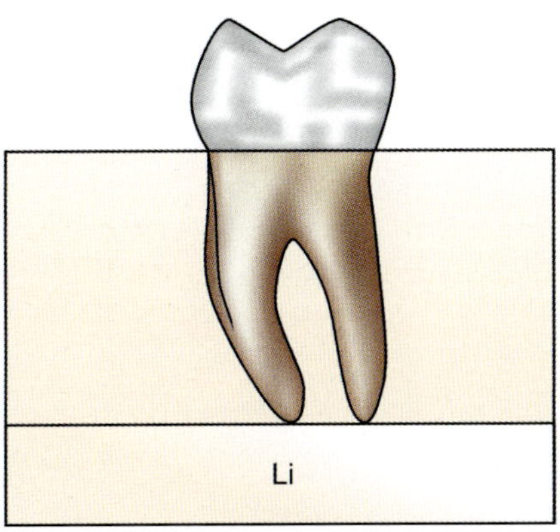

Fig. 6.31S: Step 19—Draw the lingual outline

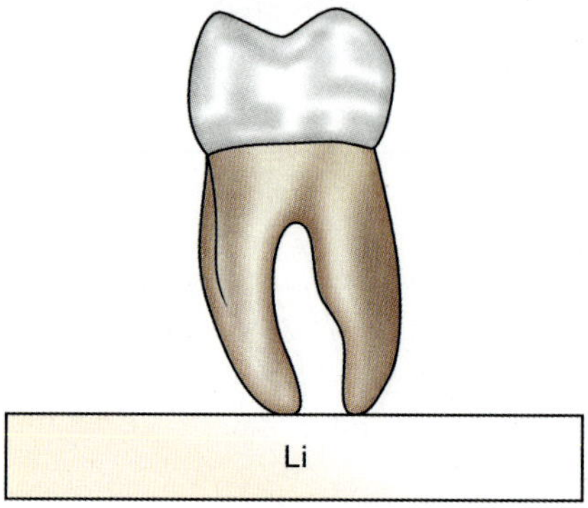

Fig. 6.31T: Step 20—Carve according to the outline

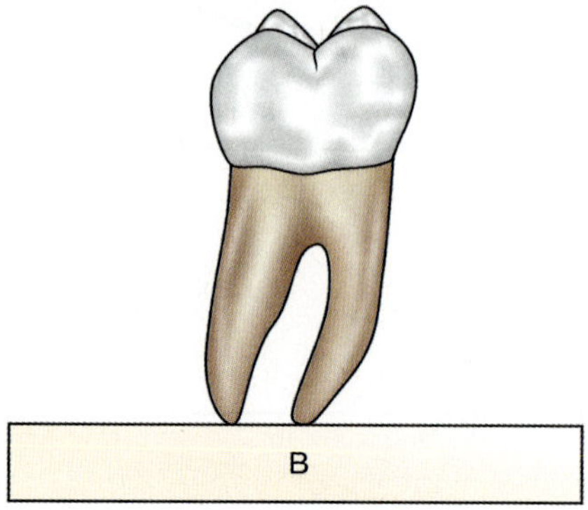

Fig. 6.31U: Step 21—Carved permanent mandibular second molar

REFERENCES

1. Woelfel JB, Scheid RC. Dental Anatomy. Williams & Wilkins. 1997.
2. Ash, Nelson. Wheelers Dental Anatomy, Physiology & Occlusion. 8th edition. Elsevier. 2003.

THE PERMANENT MANDIBULAR THIRD MOLAR

Morphology

The mandibular third molar shows greater variations considerably in different individuals.[1,2] The number of cusps might vary from 4 to 6, the roots may be two or may be fused but are smaller roots. This tooth may present anomalies both in form and in position.[2] It supplements the function of mandibular second molar and closely resembles it.

Buccal Aspect[1,2] (Fig. 6.32)

The outline in general is similar to that of all mandibular molars. The buccal cusps are short and rounded. The contact areas are placed more cervical than that of other molars. Only buccal cusps are seen from buccal aspect, i.e. the mesiobuccal and distobuccal cusp. Two roots mesial and distal roots may be seen or they might be fused sometimes. The roots are distally inclined.

Lingual Aspect[1,2] (Fig. 6.33)

The mandibular third molar, when well-developed resembles second molar.

Mesial Aspect[1,2] (Fig. 6.34)

Except for the dimensions this tooth resembles second molar. The roots are short and taper with a pointed apex.

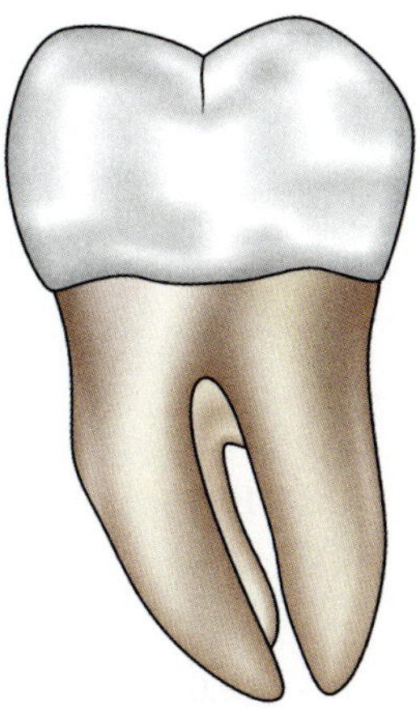

Fig. 6.32: Permanent mandibular left third molar, buccal aspect

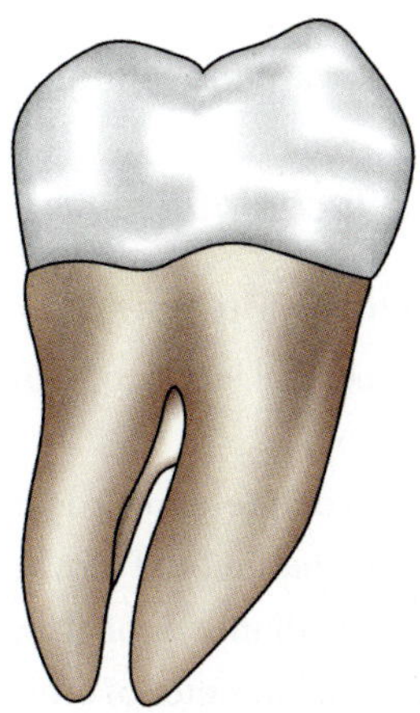

Fig. 6.33: Permanent mandibular left third molar, lingual aspect

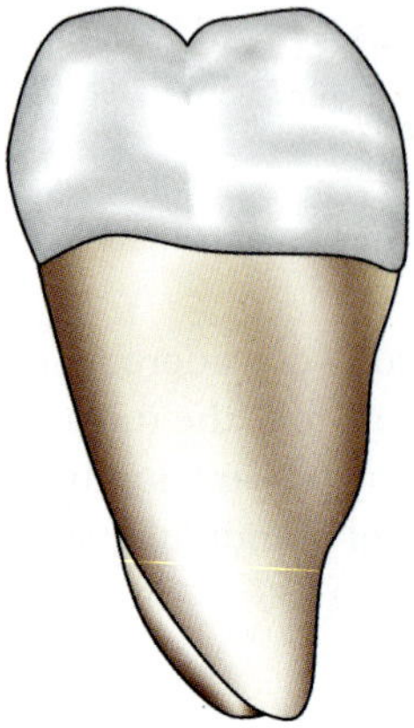

Fig. 6.34: Permanent mandibular left third molar, mesial aspect

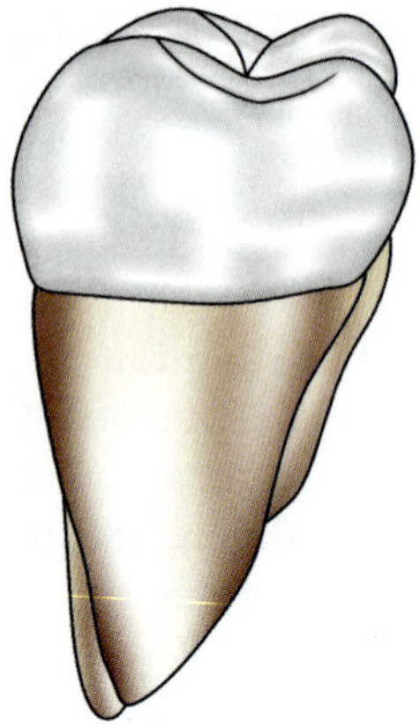

Fig. 6.35: Permanent mandibular left third molar, distal aspect

Distal Aspect[1,2] (Fig. 6.35)

The distal aspect resembles second molar except for the size. The surface of the crown is more spheroidal. The distal root is very small compared with the crown.

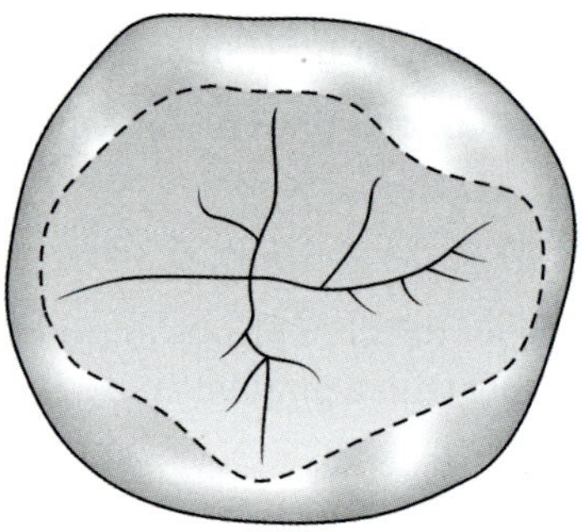

Fig. 6.36: Permanent mandibular left third molar, occlusal aspect

Occlusal Aspect[1,2] (Fig. 6.36)

The occlusal form is more rounded with a smaller buccolingual width distally. Numerous radiating supplementary grooves which are much deeper than second molar are found and they do converge toward the central pit.

Carving Technique

Measurements (in mm)

Cervico-occlusal length of crown	–	7.0
Length of root	–	11.0
Mesiodistal diameter of crown	–	10.0
Mesiodistal diameter of crown at cervix	–	7.5
Buccolingual diameter of crown	–	9.5
Buccolingual diameter of crown at cervix	–	9.0
Curvature of cervical line - mesial	–	1.0
Curvature of cervical line - distal	–	0.0

The technique of carving for third molar is similar to permanent maxillary first molar. First carve the crown and then the root. Figures 6.37A to 6.37U represent the technique for carving.

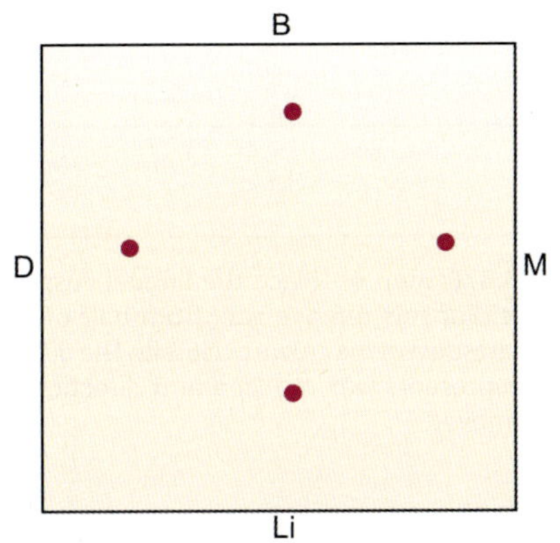

Fig. 6.37A: Step 1—Mark the buccolingual and mesiodistal width

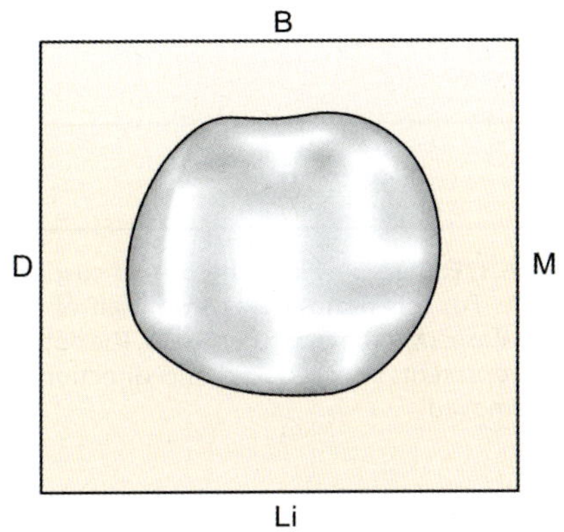

Fig. 6.37B: Step 2—Draw the occlusal outline

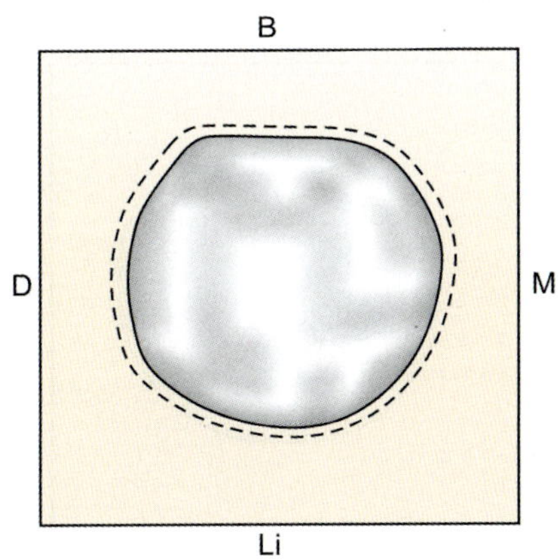

Fig. 6.37C: Step 3—Carve according to the outline leaving 0.5 mm wax extra

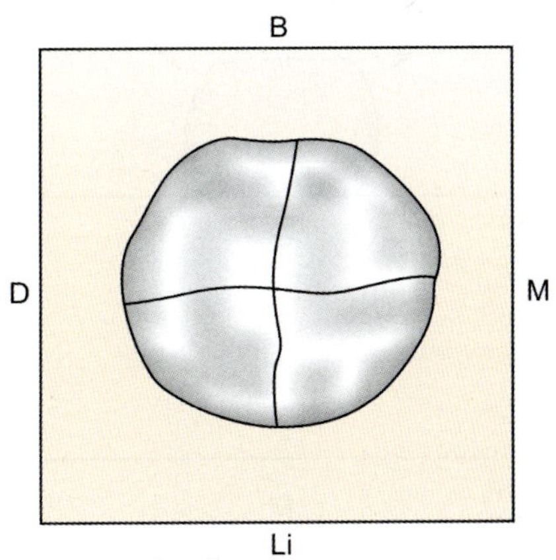

Fig. 6.37D: Step 4—Draw the outline of four cusps based on the size of the cusps

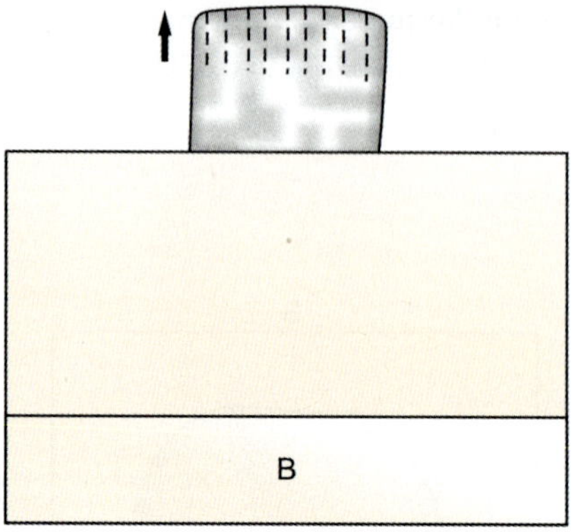

Fig. 6.37E: Step 5—Place the buccal cusp tip inside. For this remove wax from half of the buccal aspect of the crown occlusally. The dotted line represents wax reduced and direction to be removed

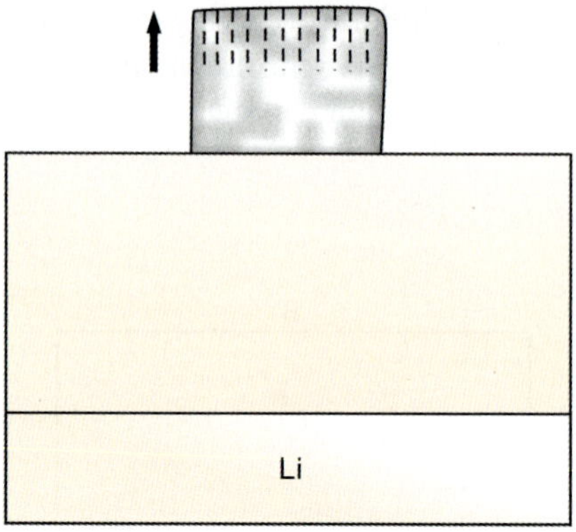

Fig. 6.37F: Step 6—Place the lingual cusp tip inside. For this remove wax from half of the lingual aspect of the crown occlusally. The dotted line represents wax reduced and direction to be removed

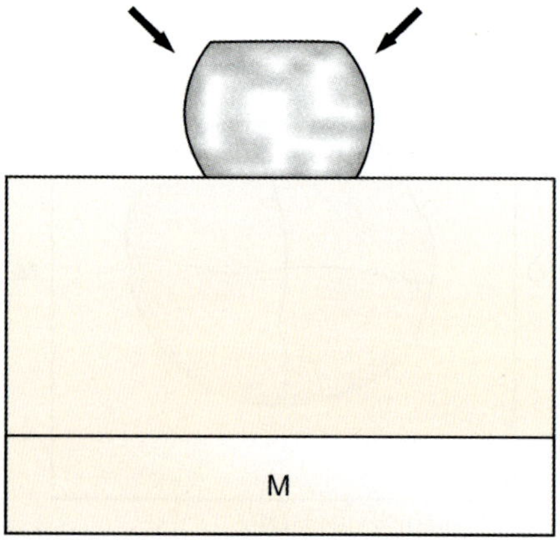

Fig. 6.37G: Step 7—The cusp tips are placed inside. The arrow mark are pointing the cusp tips

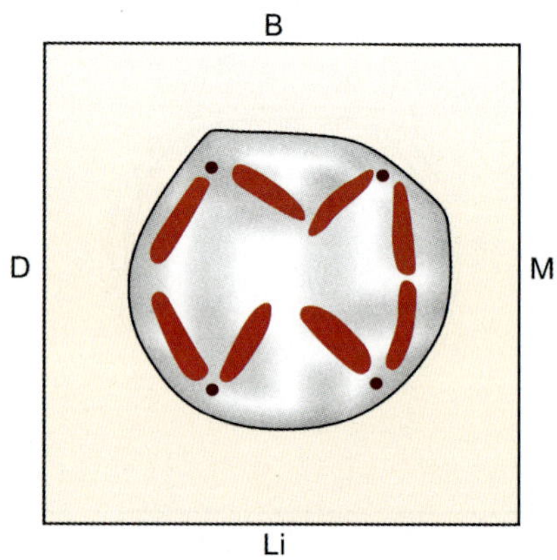

Fig. 6.37H: Step 10—Carve the triangular ridges, cusp ridges and marginal ridges. The shaded part represents the wax to be reduced

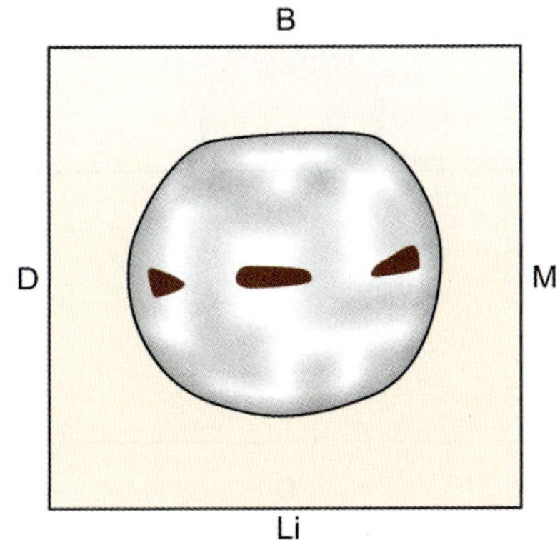

Fig. 6.37I: Step 11—Carve the central fossa, mesial triangular fossa and distal triangular fossa

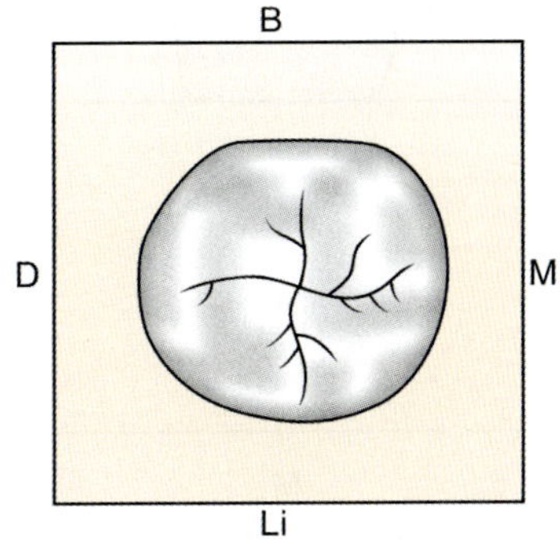

Fig. 6.37J: Step 12—Carve the central developmental groove, buccal develop-mental groove, lingual developmental groove, and the numerous supple-mental grooves

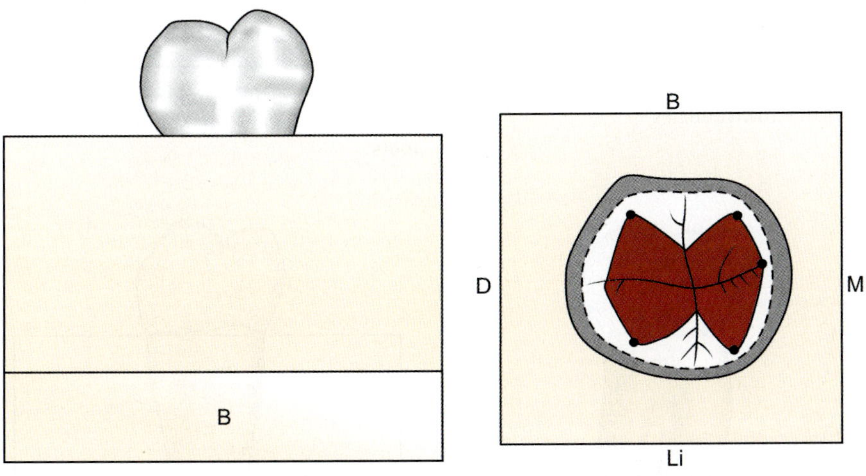

Fig. 6.37K: Step 13—Turn toward buccal aspect carve the outlines of buccal aspect. Extend the buccal groove from central developmental groove. Carve the cusp tips (The shaded part of the diagram represents the cusp ridges, marginal ridges and triangular ridges with the grooves)

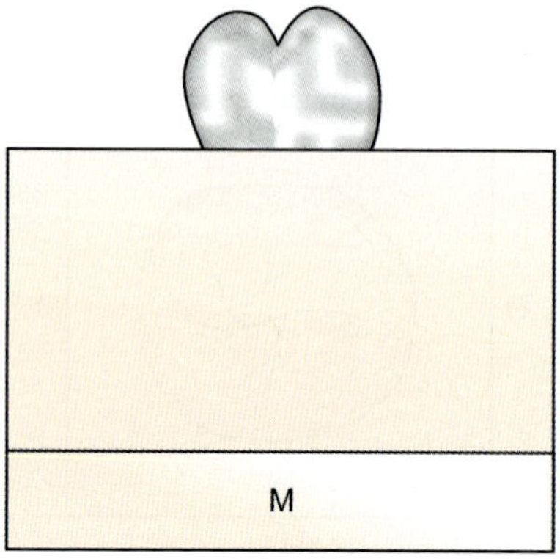

Fig. 6.37L: Step 14—Turn toward mesial aspect, carve the buccal and lingual outline of the crown. Carve the cusp tips also

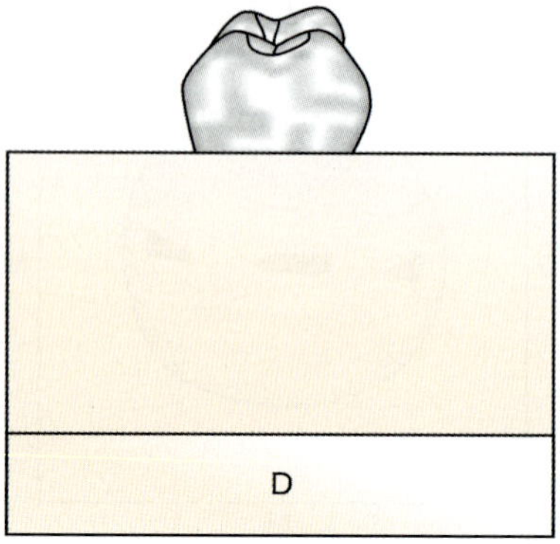

Fig. 6.37M: Step 15—Similarly carve the distal aspect of the crown

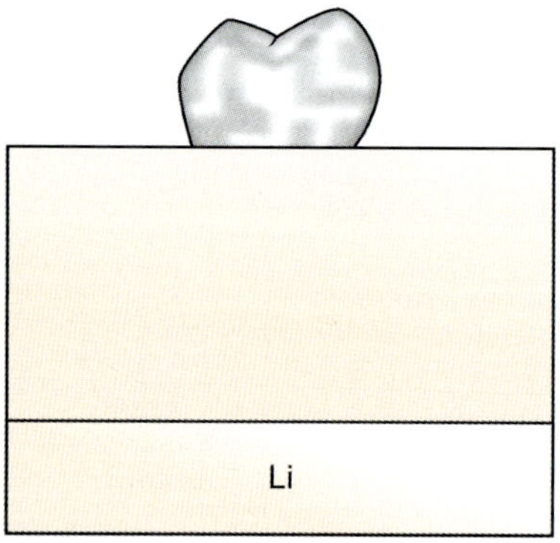

Fig. 6.37N: Step 16—Turn toward lingual aspect, carve the crown outlines

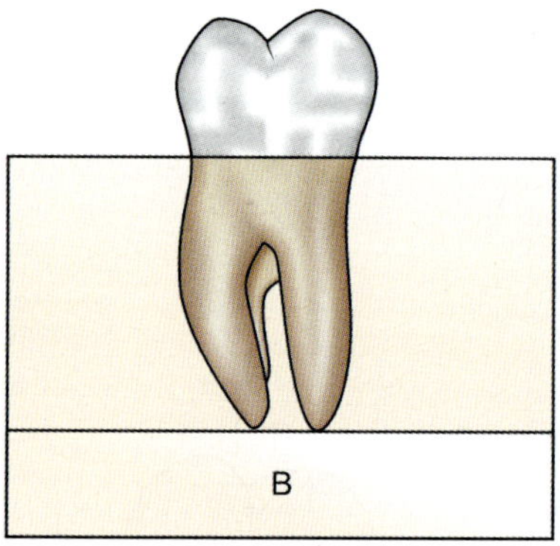

Fig. 6.37O: Step 17—Turn the carving toward buccal aspect, draw the buccal outline of the roots

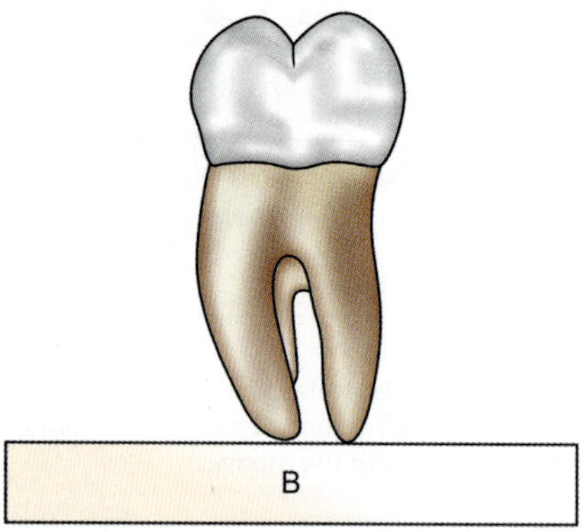

Fig. 6.37P: Step 18—Carve according to the outline

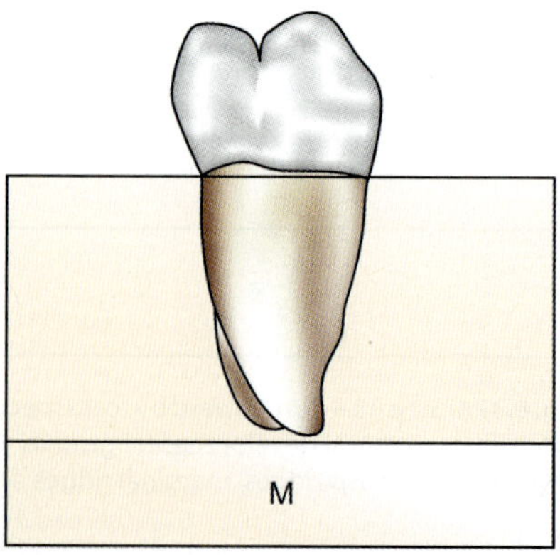

Fig. 6.37Q: Step 19—Turn toward mesial aspect. Draw the mesiobuccal and lingual outline of the root

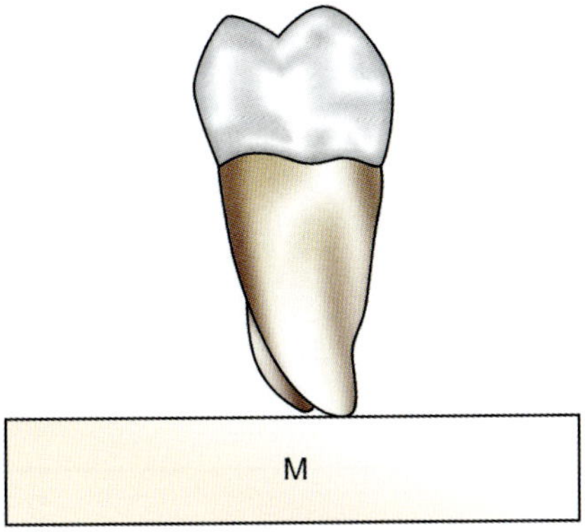

Fig. 6.37R: Step 20—Carve according to the outline

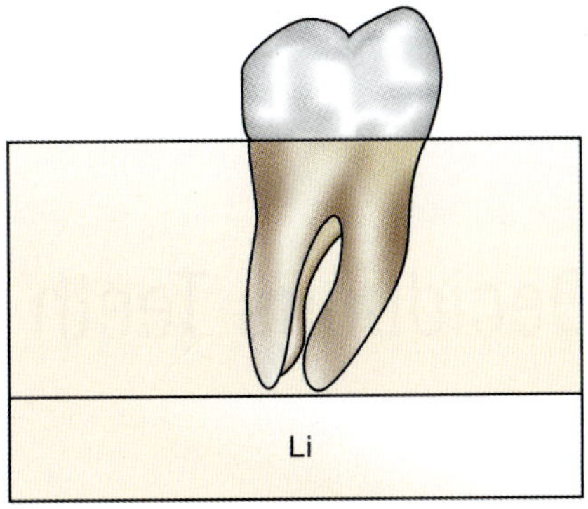

Fig. 6.37S: Step 21—Draw the lingual outline

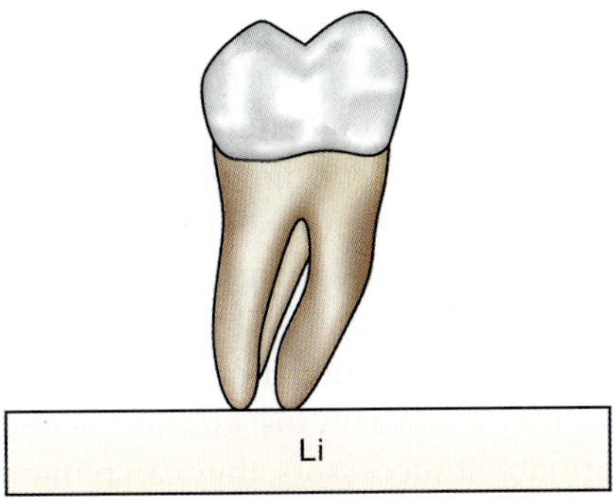

Fig. 6.37T: Step 22—Carve according to the outline

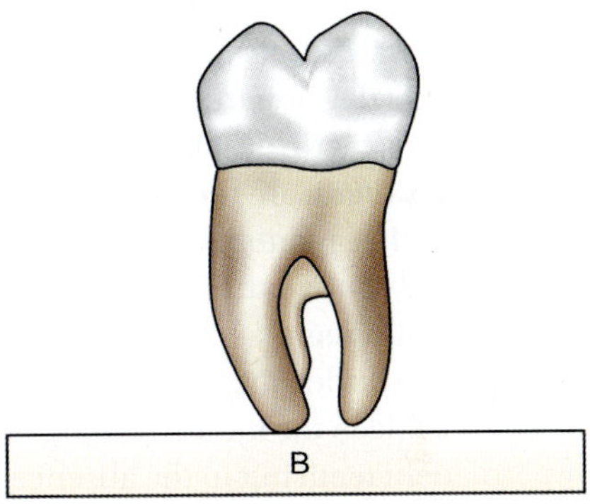

Fig. 6.37U: Carved permanent mandibular third molar

REFERENCES

1. Woelfel JB, Scheid RC. Dental Anatomy. Williams & Wilkins. 1997.
2. Ash, Nelson. Wheelers Dental Anatomy, Physiology & Occlusion. 8th edition. Elsevier. 2003.

CHAPTER

7

Deciduous Teeth

The development of deciduous teeth starts at the sixth week of development as the dental lamina.[1] The deciduous dentition is made up of central incisors, lateral incisors, canines, first molars, and second molars.[1,2,3] The permanent teeth replacements develop from the same tooth bud as the deciduous teeth.

Deciduous teeth, also known as **reborner teeth**, **baby teeth**, **temporary teeth** and **primary teeth**, are the first set of teeth in the growth development of humans and many other mammals.[4] In some Asian countries they are referred to as **fall teeth** as they will eventually fall out, while in almost all European languages they are called **milk teeth** as they exist when the child is still mainly drinking milk.[4,5] They develop during the embryonic stage of development and erupt—that is, they become visible in the mouth, during infancy. They are usually lost and succeeded by permanent teeth but in the absence of permanent successors, they can remain functional for many years.

MORPHOLOGY

Maxillary Central Incisor (Fig. 7.1)

Labial Aspect[2] *(Fig. 7.2)*

The mesiodistal diameter is greater than the cervicoincisal length. The labial surface is very smooth and the incisal edge is straight. The root length is much greater compared with the crown.

Lingual Aspect[2] *(Fig. 7.3)*

Well-developed marginal ridges and highly developed cingulum are present on the lingual surface of the crown.

The cingulum extends toward the incisal ridge giving rise to mesial and distal fossa. The root tapers lingually and presents a ridge for its full length.

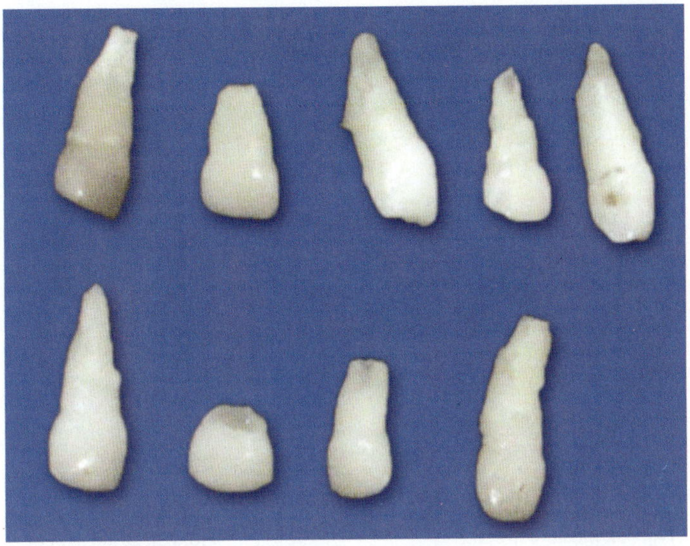

Fig. 7.1: Photograph of deciduous maxillary central incisors

(*Courtesy:* Dr Jaya Naidu, Professor, Department of Pedodontics, Vydehi Institute of Dental Sciences, Bangalore)

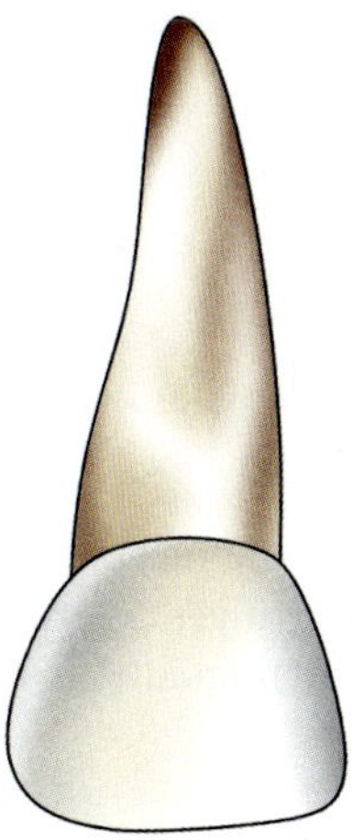

Fig. 7.2: Deciduous maxillary right central incisor, labial aspect

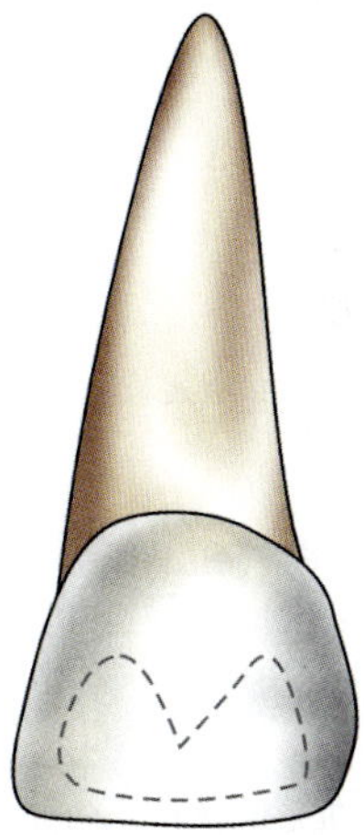

Fig. 7.3: Deciduous maxillary right central incisor, lingual aspect

Mesial (Fig. 7.4) and Distal (Fig. 7.5) Aspect[2]

The mesial and distal aspects of the primary maxillary central incisors are similar. The labiolingual width is wider as compared to its length of crown. Because of the short crown and its labiolingual measurements, the crown appears thick at the middle third. The cervical line curves toward the incisal ridge.

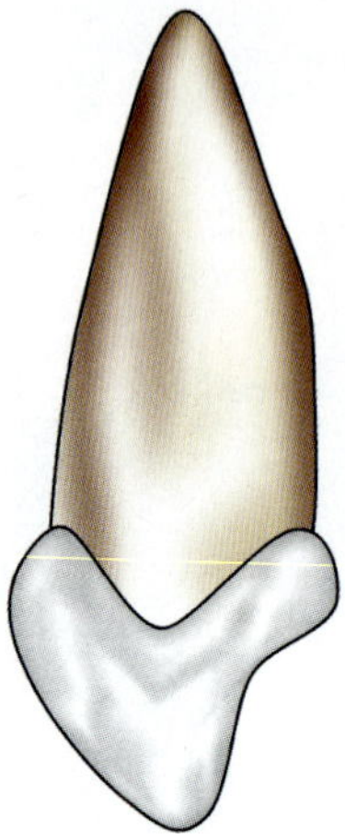

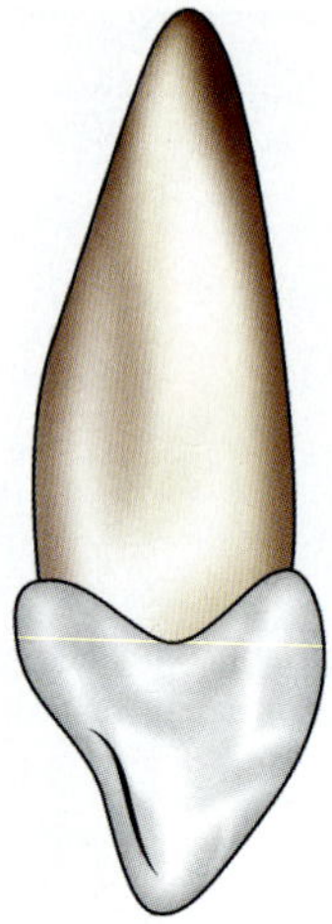

Deciduous maxillary right central incisor

Fig. 7.4: Mesial aspect

Fig. 7.5: Distal aspect

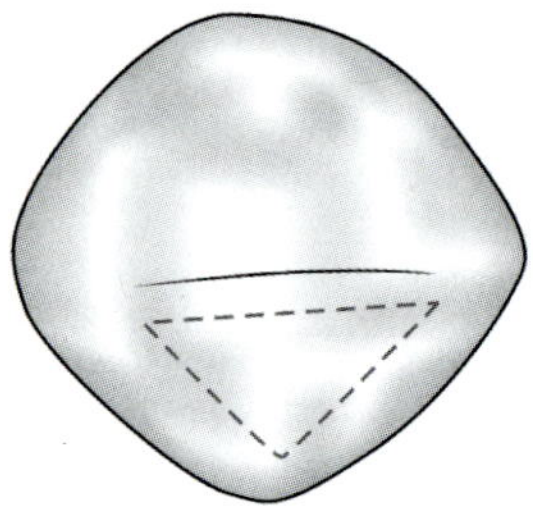

Fig. 7.6: Deciduous maxillary right central incisor, incisal aspect

The root tapers giving a shape of long cone. Usually the mesial surface of the root is concave and distal surface is convex. Cervical ridges of enamel is well developed at the cervical third of the crown labially and lingually.

Incisal Aspect[2] (Fig. 7.6)

The mesiodistal width is greater than the labiolingual width. The incisal edge is centered over the main bulk of the crown and is relatively straight. The labial surface is much broader and also smoother than the lingual surface. The lingual surface tapers toward the cingulum. The mesial and distal surfaces of this tooth are relatively broad.

Deciduous Maxillary Lateral Incisor[2] (Fig. 7.7)

The maxillary lateral incisor is similar to the deciduous maxillary central incisor from all aspects (Fig. 7.8), but its dimensions differ. Its crown is smaller

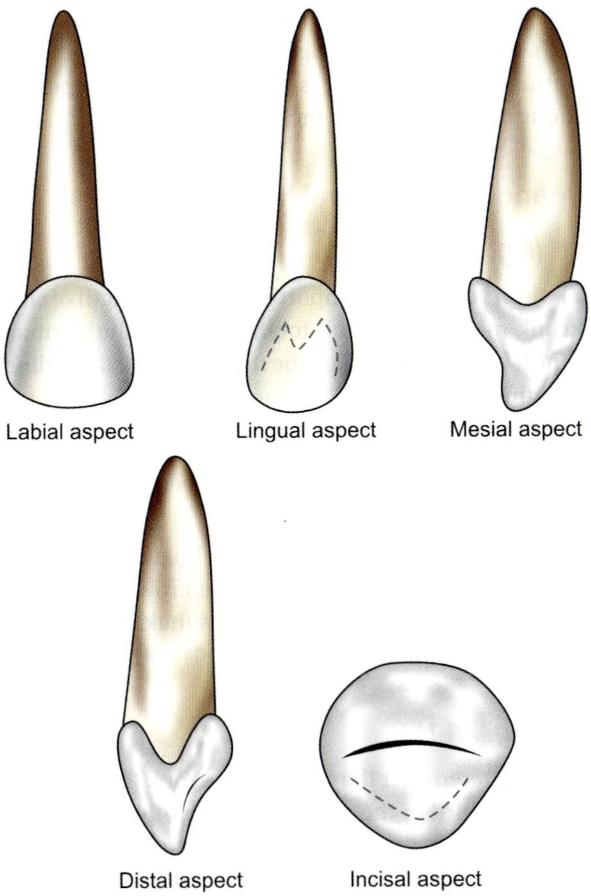

Fig. 7.7: Deciduous maxillary right lateral incisors

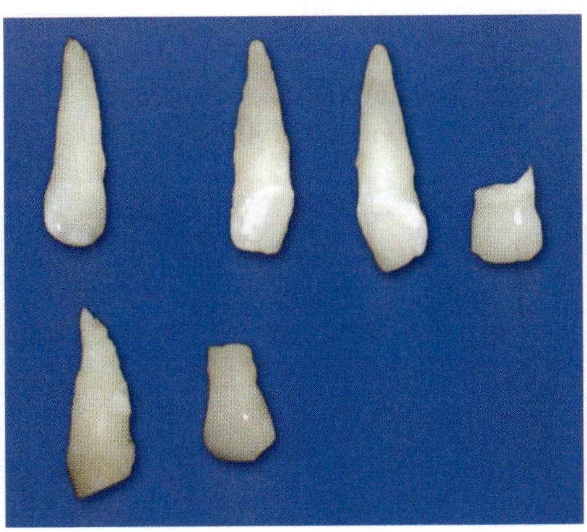

Fig. 7.8: Photograph of deciduous maxillary lateral incisors

(*Courtesy:* Dr Jaya Naidu, Professor, Department of Pedodontics, Vydehi Institute of Dental Sciences, Bangalore)

Deciduous Mandibular Lateral Incisor[2] (Fig. 7.15 and 7.16)

This tooth resembles primary mandibular central incisor. These two teeth supplement each other in function. The tooth appears somewhat larger in all measurements except labiolingual measurement. Cingulum is more prominent than the central incisor. The lingual surface is more concave. The incisal ridge slopes downward distally in a cervical direction. So the distal contact area is placed slightly at a lower level than the mesial contact area.

Deciduous Maxillary Canine (Fig. 7.22)

Labial Aspect[2] (Fig. 7.17)

This tooth has a long, well-developed sharp cusp. The mesial and distal contact areas are at the same level. In permanent canine, the contact areas are not at the same level. The mesial slope is longer than the distal slope. The crown shows a

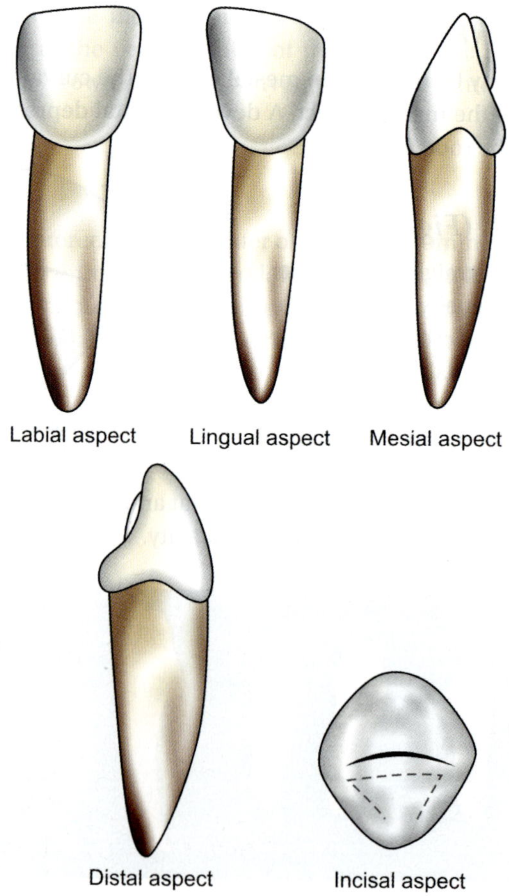

Fig. 7.15: Deciduous mandibular right lateral incisor

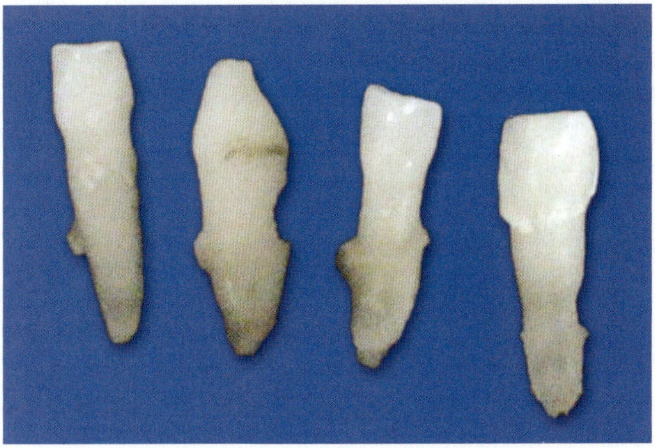

Fig. 7.16: Photograph of deciduous mandibular lateral incisors

(*Courtesy:* Dr Shubha, Lecturer, Department of Pedodontics, Vydehi Institute of Dental Sciences, Bangalore)

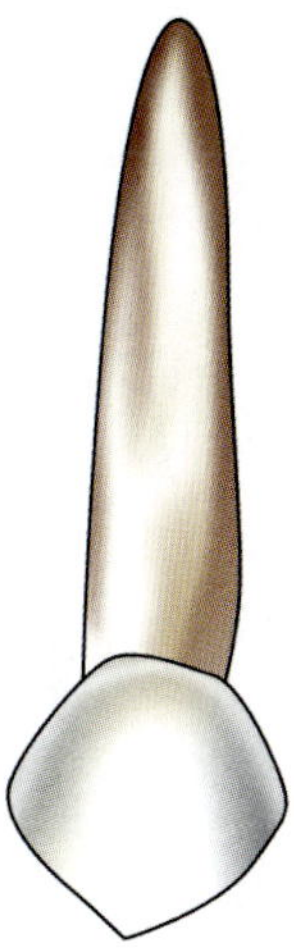

Fig. 7.17: Deciduous maxillary right canine, labial aspect

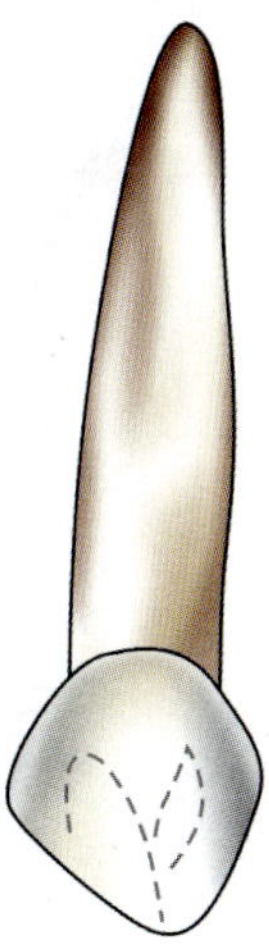

Fig. 7.18: Deciduous maxillary right canine, lingual aspect

marked constriction at the cervix, mesiodistally. The root of the primary canine is long, slender and tapering and the length is twice the crown length.

Lingual Aspect[2] (Fig. 7.18)

Prominent enamel ridges merge with each other. They are cingulum, mesial and distal marginal ridges, incisal cusp ridges and a lingual ridge from cingulum to cusp tip. This lingual ridge divides the shallow lingual fossa into mesiolingual and distolingual fossae. The root tapers lingually and it is inclined distally.

Mesial Aspect[2] (Fig. 7.19)

From mesial aspect, the outline is similar to that of lateral and central incisors. Some of the differences are the labiolingual measurements at the cervical third is much greater. This greater width in conjunction with the root width and length adds up resistance against forces that the tooth could withstand during function.

Distal Aspect[2] (Fig. 7.20)

The distal outline of this tooth is the reverse of the mesial aspect. The difference is only with respect to the curvature of cervical line which is toward the cusp ridge and is less than that of the mesial surface.

Incisal Aspect[2] (Fig. 7.21)

The occlusal form is diamond shaped. The line angles, mesially and distally and the outlines labially and lingually is more pronounced and less rounded than those found on the permanent canines. The cusp tip is distally placed to the center and the mesial cusp slope is longer than the distal cusp slope.

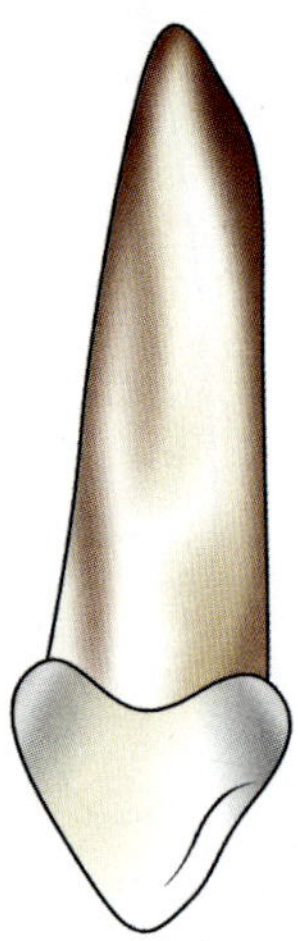

Fig. 7.19: Deciduous maxillary right canine, mesial aspect

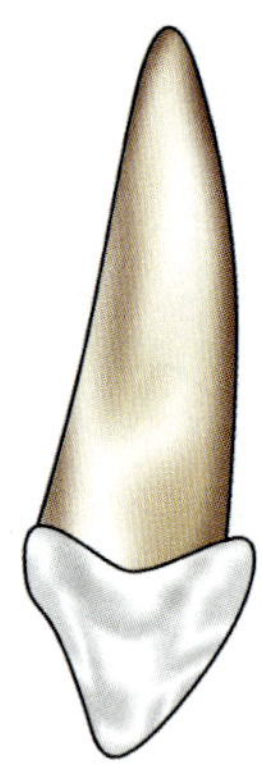

Fig. 7.20: Deciduous maxillary left canine, distal aspect

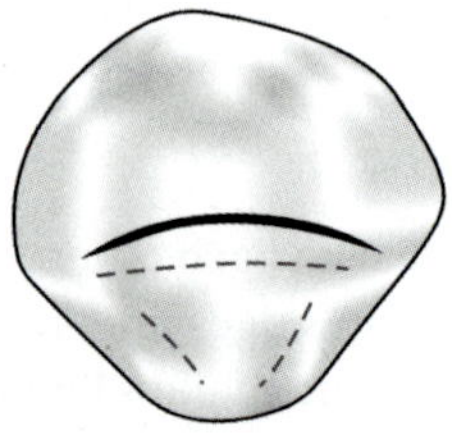

Fig. 7.21: Deciduous maxillary left canine, incisal aspect

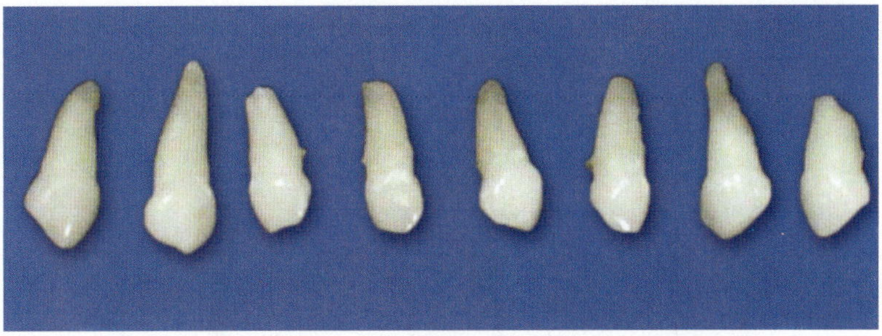

Fig. 7.22: Photograph of deciduous maxillary canines

(*Courtesy:* Dr Shubha, Lecturer, Department of Pedodontics, Vydehi Institute of Dental Sciences, Bangalore)

Deciduous Mandibular Canine[2] (Fig. 7.23 and 7.24)

Little difference may be noted from deciduous maxillary canine. The difference is mainly in the dimensions. The crown is 0.5 mm shorter and the root is 2 mm shorter. The mesiodistal width of mandibular canine at the root trunk is greater when compared with its mesiodistal width at its contact areas than that of the maxillary canine, that is thicker accordingly at the neck of the tooth. The labiolingual width of mandibular canine is much lesser than that of the maxillary canine.

The cervical bulges of the crown labially and lingually is less pronounced. The distal cusp slope is longer than the mesial cusp slope. This makes proper intercuspation of maxillary and mandibular canine during mastication.

Deciduous Maxillary First Molar (Fig. 7.30)

Buccal Aspect[1-3] (Fig. 7.25)

The mesiodistal measurement at contact areas is greater by 2 mm than the measurement at the cervix. This furnishes a narrower look to the cervical portion of the crown and root of this tooth than that of the same portion of the permanent maxillary first molar.

The occlusal line is slightly scalloped but with no definite cusp form. The buccal surface is smooth and there is little evidence of developmental grooves. From this aspect the relative size of the primary maxillary first molar may be judged when it is compared with the second molar. The tooth is smaller in all measurements than the primary second molar. Its relative size and shape suggests that it was designed to be the premolar section of the primary dentition.

The roots of the maxillary first molar are slender and long and they spread widely. The distal root is shorter than the mesial one. The bifurcation of the roots begins almost immediately at the site of the cervical line. This is characteristic of all primary maxillary and mandibular molars. Permanent molars do not possess this characteristic feature.

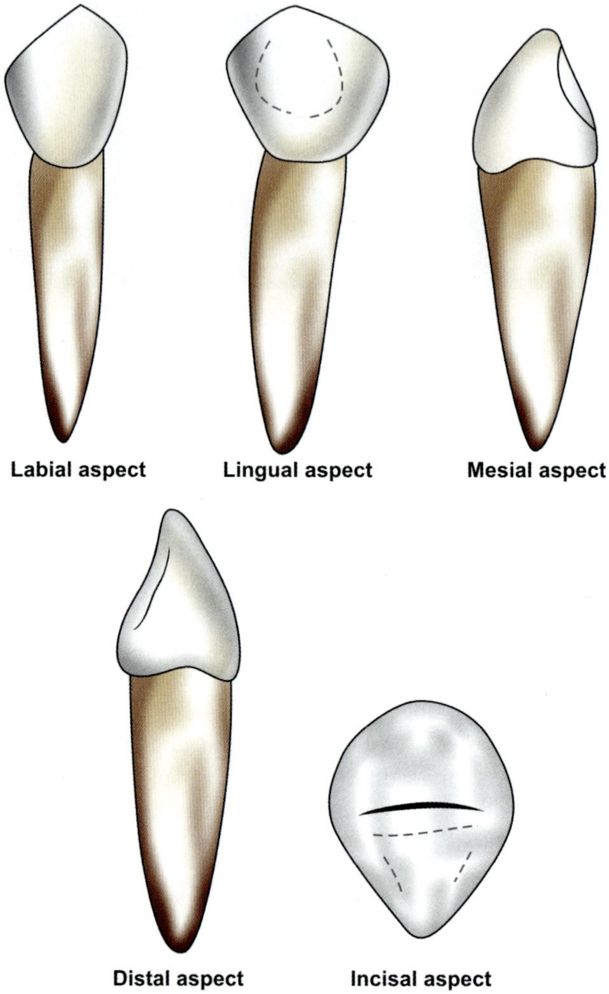

Fig. 7.23: Deciduous mandibular left canine

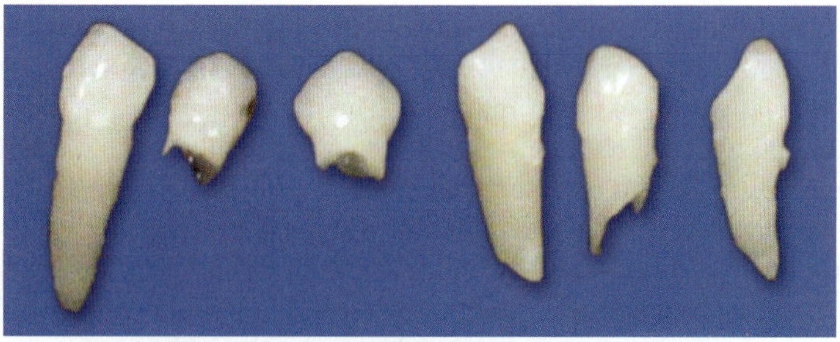

Fig. 7.24: Photograph of deciduous mandibular canines

(*Courtesy:* Dr Shubha, Lecturer, Department of Pedodontics, Vydehi Institute of Dental Sciences, Bangalore)

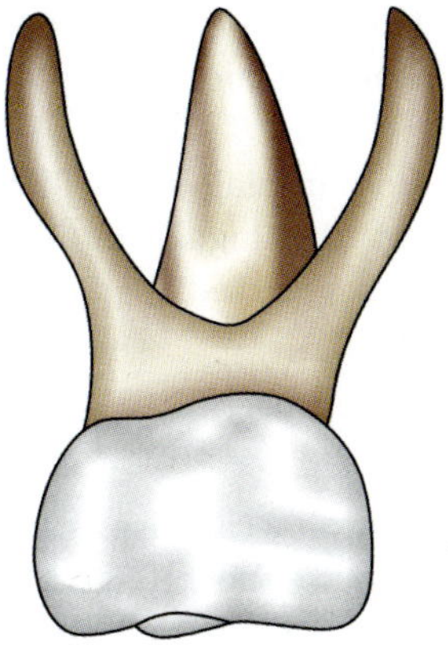

Fig. 7.25: Deciduous maxillary left first molar, buccal aspect

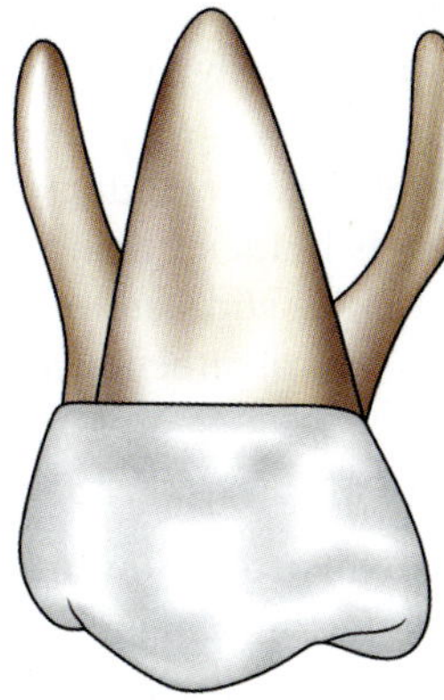

Fig. 7.26: Deciduous maxillary left first molar, lingual aspect

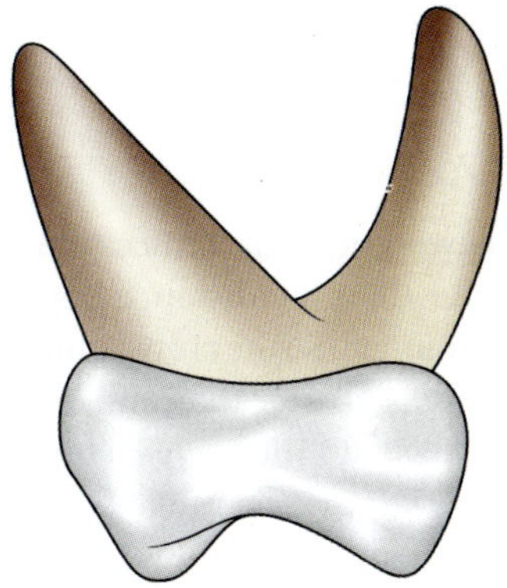

Fig. 7.27: Deciduous maxillary left first molar, mesial aspect

Lingual Aspect[1-3] (Fig. 7.26)

The outline is similar to buccal aspect. The crown converges considerably in a lingual direction, making mesiodistal width of lingual aspect less than that of the buccal aspect.

The mesiolingual cusp is the most prominent cusp. It is the longest and sharpest cusp. The distolingual cusp is poorly defined, small and rounded. The distobuccal cusp may be seen since it is longer and better developed than the distolingual cusp. Sometimes in three cusped molar, a large lingual cusp may be evident. All the three roots are seen from this aspect, being the lingual root larger.

Mesial Aspect[1-3] (Fig. 7.27)

The dimension at the cervical third is greater than the dimension at the occlusal third. This is true for all molars, but it is more pronounced on primary than on permanent teeth. The mesiolingual cusp is longer and sharper than the mesiobuccal cusp. A pronounced convexity is evident on the buccal outline of the cervical third. This convexity is an outstanding characteristic of this tooth. The cervical line mesially shows some curvature in the direction of the occlusal surface.

The mesiobuccal and lingual roots are visible from mesial aspect. The distobuccal root is hidden behind the mesiobuccal root. The lingual root from this aspect looks long and slender and extends lingually to a marked degree. It curves sharply in a buccal direction above the middle third.

Distal Aspect[1-3] (Fig. 7.28)

The crown is narrower toward distal aspect. The distobuccal cusp is long and sharp and the distolingual cusp is poorly developed. The prominent bulge seen from the mesial aspect at the cervical third does not continue distally. The cervical line may curve occlusally or it may extend straight across from the buccal to lingual surface. All the three roots are visible as part of mesiobuccal root is seen. The point of bifurcation of the distobuccal root and the lingual root is near the cementoenamel junction (CEJ).

Occlusal Aspect[1-3] (Fig. 7.29)

Dimension: The distance between the mesiobuccal line angle and the distobuccal line angle is definitely greater than the distance between the mesiolingual line angle and the distolingual line angle. So the crown outline converges lingually. The mesial portion buccolingually is greater than the distal portion buccolingually. So the crown also converges distally. The occlusal form is somewhat rectangular. The mesiolingual cusp is the largest cusp followed by mesiobuccal cusp then distobuccal and distolingual cusp.

Ridges: The mesial and distal cusp ridges of all the four cusps are present. The triangular ridges of four cusps, the mesial marginal ridge and the distal marginal ridge are also seen. Sometimes a well-defined triangular ridge connecting the mesiolingual cusp with distobuccal cusp called as the oblique ridge is seen.

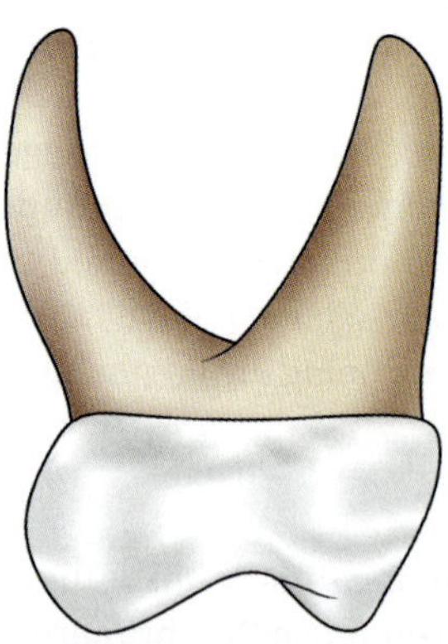

Fig. 7.28: Deciduous maxillary left first molar, distal aspect

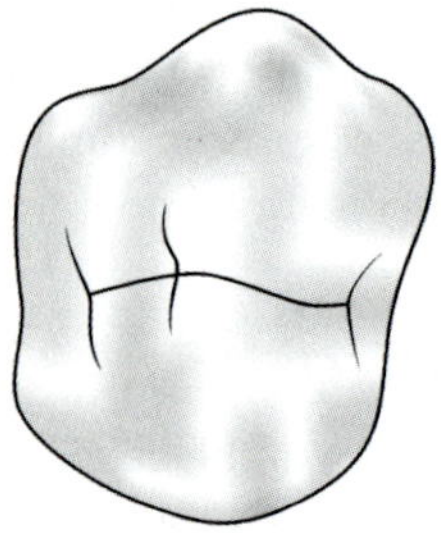

Fig. 7.29: Deciduous maxillary left first molar, incisal aspect

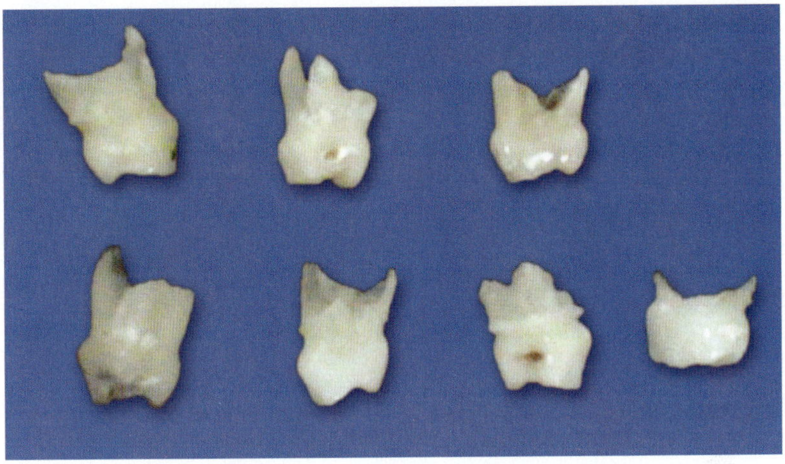

Fig. 7.30: Photograph of deciduous maxillary first molars

(*Courtesy:* Dr Shubha, Lecturer, Department of Pedodontics, Vydehi Institute of Dental Sciences, Bangalore)

Fossae: Central fossa, mesial triangular fossa and distal triangular fossa are seen.

Grooves: Central developmental groove runs mesially and distally over the occlusal surface called as the mesial developmental groove and distal developmental groove. The mesial developmental groove gives supplemental grooves within the mesial triangular fossa. A buccal developmental groove is present in between the mesiobuccal and distobuccal cusp extending from central developmental groove.

Pits: Mesial pit is seen within the mesial triangular fossa.

Deciduous Maxillary Second Molar (Fig. 7.36)

Buccal Aspect[1-3] (Fig. 7.31)

From buccal aspect, this tooth resembles the permanent maxillary first molar, but it is smaller. Two well defined cusps and three roots are seen, the mesiobuccal, and distobuccal cusps and the roots are mesiobuccal, distobuccal and lingual roots. The two buccal cusps are nearly equal in size. A buccal developmental groove is present in between mesiobuccal and distobuccal cusp. The crown is narrow at the cervix than at the mesial and distal contact areas. The roots are much slender, longer and heavier than that of the deciduous maxillary first molar.

Lingual Aspect[1-3] (Fig. 7.32)

The cusps seen from lingual aspect are the mesiolingual cusp, which is large and well developed; the distolingual cusp which is well developed than the primary maxillary first molar and the fifth cusp (tubercle of Carabelli) is present apical to the mesiolingual cusp.

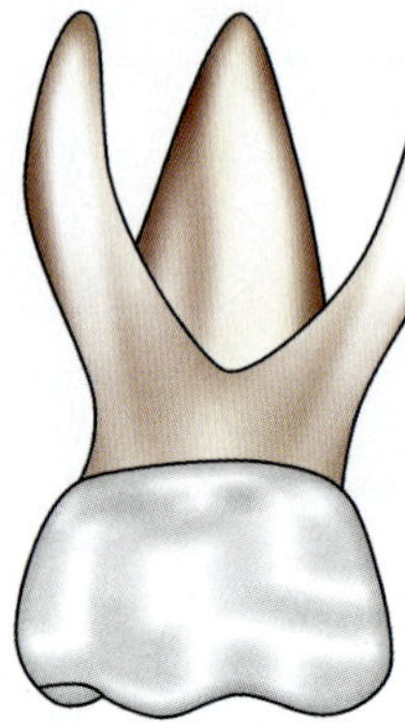

Fig. 7.31: Deciduous maxillary right second molar, buccal aspect

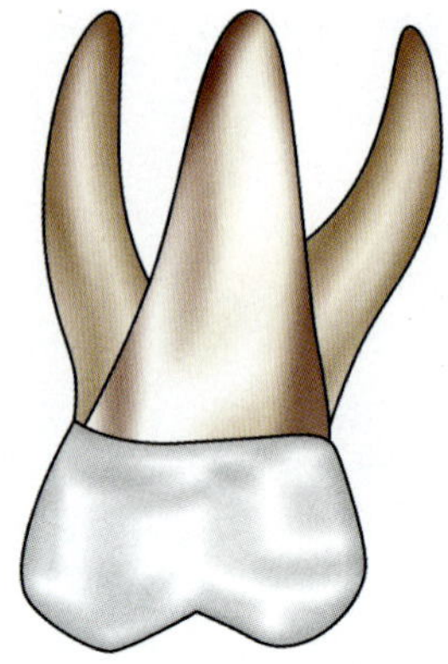

Fig. 7.32: Deciduous maxillary right second molar, lingual aspect

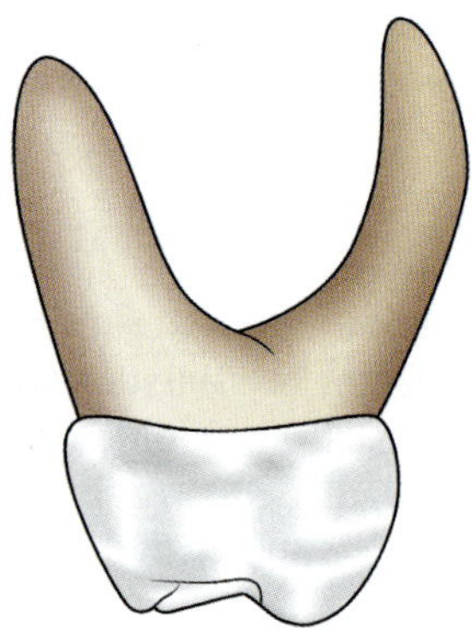

Fig. 7.33: Deciduous maxillary right second molar, mesial aspect

Mesial Aspect[1-3] (Fig. 7.33)

The mesial outline is typical which resembles that of the permanent molars. Since the buccolingual width is greater, the crown appears short.

The crown is 0.5 mm longer than the crown of the first deciduous molar, but the buccolingual measurement is 1.5 to 2 mm greater. The roots are 1.5 to 2 mm longer. The mesiolingual cusp with the fifth cusp is larger than the mesiobuccal cusp. The mesiobuccal cusp is short and sharp. Slight curvature is seen on the mesial aspect.

The mesiobuccal root is broad and flat. The lingual root is long and slender and extends lingually. The outline of mesiobuccal root curves out lingually than that of the mesial outline of the crown. The point of bifurcation between the mesiobuccal root and the lingual root is 3 mm apical to the cervical line. The mesiobuccal root is wider about two-third of the width of the root trunk. The mesiolingual cusp is directly below the bifurcation. The crest of curvature at the cervical third lingually is prominent than on the buccal surface. This less pronounced crest of curvature at the cervical third buccally resembles that of the permanent maxillary first molar.

Distal Aspect[1-3] (Fig. 7.34)

The distal calibration is less than the mesial measurement. From both the mesial and distal aspects, the outline of the crown lingually creates a smooth rounded line, whereas the buccal outline is almost straight from the crest of curvature to the tip of the buccal cusp. The height of distobuccal and distolingual cusp is same in length. The cervical line is straight. All three roots, i.e. the lingual root, distobuccal root and part of the outline of the mesiobuccal root are seen. Since the distobuccal root is superimposed over mesiobuccal root, only part of this root is seen. The distobuccal root is shorter and narrower than the other roots. The point of bifurcation between the distobuccal root and the lingual root is more apical in location than any of the other points of bifurcation and the point of bifurcation is more distal.

Occlusal Aspect[1-3] (Fig. 7.35)

From the occlusal aspect, this tooth resembles the permanent first molar. The occlusal outline form is rhomboidal and has four well developed cusps and one supplemental cusp. The mesiobuccal, distobuccal, mesiolingual, distolingual

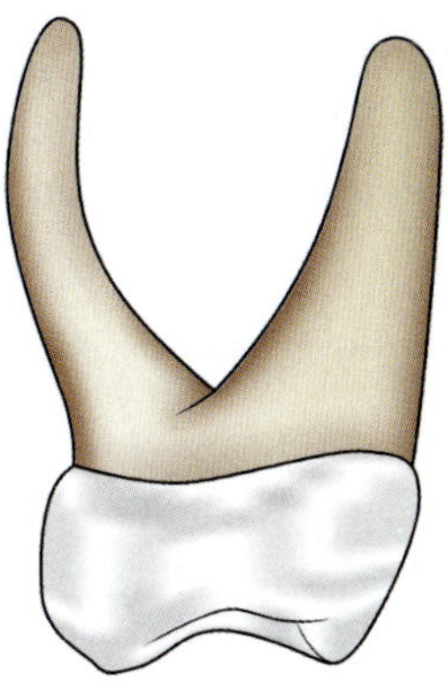

Fig. 7.34: Deciduous maxillary right second molar, distal aspect

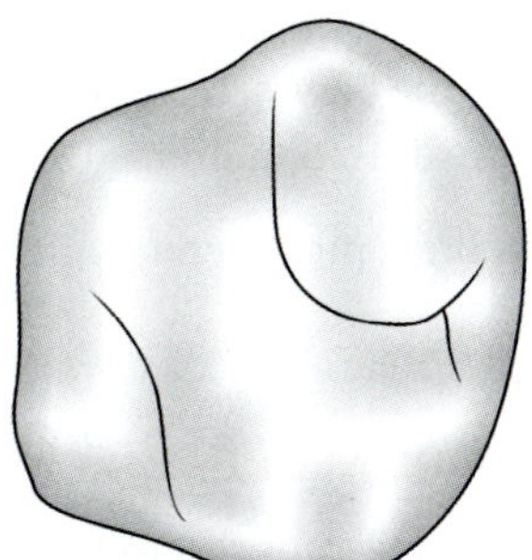

Fig. 7.35: Deciduous maxillary right second molar, occlusal aspect

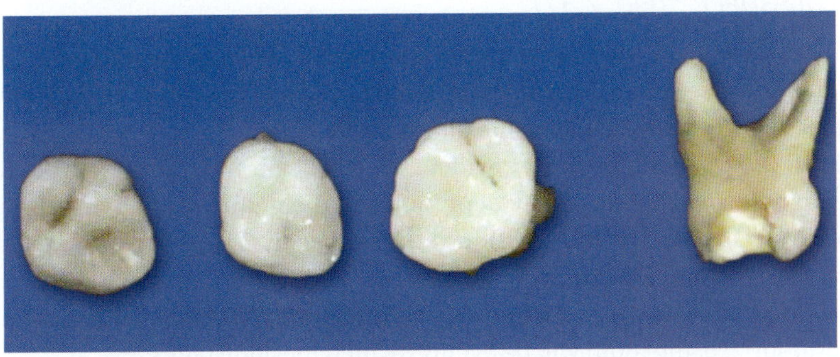

Fig. 7.36: Photograph of deciduous maxillary second molars

(*Courtesy:* Dr Shubha, Lecturer, Department of Pedodontics, Vydehi Institute of Dental Sciences, Bangalore)

and fifth cusps are seen from occlusal aspect. The buccal surface is flat with the develop-mental groove between the cusps. The cusps are less marked than that found on the first permanent molar. The character of the mold is constant.

Dimensions: The buccolingual width is greater than the mesiodistal width. The mesiolingual cusp is the largest cusp followed by mesiobuccal, distobuccal, distolingual and then the fifth cusp.

Ridges: The mesial and distal cusp ridges of all the five cusps, the triangular ridges of the cusps and the mesial and distal marginal ridges are seen from this aspect. The oblique ridge is prominent and connects the mesiolingual cusp with the distobuccal cusp. The distal marginal ridge is well developed as the mesial marginal ridge. The marginal ridges are not developed equally as on the primary maxillary first molar.

Fossae: Central fossa, mesial triangular fossa present distal to mesial marginal ridge and distal triangular fossa seen mesial to distal marginal ridge are seen.

Grooves: A central developmental groove is found at the bottom of a sulcus connecting the mesial triangular fossa with the central fossa. The buccal developmental groove extends buccally from the central pit, separating the triangular ridges of mesiobuccal and distobuccal cusps. A distal groove is seen in between the mesiolingual and distolingual cusp and continues to the lingual surface as the lingual developmental groove. Supplemental grooves often radiate from these developmental grooves.

Pit: A central pit is seen from which the central groove extends buccally and mesially.

Deciduous Mandibular First Molar (Fig. 7.42)

This tooth does not resemble any of the other teeth, deciduous or permanent, because of its greater variation in form.

Buccal Aspect[1-3] (Fig. 7.37)

The mesial outline of the buccal aspect is straight from contact area to the cervix. The distal outline is more curved. The distal portion of the crown is shorter than the mesial portion, the cervical line dipping apically.

No developmental groove is evident between the two buccal cusps, but a developmental depression is evident between them. The mesial cusp is larger than the distal cusp. The roots are long and slender and they spread greater at the apical third beyond the outline of the crown.

From the buccal aspect, if a line drawn from the bifurcation of the roots to the occlusal surface, the tooth will be evenly divided mesiodistally.

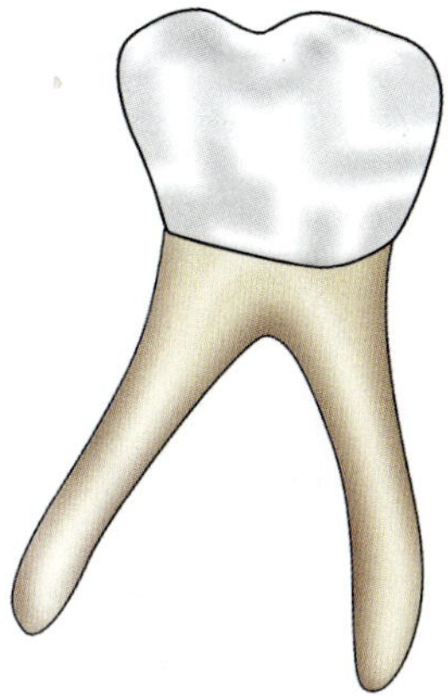

Fig. 7.37: Deciduous mandibular right first molar, buccal aspect

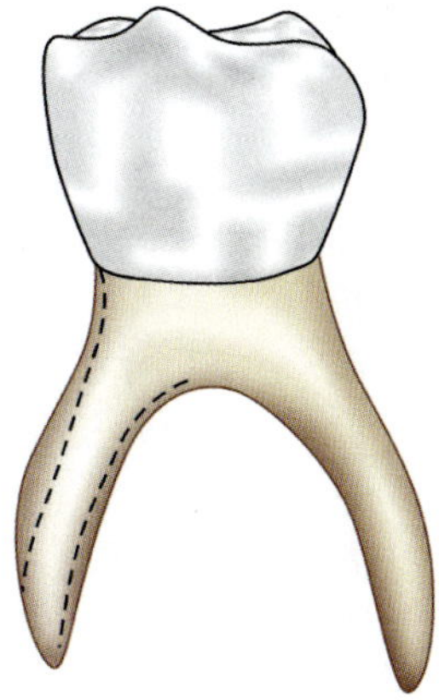

Fig. 7.38: Deciduous mandibular right first molar, lingual aspect

Lingual Aspect[1-3] (Fig. 7.38)

The crown and root converge on the lingual surface. The distolingual cusp is rounded and suggests a developmental groove between this cusp and the mesiolingual cusp. The mesiolingual cusp is long and sharp at the tip, more so than any of the other cusps. The sharp and prominent mesiolingual cusp is an outstanding characteristic found occlusally on the primary first mandibular molar. The mesial marginal ridge is very well developed that it might almost be considered another small cusp lingually. Part of the two buccal cusps may be seen from this angle. The cervical line is straighter.

Mesial Aspect[1-3] (Fig. 7.39)

A well noticeable detail is extreme curvature buccally at the cervical third. Except for this detail, the crown outline of this tooth from this aspect resembles the mesial aspect of the primary second molar and mesial aspect of the permanent mandibular molars.

In this comparison, the buccal cusps are placed over the root base and the lingual outline of the crown extends out lingually beyond the confines of the root base. Both mesiobuccal and mesiolingual cusp are seen from this aspect. The cervical line slants upward buccolingually because the mesiobuccal crown length is greater than the mesiolingual crown length. The buccal outline of the crown is straight from the crest of curvature of the buccal surface at the cervical third to the tip of the mesiobuccal cusp. All of the primary molars have flattened buccal surfaces above this cervical ridge.

The buccal and lingual outline of the root drop straight down from the crown and are approximately parallel for more than half of their length, tapering only slightly at the apical third. The root end is flat and almost square. A developmental depression usually extends almost the full length of the root on the mesial side.

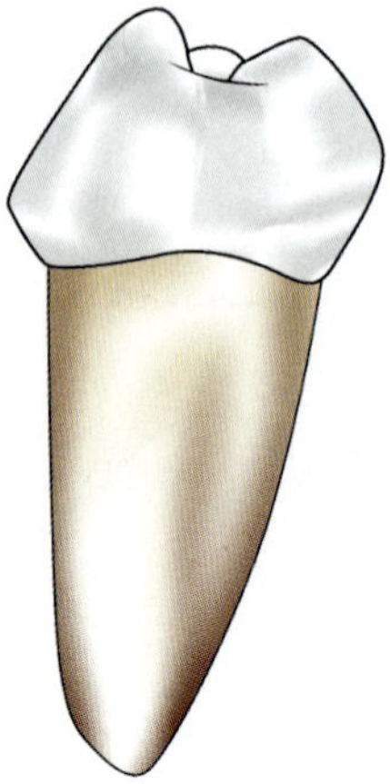

Fig. 7.39: Deciduous mandibular right first molar, mesial aspect

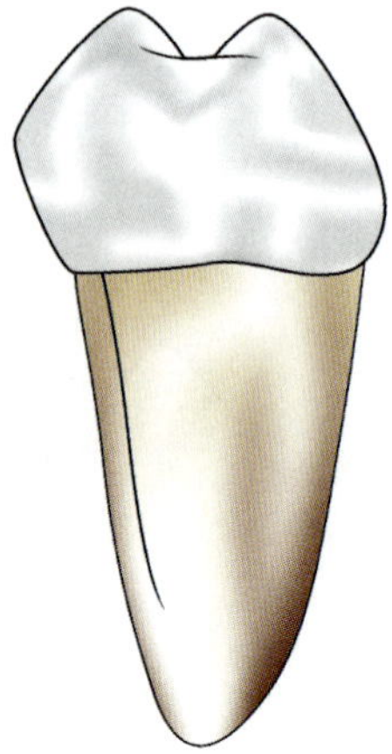

Fig. 7.40: Deciduous mandibular right first molar, distal aspect

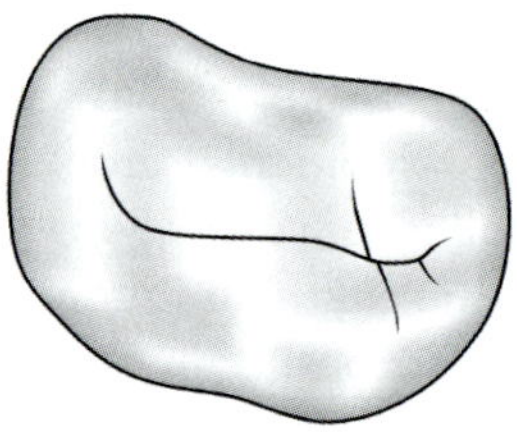

Fig. 7.41: Deciduous mandibular right first molar, occlusal aspect

Distal Aspect[1-3] (Fig. 7.40)

The differences from mesial aspect are the cervical line which does not drop buccally. The length of crown buccally and lingually is more uniform and the cervical line is almost straight. The distobuccal cusp and the distolingual cusp is not as long or as sharp as the mesial cusps. The distal marginal ridge is not as straight and well defined as the mesial marginal ridge. The distal root is rounder and shorter and tapers more apically.

Occlusal Aspect[1-3] (Fig. 7.41)

The occlusal outline form is rhomboidal. The prominence present mesiobuccally is noticeable from this aspect. The mesiolingual cusp may be seen as the largest and well-developed of all the cusps.

The central developmental groove extends buccally called as the buccal developmental groove in between the buccal cusps, when it extends mesially termed as mesial developmental groove and extends distally called as distal developmental groove. A central pit and mesial pit is seen on the occlusal surface. Supplemental grooves extend from these pits.

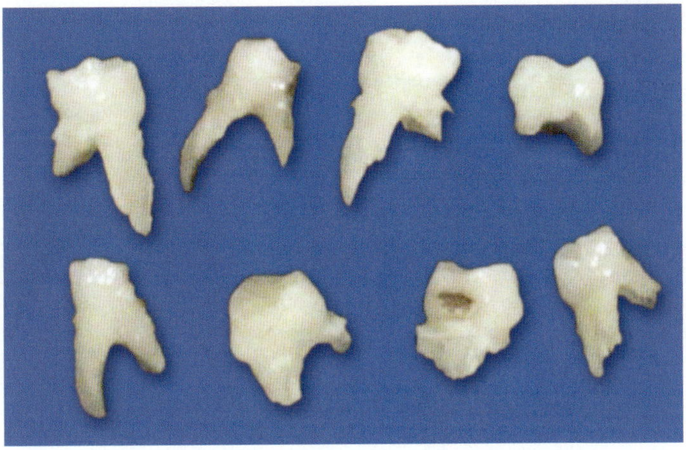

Fig. 7.42: Photograph of deciduous mandibular first molar

(*Courtesy:* Dr Jaya Naidu, Professor, Department of Pedodontics, Vydehi Institute of Dental Sciences, Bangalore)

The fossae are mesial triangular fossa and distal triangular fossa. The buccal and lingual developmental grooves do not extend on the surfaces but stop at the junction of respective cusp ridges.

Triangular ridges may not be well developed.

Deciduous Mandibular Second Molar (Fig. 7.48)

This tooth resembles that of the permanent mandibular first molar.

Buccal Aspect[1-3] (Fig. 7.43)

The mesiodistal width at the cervical portion is less than at the contact level. The mandibular first permanent molar, accordingly, is wider at the cervical portion. Three cusps are seen from buccal aspect—mesiobuccal, distobuccal and buccal cusp. All the three cusps are equal in size. This arrangement forms a straight buccal surface presenting a mesiobuccal, a buccal and distobuccal cusp. It differs, therefore, from the mandibular first permanent molar, which has an uneven distribution buccally, presenting two buccal cusps and one distal cusp. Mesiobuccal and distobuccal grooves are present in between the three cusps.

The roots of the primary second molar from this angle are slender and long. They have a characteristic flare mesiodistally at the middle and apical thirds. The point of bifurcation of the roots starts immediately below the CEJ of crown and root.

Lingual Aspect[1-3] (Fig. 7.44)

Two cusps, i.e. mesiolingual and distolingual cusps almost equal in dimensions may be noticed. A short lingual groove is seen between them. The crown narrows lingually. The cervical line is straight and the crown extends out over the root

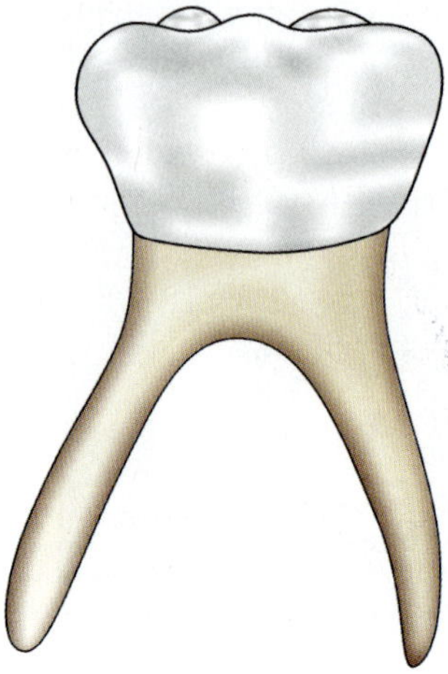

Fig. 7.43: Deciduous mandibular right second molar, buccal aspect

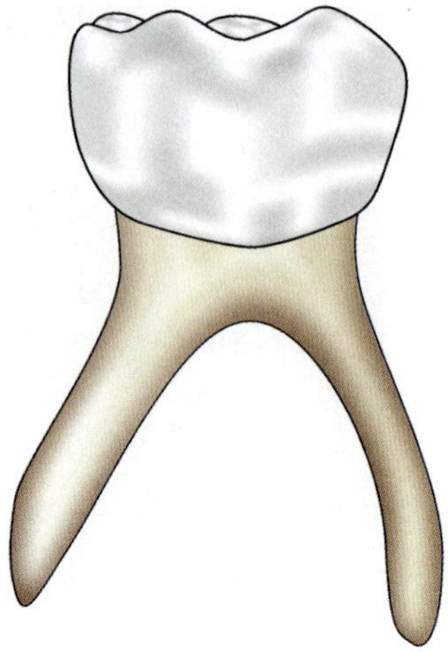

Fig. 7.44: Deciduous mandibular right second molar, lingual aspect

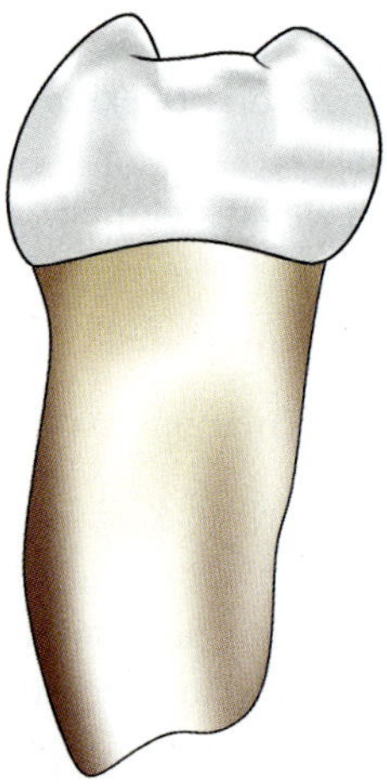

Fig. 7.45: Deciduous mandibular right second molar, mesial aspect

more distally than it does mesially. The mesial portion of the crown seems to be a little higher than the distal portion of the crown when viewed from the lingual aspect. It gives the impression of being tipped distally. Part of three buccal cusps may be seen from this aspect. The roots from this aspect give somewhat the same appearance as from the buccal aspect.

Mesial Aspect[1-3] (Fig.7.45)

The outline of the crown from mesial aspect resembles the permanent mandibular first molar. The crest of contour buccally is more prominent on the primary molar and the tooth seems to be more constricted occlusally because of the flattened buccal surface above this cervical ridge.

The crown is poised over the root of this tooth in the same manner as all mandibular posteriors. Its buccal cusp is over the root and the lingual outline of the crown extending out beyond the root line. The marginal ridge is high, a characteristic that makes the mesiobuccal cusp and the mesiolingual cusp appear short. The lingual cusp is longer than the buccal cusp. The cervical line is regular, although it extends upward buccolingually, making up for the difference in length between the buccal and lingual cusps. The mesial root is unusually broad and flat with a blunt apex that is sometimes serrated.

Distal Aspect[1-3] (Fig. 7.46)

The crown is not as wide distally as it is mesially. So part of mesiobuccal and distobuccal cusps are seen from the distal aspect. The distolingual cusp appears well developed and triangular ridge of this cusp is seen through the distal marginal ridge.

The distal marginal ridge bends down more sharply and is shorter buccolingually than the mesial marginal ridge. The cervical line of the crown is regular.

The distal root is almost as broad as the mesial root and is flattened on the distal surface. The distal root tapers more at the apical end than does the mesial root.

Occlusal Aspect[1-3] (Fig. 7.47)

The occlusal outline form is somewhat rectangular. The three buccal cusps are similar in size. The two lingual cusps are also equally matched. But the total mesiodistal width of the lingual cusps is less than the total mesiodistal width of the three buccal cusps.

Ridges: The highly placed mesial marginal ridge and a slightly lower distal marginal ridge. Well formed triangular ridges extend occlusally from each one of the cusp tips. The mesial and distal cusp ridges of all the cusps are seen.

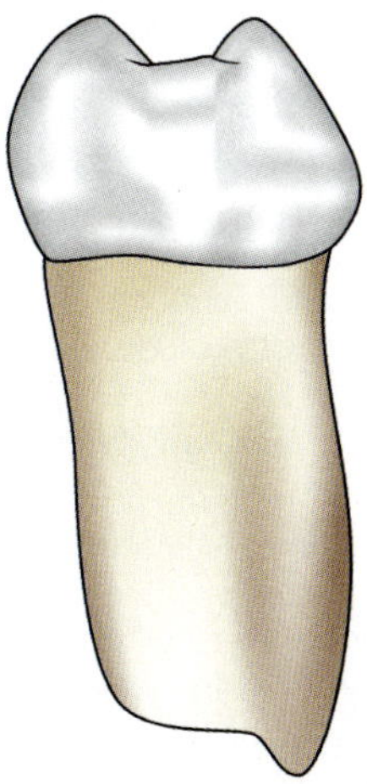

Fig. 7.46: Deciduous mandibular right second molar, distal aspect

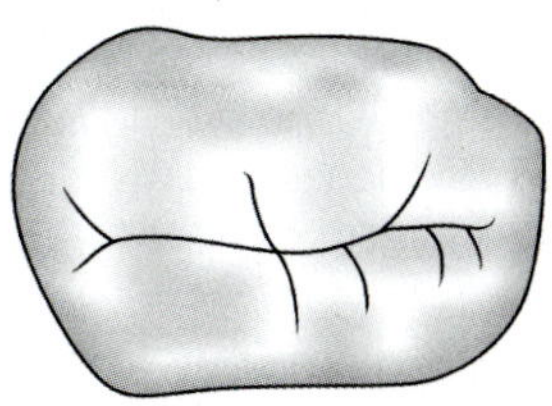

Fig. 7.47: Deciduous mandibular right second molar, occlusal aspect

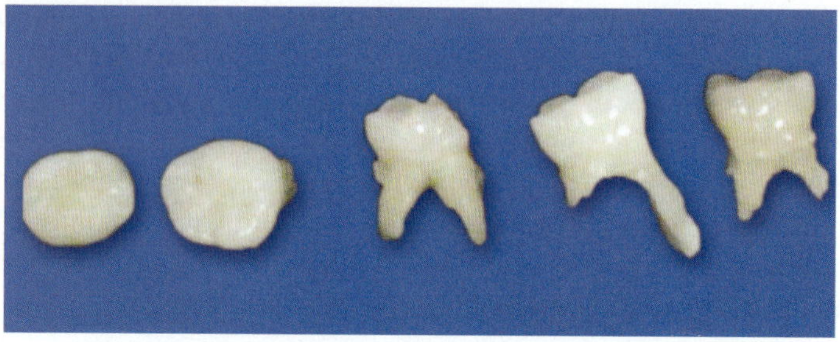

Fig. 7.48: Photograph of deciduous mandibular second molar

(*Courtesy:* Dr Shubha, Lecturer, Department of Pedodontics, Vydehi Institute of Dental Sciences, Bangalore)

Grooves: A central developmental groove which extends mesially is called as mesial developmental groove; when it extends distally it is called as distal developmental groove. It also extends buccally in between the cusps called as distobuccal and mesiobuccal groove and lingual extension is called as lingual developmental groove.

Fossa: Mesial and distal triangular fossa are present on the occlusal surface. The difference between the deciduous mandibular second molar and the permanent mandibular first molar is as follows. The deciduous molar has its mesiobuccal, distobuccal and distal cusps almost equal in size and development. The distal cusp of the permanent molar is smaller than the other two. Because of the small buccal cusps, the deciduous tooth crown is much narrower buccolingually, in comparison with its mesiodistal measurements than that of the permanent tooth.

Carving Technique for Deciduous Teeth

The carving technique for deciduous teeth may be followed as the steps in carving as given with illustrations in the respective chapters of permanent teeth. Carving of deciduous anterior teeth can be followed as per that of permanent anteriors and for carving of deciduous molars, the technique as given as in permanent molars.

REFERENCES

1. Finn SB. Clinical Pedodontics. 4th Edition. Philadelphia. WB Saunders Co. 2003.
2. Wheeler RC. Dental Anatomy, Physiology and Occlusion. 8th edition. Philadelphia. WB Saunders Co. 2003.
3. Damle SG. Textbook of Pediatric Dentistry. 2nd edition. Arya Publishing House. Delhi. 2002.
4. Pediatric Dentistry for Children. http://www.theultimatedentistryguide.com/pediatric-dentistry/. 2010.
5. Primary Teeth. Concise Medical Dictionary. Ed. Oxford University Press. 2002 edition. Oxford Reference Online. 2002. Oxford University. 31 Jan. 2006 <http://www.oxfordreference.com>.

CHAPTER

8

Differences Between Primary and Permanent Teeth

In general comparison with permanent dentition, the primary teeth are smaller in overall size and crown dimension.

MORPHOLOGIC DIFFERENCES[1]

Number

1. Primary teeth are 20 in number. Permanent teeth are 32 in number.

Color[2,3]

2. The primary teeth are lighter in color and less pigmented because of thinner enamel and different refractive index of the enamel whereas the permanent teeth are yellowish in color because of thicker and more translucent enamel.

Size and Shape[2,3]

3. The mesiodistal width is greater than the cervico-incisal length of crown in primary dentition, giving the anterior teeth a cup-shaped appearance and the molars a squat appearance. In permanent anteriors, the cervico-incisal dimension is greater than the mesiodistal dimension.
4. The crown and roots of primary teeth show marked cervical constriction. The permanent teeth do not possess this cervical constriction.
5. The buccal cervical ridge is more prominent in primary molars than on the permanent molars.
6. Contact areas in primary teeth are broader and flatter. In permanent teeth, contact areas are less broader.
7. The buccal and lingual surfaces of primary molars are flatter above the cervical ridges than those of permanent molars.

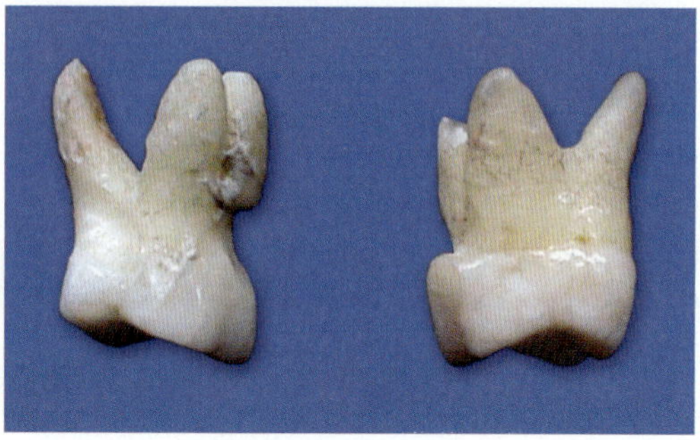

Fig. 8.1: Photograph showing narrow and flaring roots of deciduous molars
(*Courtesy:* Dr Jaya Naidu, Professor, Department of Pedodontics, Vydehi Institute of Dental Sciences, Bangalore)

Roots (Fig. 8.1)[2,3]

8. The roots of primary molars are more narrower mesiodistally at the cervical third than the permanent molars.
9. The roots of primary molars flare more, extending out beyond projected outlines of the crown. This flare allows more room between the roots for the development of permanent tooth crowns (Fig. 8.1).
10. The furcation is close to the cervical line resulting in a shorter root trunk in primary teeth whereas in permanent teeth the root trunk width is greater.

Pulp Chambers and Pulp Canals[1,2,3]

11. Pulp chambers are larger in size in primary teeth compared to permanent teeth.
12. The pulp horns are at a higher level in primary teeth. In permanent teeth, the pulp horns are at a lower level.
13. Number of accessory canals are more in primary teeth.

Histological Differences[1,3]

14. The thickness of enamel and dentin is less in primary teeth as compared to the permanent teeth.
15. Enamel rods are inclined occlusally in the cervical third of crown of primary teeth. In permanent teeth, enamel rods are inclined cervically in the cervical third of crown.

REFERENCES

1. Finn SB. Clinical Pedodontics. 4th Edition. Philadelphia. WB Saunders Co. 2003.
2. Wheeler RC. Dental Anatomy, Physiology and Occlusion. 8th edition. Philadelphia. WB Saunders Co. 2003.
3. Damle SG. Textbook of Pediatric Dentistry. 2nd edition. Arya Publishing House. Delhi. 2002.

CHAPTER

9

Ground Section of Tooth: A Grinding Process

DEFINITION

Ground section of tooth is a process in which tooth grinding is done to its thinnest section for microscopic examination of dental hard tissues.

Grinding Process (Fig. 9.1)

There are 2 alternative methods for preparing hard dental tissues for microscopic examination 1. Grinding 2. Decalcification

Ground Sections

Enamel contains such a small percentage of organic matter that is, it disappears during the process of decalcification. There is therefore only one method, namely grinding, that can be employed to prepare enamel for microscopic examination.

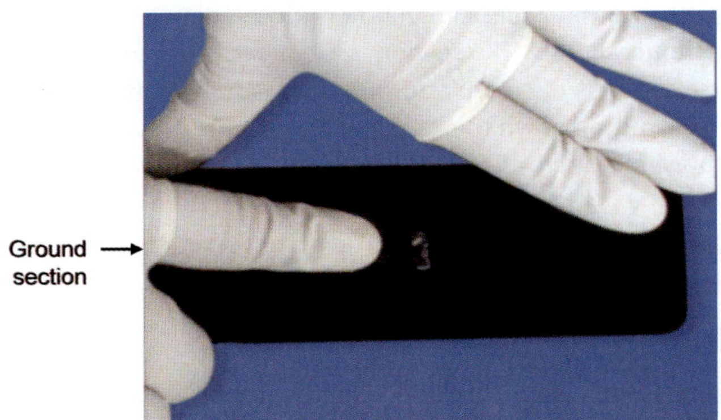

Fig. 9.1: Photograph showing the method of grinding process
(*Courtesy:* Mrs Dorothy Anitha, Sr Technician, Department of Oral Pathology, Vydehi Institute of Dental Sciences, Bangalore)

Materials Required

File, dental lathe with carborundum stone, one large and one smaller glass slab, ground on one side are required.

Procedure

An extracted human tooth is taken, which should be kept constantly moist throughout the grinding process to avoid charring of the tissues. Place it upon the bench pin and file one proximal side of the root portion flat, until the pulp canal is almost exposed throughout its entire length, using a fine metal file.

Place the flattened root surface against a flat piece wood or cork, so that it can be held firmly between the fingers and still continuing to keep it moist, grind down the enamel. On the same side with a corborundum stone on the lathe, file until the pulp chamber is exposed and the entire side of the tooth is flattened.

Water and powdered pumice are then sprinkled on the roughened side of the larger glass slab. The flattened surface of the tooth is rubbed vigorously over the glass surface with a rotary movement until all the file marks and irregularities are removed from the surface of the tooth and it is entirely flat and smooth from the apex of the root to the incisal tip.

The flattened surface is then placed against the piece of wood or cork and the rounded side of the root is filed down until the root portion is about twice the thickness of a visiting card. Still supporting the tooth against the cork and keeping it wet to avoid charring, the crown portion is stoned down on the rounded side by means of a corborandum stone on the lathe until it is thinner than the stoned down until the tooth thickness is of a visiting card and polished in the same manner as the other side.

Pumice and water are then sprinkled on the ground surface of the larger of the glass slabs. The tooth is placed upon this surface and the smaller glass slab is then placed on top, ground downwards.

The smaller slab is rotated gently over the tooth until the latter is sufficiently thin. A simple test is done, i.e. the section is placed between the fingers until the root portion bends slightly. The section is then ready for mounting.

Transverse sections of crown and root are made by cutting through the neck of a tooth and grinding down the 2 parts at the required levels of crown or root as described above for longitudinal sections.

Different Mounting Methods given by Noyes's and Charters White

Noyes's Method

- He advocates placing a drop of xylol balsam on a slide and another drop on a coverslip and heating them over a Bunsen flame to drive off the xylol.
- Then place the section between the 2 balsam surfaces, heat gently until the balsam flows. Squeeze the slide and cover slip together to express the excess balsam.

- The cover slip and slide are then held together by a clip or weight until the balsam sets.
- He advises to employ soft xylol balsam for mounting all sections whether calcified or soft tissues.

Before mounting, the section is stained in 1% eosin for 2 minutes, quickly washed, dehydrated and mounted in xylol balsam.

Charters White Method

The main purpose of the *Charters White method* is to fill the internal cavities in the hard dental tissues such as enamel spindles, interglobular spaces, etc. with stained celloidin in order to show them clearly in microscopic sections.

Procedure

1. Cut a tooth into slices about $^{1}/_{25}$ inch thick with a watch spring saw.
2. Soak the pieces in absolute alcohol for a short time.
3. Soak for a corresponding period in methylated ether.
4. Saturate the impregnated pieces of tooth in stained celloidin solution.
5. Remove the pieces and allow them to dry by evaporation.
6. Grind sections by grinding and polishing one side by means of heated Canada balsam, which takes about 2 days to set. The other side of the dental slice is then ground down to the required thickness.
7. The section is then removed from the slide by immersing in absolute alcohol, which is wiped off with a camel's hair brush.
8. When clean, the section is placed in distilled water until it is completely dehydrated.
9. The surfaces are dried quickly on a thin cloth.
10. The section is mounted in stiff Canada balsam by placing a drop of stiff balsam on both the cover slip and slide, heating both to fix the balsam. The section is then placed between the two balsam surfaces, which are again heated to make the balsam flow. Cover slip and slide are then clamped together to express the excess balsam and to retain the cover slip and slide closely together until the balsam sets, the process of which is completed within 2 days.

CHAPTER

10

Tooth Traits

Trait categories help in describing tooth similarities and differences between them.[1]

Definition: "A trait is a distinguishing characteristic, quality, peculiarity or attribute."[1]

Traits are classified as:[1]

A. **Set traits:** Set traits (dentition traits) distinguish teeth in the **primary** (deciduous) from **secondary** (permanent dentition).
B. **Arch traits:** Arch traits distinguish **maxillary** from **mandibular** teeth.
C. **Class traits:** Class traits distinguish the four categories (or classes) of teeth described in the introduction; namely incisors, canines, premolars and molars. Examples of class traits: **incisors** have crown compressed labiolingually for efficient cutting; **canines** have single pointed cusps for piercing food; **premolars** have two or three cusps for shearing and grinding; **molars** have three to five somewhat flattened cusps, ideally suited for grinding food morsels.
D. **Type traits**: Type traits differentiate teeth within one class (such as differences between central and lateral incisors, or between first and second premolars, or amongst first, second and third molars).

MAXILLARY INCISORS TYPE TRAITS AND OTHER CHARACTERISTICS

Permanent Maxillary Central Incisor[1,2]

1. Mesial outline is straight, distal outline is convex from labial aspect.
2. Incisal outline is straight.
3. Mesioincisal angle is a sharp right angle, distoincisal angle is curved.
4. Cervical third of labial surface shows convexity.

5. The characteristic feature of this tooth from mesial or distal aspect is that when a line drawn through the center of the tooth, the line will bisect the tooth into two equal halfs, i.e. the line that touches the root apex, crest of curvature of cervical line and the incisal edge.
6. Linguoincisal ridge is present.
7. Develops from four lobes.
8. Contour height on both labial and lingual aspect is at cervical third.
9. Eruption: 7 to 8 years.
10. Tooth notations - refer Chapter 2.

Permanent Maxillary Lateral Incisor[1,2]

1. Mesiodistal width and length of crown is less.
2. Both mesioincisal and distoincisal angles are curved.
3. Incisal ridge is curved.
4. The complete labial surface is convex.
5. The root apex is inclined distally.
6. Lingual fossa is very deep.
7. The characteristic feature of this tooth from mesial or distal aspect is that when a line drawn through the center of the tooth, the line will bisect the tooth into two equal halfs, i.e. the line that touches the root apex, the crest of curvature of cervical line and the incisal edge.
8. Develops from four lobes.
9. Contour height on both labial and lingual aspect is at cervical third.
10. Eruption: 8 to 9 years.
11. Tooth notations - refer Chapter 2.

MANDIBULAR INCISORS—TYPE TRAITS AND OTHER CHARACTERISTICS[1,2]

Permanent Mandibular Central Incisor

1. The crown and root appear narrower.
2. The mesial outline of the crown is straight and it is continuous with the outline of the root.
3. Both mesioincisal and distoincisal angles are sharp.
4. The characteristic feature of this tooth is that the incisal ridge is straight and is perpendicular to the long axis of the tooth.
5. The labial outline inclines lingually in a cervical direction, so that the incisal edge is placed lingually when viewed from mesial aspect or distal aspect.
6. The cingulum and marginal ridges are poorly developed.
7. Develops from four lobes.
8. Contour height on both labial and lingual aspect is at cervical third.
9. Eruption: 6 to 7 years.
10. Tooth notations - refer Chapter 2.

Permanent Mandibular Lateral Incisor

1. The crown appears slightly larger than the central incisor.
2. The mesioincisal angle is sharp.
3. The characteristic feature is that the incisal ridge slopes distally in a cervical direction. So, the distal contact area is placed more cervically than the mesial contact area.
4. The incisal ridge is curved from the incisal aspect and is not perpendicular to the long axis of the tooth.
5. The cingulum and marginal ridges are poorly developed.
6. Develops from four lobes.
7. Contour height on both labial and lingual aspect is at cervical third.
8. Eruption: 7 to 8 years.
9. Tooth notations - refer Chapter 2.

MAXILLARY AND MANDIBULAR INCISORS—ARCH TRAITS AND OTHER CHARACTERISTICS[1,2]

Maxillary Incisors

The central incisor is wider than the lateral incisor, wider than the mandibular central incisors. Marginal ridges and cingulum are more prominent. Lingual fossa is pronounced, often with a lingual pit. The crown width is greater mesiodistally than labiolingually. Incisor edge is labial to root axis. Roots are rounded.

Mandibular Incisors

The lateral incisor is wider than the central incisor. It is the narrowest tooth of the incisor class. The marginal ridges and cingulum are not prominent. The lingual fossa is shallow without grooves or pits. The crown width is greater labiolingually than mesiodistally. Incisal ridge is placed lingual to root axis. The roots are thin mesiodistally.

CANINE—ARCH TRAITS AND OTHER CHARACTERISTICS[1,2]

Permanent Maxillary Canine

1. Presence of mesial and distal slope. The mesial slope is short and straight than the distal slope which is long and curved. The cusp tip is placed mesially.
2. The labial ridge is present which curves mesially starting from the center of cervical line to the cusp tip.
3. The root is longer and slender.
4. Buccolingually the crown appears bulky.
5. Cingulum is very prominent. A lingual ridge is continuous from cingulum to the cusp tip.

6. The cusp tip from the mesial or distal aspect is placed labially.
7. Distal portion from occlusal aspect appears to be stretched to make contact with the first premolar.
8. Develops from four lobes.
9. Contour height on both labial and lingual aspect is at cervical third.
10. Eruption: 11 to 12 years.
11. Tooth notations - refer Chapter 2.

Permanent Mandibular Canine

1. Both the mesial slope and distal slope are straight even though the distal slope is longer.
2. The mesioincisal and distoincisal angle is sharp.
3. The mesial outline is straight and is continuous with the outline of the root.
4. The labial ridge is straight and thin from cusp tip to the center of cervical line.
5. The cusp tip is lingually placed from mesial or distal aspect.
6. Labiolingually the cervical third thickness is very thin from mesial or distal aspect.
7. Lingual ridge is confined only to the incisal third of crown.
8. Poorly developed cingulum is seen.
9. Develops from four lobes.
10. Contour height on both labial and lingual aspect is at cervical third.
11. Eruption: 9 to 10 years.
12. Tooth notations - refer Chapter 2.

MAXILLARY PREMOLARS—TYPE TRAITS AND OTHER CHARACTERISTICS[1,2]

Permanent Maxillary First Premolar

1. The lingual cusp is shorter by 1 mm than the buccal cusp.
2. This is the only tooth which has mesial slope longer than the distal slope.
3. This tooth has 2 roots: buccal and lingual roots.
4. The characteristic feature of this tooth is that, presence of mesial marginal developmental groove on the mesial aspect which is the extension of central developmental groove from occlusal aspect.
5. The second characteristic feature is presence of mesial developmental depression on the mesial aspect of the crown. It crosses the cervical line and ends at the bifurcation of root.
6. The shape of occlusal aspect is hexagonal and all the line angles are more angular.
7. The cusp tips are confined to the width of root trunk and the distance between the cusp tips is less.

8. Buccal ridge is present on buccal cusp.
9. Develops from four lobes.
10. Contour height on buccal is at cervical third and on lingual aspect is at middle third.
11. Eruption: 10 to 11 years.
12. Tooth notations - refer Chapter 2.

Permanent Maxillary Second Premolar

1. Both the buccal and lingual cusps are of same height.
2. The buccal cusp appears broader.
3. The mesial slope is straight and shorter than the distal slope which is long and curved. So the buccal cusp tip is placed mesially.
4. All the line angles are rounded.
5. A single root is present.
6. There is no mesial marginal developmental groove and no mesial developmental depression present on mesial aspect.
7. The distance between the two cusp tips is greater.
8. The shape of occlusal outline is oval.
9. Numerous supplemental grooves are present on occlusal aspect which makes the occlusal surface appear wrinkled.
10. The grooves on occlusal aspect are deeper.
11. Develops from four lobes.
12. Contour height on buccal is at cervical third and on lingual aspect is at middle third.
13. Eruption: 10 to 12 years.
14. Tooth notations - refer Chapter 2.

MANDIBULAR PREMOLARS—TYPE TRAITS AND OTHER CHARACTERISTICS[1,2]

Permanent Mandibular First Premolar

1. The buccal cusp is large and the lingual cusp is small or rudimentary.
2. The buccal cusp tip is more pointed.
3. The mesial slope is shorter than the distal slope.
4. At the cervical third of buccal aspect, the mesial and distal outline converges toward the cervical line.
5. The broader buccal ridge extends from cusp tip to cervical line.
6. Since the lingual cusp is small, much of the occlusal part can be seen from lingual aspect.
7. The characteristic feature of this tooth is presence of mesiolingual developmental groove within the mesiolingual depression.
8. The buccal outline inclines lingually when viewed from mesial or distal aspect.

9. The shape of occlusal outline is diamond.
10. Develops from four lobes.
11. Contour height on buccal is at cervical third and on lingual aspect is at middle third.
12. Eruption: 10 to 12 years.
13. Tooth notations - refer Chapter 2.

Permanent Mandibular Second Premolar

Two cusp type:

1. The buccal cusp length is slightly shorter. The lingual cusp is about 1mm shorter than the buccal cusp.
2. The buccal cusp tip is more pointed with a broader buccal ridge.
3. At the cervical third of buccal aspect, the mesial and distal outline converges cervically.
4. The buccal outline inclines lingually in a cervical direction from mesial or distal aspect.
5. The occlusal aspect is oval in shape.
6. All the line angles are round.
7. A single root is present.

Three cusp type:

1. The tooth hase three cusps—the buccal, mesiolingual and distolingual cusp.
2. The length of lingual cusps is shorter by 1 mm than the buccal cusp.
3. The cusp tip is pointed with broader buccal ridge.
4. The mesiolingual cusp is longer and broader than the distolingual cusp.
5. The mesiolingual cusp tip is more pointed than the distolingual cusp tip.
6. A lingual groove is present in between the lingual cusps.
7. The shape of occlusal aspect is square.
8. The characteristic feature from occlusal aspect is presence of Y-shaped groove.

Common to both types of premolars:

1. Develops from four or five lobes.
2. Contour height on both buccal and lingual aspect is at middle third.
3. Eruption: 11 to 12 years.
4. Tooth notations - refer Chapter 2.

PREMOLARS[1,2]

Arch traits and other chracteristics.

Maxillary Premolars

Crowns are trapezoidal in shape. Buccal and lingual cusps are almost equal in height. Two major cusps of almost equal size and prominence are seen from the occlusal aspect. Cusps are relatively wider buccolingually.

Mandibular Premolars

Crowns are rhomboidal in shape, lingual cusp tips may be placed lingual to the root. The lingual cusps are comparatively much shorter than the maxillary lingual cusps. The buccal and lingual cusps are of uneven height and prominence.

MAXILLARY MOLARS—TYPE TRAITS AND OTHER CHARACTERISTICS[1,2]

Permanent Maxillary First Molar

1. Five cusps and three roots are present. The cusps are mesiobuccal, distobuccal, mesiolingual, distolingual and fifth cusp (cusp of Carabelli). The roots are mesiobuccal, distobuccal and lingual root.
2. The mesiolingual cusp is the largest, smallest is distobuccal and the lingual root is longest.
3. Buccal groove and lingual groove is present.
4. The distance between the three roots is greater.
5. The bifurcation level is different for all the three aspects, i.e. root trunk length on buccal aspect is 4 mm, mesial aspect is 3 mm and on distal aspect is 5 mm.
6. The occlusal outline shape is rhomboidal, i.e. it is wider lingually and mesially.
7. The oblique ridge is present.
8. Transverse groove of oblique ridge is present.
9. Develops from five lobes.
10. Contour height on buccal is at cervical third and on lingual aspect is at middle third.
11. Eruption: 6 years.
12. Tooth notations - refer Chapter 2.

Permanent Maxillary Second Molar

1. Four cusps and three roots are present. The cusps are mesiobuccal, distobuccal, mesiolingual and distolingual cusp. The roots are mesiobuccal, distobuccal and lingual root.
2. No fifth cusp is evident.
3. Line angles are more obtuse.
4. Occlusal outline form is rhomboidal.
5. Distally, the crown convergence is greater.
6. Numerous supplemental grooves are present on the occlusal surface and are much deeper comparatively.
7. The distance between the three roots is reduced.
8. Develops from four lobes.

9. Contour height on buccal aspect is at cervical third and on lingual aspect is at middle third.
10. Eruption: 12 to 13 years.
11. Tooth notations - refer Chapter 2.

Permanent Maxillary Third Molar

1. Three cusps and three roots are seen. The mesiobuccal, distobuccal and lingual cusps; roots are mesiobuccal, distobuccal and lingual root.
2. The distance between the roots are highly reduced and may be fused sometimes.
3. The level of bifurcation of roots is more toward the apices of roots.
4. Distolingual cusp is less distinct.
5. Both crown and root are poorly developed and has a small crown and root.
6. The occlusal outline shape is heart shaped.
7. Numerous, deeper supplemental grooves are seen on the occlusal surface.
8. Develops from three to four lobes.
9. Contour height on buccal aspect is at cervical third and on lingual aspect is at middle third.
10. Eruption: 17 to 21 years.
11. Tooth notations - refer Chapter 2.

MANDIBULAR MOLARS—TYPE TRAITS AND OTHER CHARACTERISTICS[1,2]

Permanent Mandibular First Molar

1. Five cusps and two roots are present. The cusps are mesiobuccal, distobuccal, mesiolingual, distolingual, and distal cusp. The roots are mesial and distal root.
2. Mesiobuccal and distobuccal grooves are present on the buccal surface. The distobuccal groove is longer than mesiobuccal groove.
3. The buccal cusp tips are flat and the lingual cusp tips are pointed and are highly placed than the buccal cusps.
4. Cervical ridge is prominent on the buccal surface.
5. The occlusal outline form is hexagonal.
6. The developmental grooves on the occlusal surface are the central developmental groove, the mesiobuccal developmental groove, the distobuccal developmental groove and the lingual developmental groove.
7. Develops from five lobes.
8. Contour height on buccal is at cervical third and on lingual aspect is at middle third.
9. Eruption: 6 to 7 years.
10. Tooth notations - refer Chapter 2.

Permanent Mandibular Second Molar

1. Four cusps and two roots are present. The cusps are mesiobuccal, distobuccal, mesiolingual and distolingual cusp. The roots are mesial and distal root.
2. Only buccal developmental groove is present on the buccal surface of the crown.
3. The buccal cusp tips are flat and the lingual cusp tips are pointed and are slightly placed higher than the buccal cusps.
4. The occlusal outline form is rectangular.
5. The central developmental groove, buccal developmental groove, and lingual developmental grooves are present.
6. The distance between the two roots is reduced.
7. Numerous supplemental grooves radiate from the central developmental groove and are much deeper.
8. Develops from four lobes.
9. Contour height on buccal is at cervical third and on lingual aspect is at middle third.
10. Eruption: 11 to 13 years.
11. Tooth notations - refer Chapter 2.

Permanent Mandibular Third Molar

1. The number of cusps varies from five or more cusps. The roots present are mesial and distal roots and they may be fused.
2. The buccal cusps are short and rounded. The lingual cusp's height is lesser than the buccal cusp height.
3. The root apices are more pointed.
4. The occlusal outline form is rectangular.
5. The grooves are less distinct. Numerous supplemental grooves, which are much deeper toward central part of the occlusal surface, are seen.
6. Develops from four lobes.
7. Contour height on buccal aspect is at cervical third and on lingual aspect is at middle third.
8. Eruption: 17 to 21 years.
9. Tooth notations - refer Chapter 2.

MANDIBULAR MOLARS—ARCH TRAITS AND OTHER CHARACTERISTICS[1,2]

Maxillary Molars

Dimensions: Crowns of maxillary molars are wider buccolingually than mesiodistally.

Height of contour: Buccal crest is at cervical third; lingual crest is at the middle third of the crown. *Proximal Contacts*: Mesial contact area is at almost at middle third; the distal contact area is at the middle third, slightly toward cervical third.

Mandibular Molars

Dimensions: Crowns of mandibular molars are wider mesiodistally than buccolingually.

Height of Contour: Buccal crest is at cervical third; lingual crest is at the middle third of the crown. *Proximal Contacts*: Mesial contact area is almost at middle third; the distal contact area is at the middle third, slightly toward cervical third.

REFERENCES

1. Woelfel JB, Scheid RC. Dental Anatomy. Williams & Wilkins. 1997.
2. Ash, Nelson. Wheelers Dental Anatomy, Physiology & Occlusion. 8th edition. Elsevier. 2003.

CHAPTER

11

Vasculature and Innervation of the Teeth

BLOOD SUPPLY: INTRODUCTION

The face is supplied mainly through the facial artery, a branch of the external carotid artery in the neck. The facial artery first appears on the face as it hooks round the lower border of the mandible, at the anterior edge of the masseter. It then runs a tortuous course between the facial muscles toward the medial angle of the eye. There is a rich anastomosis with the artery of the opposite side with additional vessels supplying the face (transverse facial branch of the superficial temporal artery; infraorbital and mental branches of the maxillary artery; dorsal nasal branch of the ophthalmic artery).[1]

The main arteries of the teeth and jaws are derived from the maxillary artery, a terminal branch of the external carotid, which runs in the infra-temporal fossa. The alveolar arteries follow essentially the same course as the alveolar nerves.[2,3]

THE ARTERIAL SUPPLY TO THE MAXILLARY TEETH[1,2,3]

The posterior superior alveolar artery arises from the maxillary artery in the pterygopalatine fossa. Occasionally, the posterior superior alveolar artery is derived from the buccal artery. It courses tortuously over the maxillary tuberosity before entering bony canals to supply molar and premolar teeth. The artery also gives off branches to the adjacent buccal, gingiva, maxillary sinus and cheek.

The middle superior alveolar artery, when present, arises from the infra-orbital artery (which is itself a branch of the third part of the maxillary artery in the pterygopalatine fossa). The middle superior alveolar artery runs in the lateral wall of the maxillary sinus, terminating near the canine tooth where it anastomoses with the anterior and posterior superior alveolar arteries. The anterior superior alveolar artery also arises from the infraorbital artery and runs downwards in the anterior wall of the maxillary sinus to supply the anterior teeth. As for the superior alveolar nerves, the superior alveolar arteries form plexuses above the root apices.

THE ARTERIAL SUPPLY TO MANDIBULAR TEETH

The inferior alveolar artery, which supplies the mandibular teeth, is derived from the maxillary artery before it crosses the lateral pterygoid muscle in the infratemporal fossa. A mylohyoid branch is given off before the inferior alveolar artery enters the mandibular foramen in the ramus of the mandibular foramen to enter the mandibular canal and terminates as the mental and incisive arteries. The anastomosis of the mental and incisive branches furnishes a good collateral blood supply for the mandible and teeth. In their canals, the inferior alveolar and incisive arteries give off dental branches to the individual tooth roots for the supply of the pulp and periodontal membrane at the root apex. Other branches enter the interdental septa, supply bone, and adjacent periodontal membrane and terminate in the gingiva. Numerous small anastomoses connect these vessels with those supplying the neighboring alveolar mucosa.

Descending palatine and sphenopalatine arteries: The palatal blood supply comes from two sources but chiefly from the descending palatine artery, which descends from its origin from the maxillary through the greater canal. Its greater palatine branch enters the palate through the greater palatine foramen and runs forward with its accompanying vein and nerve in a groove at the junction of the palatine and alveolar processes. It is distributed to the bone, glands and mucosa of the hard palate and to the bone and mucosa of the alveolar process. Minor branches of the descending palatine artery pass to the soft palate through lesser palatine foramina in the palatine bone.

The nasopalatine branch of the sphenopalatine artery courses, obliquely forwarded and downward on the septum and enters the palate through the incisive canal. It distributes incisive papilla and adjacent palate and forms an anastomosis with the greater palatine.

VENOUS DRAINAGE OF ORODENTAL TISSUES[1,2,3]

The venous drainage of this region is extremely variable. The facial vein is the main vein draining the face. It begins at the medial corner of the eye by confluence of the supraorbital and supratrochlear veins and passes across the face behind the facial artery. Below the mandible, it receives the anterior branch of the retromandibular vein before draining into the internal lingular vein.

Teeth: Small veins from the teeth and alveolar bone pass into larger veins running in the interdental septa. In the mandible, veins are then collected into one or more inferior alveolar veins, which themselves may drain anteriorly through the mental foramen to join the facial vein or posteriorly through the mandibular foramen to join the pterygoid plexus of veins in the infratemporal fossa. In the maxilla, the veins may drain anteriorly into the facial vein or posteriorly into the pterygoid plexus.

LYMPHATIC DRAINAGE OF ORODENTAL TISSUES

Figure 11.1 provides the consensus view of the lymphatic drainage of the oral structures.

INNERVATION OF MANDIBULAR TEETH[1]

Inferior Alveolar Nerve: It is the chief branch of mandibular nerve, which leaves the skull through the foramen ovale and almost immediately breaks up into its several branches. The inferior alveolar nerve, which at first runs directly downward across the medial surface of the lateral pterygoid, at the lower border of which it is directed laterally and downward across the medial surface of the lateral pterygoid, at the lower border of which, it is directed laterally and downward across the outer surface of the medial pterygoid muscle to reach the mandibular foramen. The course of the nerve is shown in Figure 11.2.

The inferior alveolar nerve continues forward through the mandibular canal beneath the roots of the molar teeth to the level of the mental foramen. During this part of its course, it gives off branches to the molar and premolar teeth and their supporting bone and soft tissues. The nerve to the teeth does not arise as individual branches but as two or three larger branches that form a plexus from which inferior dental branches enter individual tooth roots and

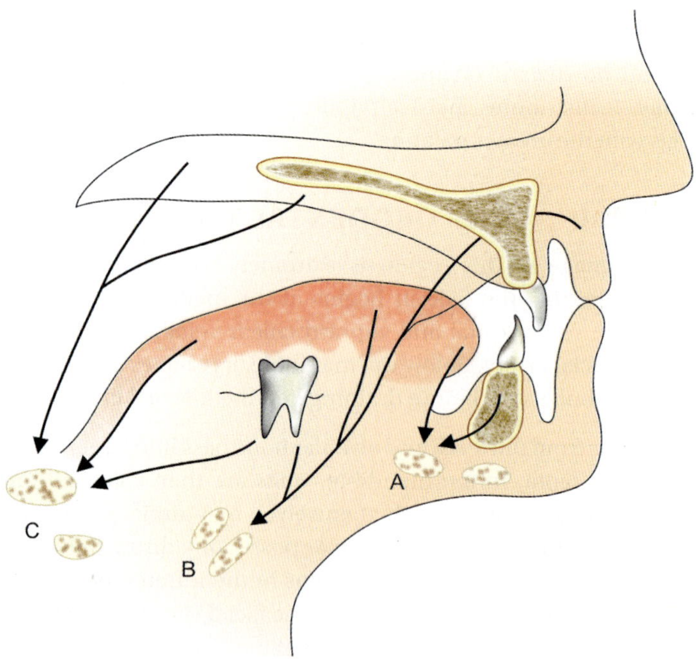

Fig. 11.1:[1] Lympatic drainage of oral structures. A = Submental nodes; B = Submandibular nodes, C = Jugulodigastric nodes

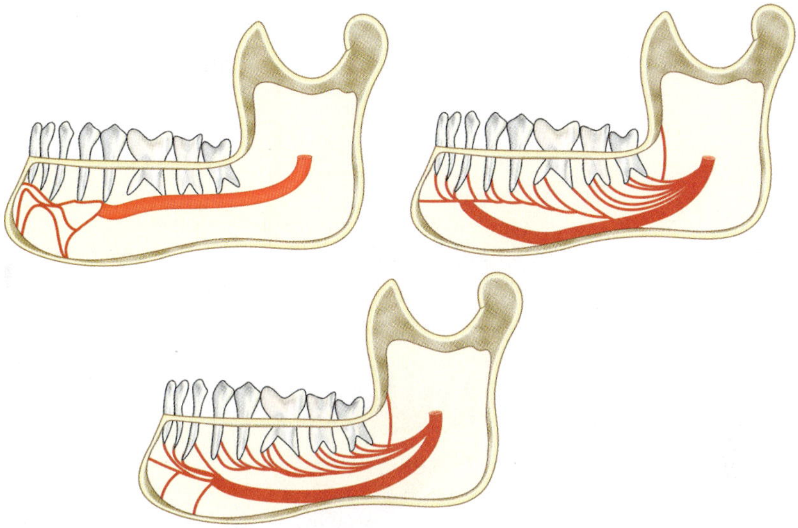

Fig. 11.2:[1] Schematic diagrams showing variation in the course of the inferior alveolar nerve through the mandible

interdental branches supply alveolar bone, periodontal membrane, and gingiva. At the mental foramen, the nerve divides and a smaller incisive branch continues forward to supply the anterior teeth and bone, and a larger mental branch emerges through the foramen to supply the skin of the lower lip and chin.

The buccal nerve, a branch of mandibular nerve distributed to the mucosa of the cheek, also distributed to a small area of the buccal gingiva in the first molar area, sometimes it may distribute from canine to the third molar.

The lingual nerve, as it enters the floor of the mouth, lies against the body of the mandible, and has mucosal branches to a variable area of lingual mucosa and gingiva.

The mylohyoid nerve continue its course forward on the lower surface of the mylohyoid muscle and enter the mandible through small foramina on either side of the midline. It is thought to innervate central incisors and periodontal ligament (Fig. 11.3).

INNERVATION OF MAXILLARY TEETH[1,2,3]

The **maxillary nerve** course forward through the wall of the cavernous sinus and leaves the skull through the foramen rotundum. It crosses the pterygopalatine fossa, where it gives branches to pterygopalatine ganglion, a parasympathetic ganglion. This ganglion gives off several branches, now containing visceral motor and sensory fibers, to the mucous membrane of the mouth, nose and pharynx.

The branches of this nerve include a greater palatine branch that enters the hard palate through the greater palatine foramen and is distributed to the hard palate and palatal gingiva as far forward as the canine tooth, a lesser palatine

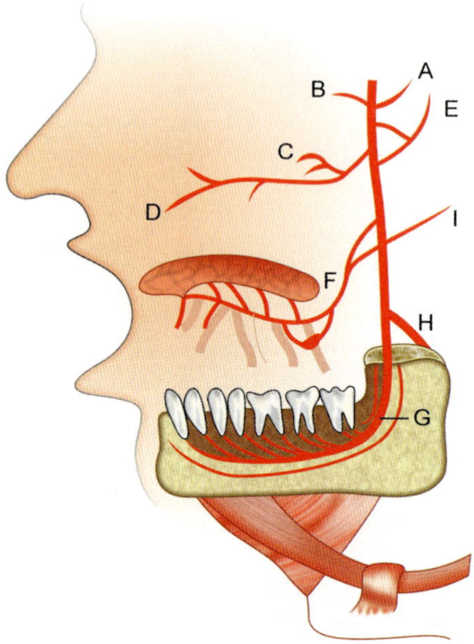

Fig. 11.3:[1] Schematic diagram of the mandibular division of the trigeminal nerve.
A = meningeal branch
B = nerve to medial pterygoid
C = anterior trunk giving motor branches to masseter, temporalis and lateral pterygoid muscles
D = buccal nerve
E = auriculotemporal nerve
F = lingual nerve
G = inferior alveolar nerve
H = mylohyoid nerve
I = chorda tympani branch of facial nerve joining the lingual nerve

branch from the ganglion that enters the soft palate through the lesser palatine foramina; a nasopalatine branch of the posterior or superior lateral nasal branch of the ganglion. It enters the palate through the incisive canal; it is distributed to the incisive papilla and to the palate anterior to the anterior palatine nerve.

The posterior superior alveolar nerve is also branch of maxillary nerve from its pterygopalatine portion. This nerve enters the alveolar canals on the infratemporal surface of the maxilla and forming a plexus, is distributed to the molar teeth and the supporting tissues.

The infraorbital nerve is another branch of maxillary nerve which enters the orbit, runs forward in its floor first in the infraorbital groove and then in the infraorbital canal. It terminates at the infraorbital foramen in branches distributed to the upper face. At a variable distance after it enters the orbit, a middle superior alveolar branch arises from the infraorbital nerve and runs through the lateral wall of the maxillary sinus. It is distributed to the premolar teeth and surrounding tissues and joins the alveolar plexus.

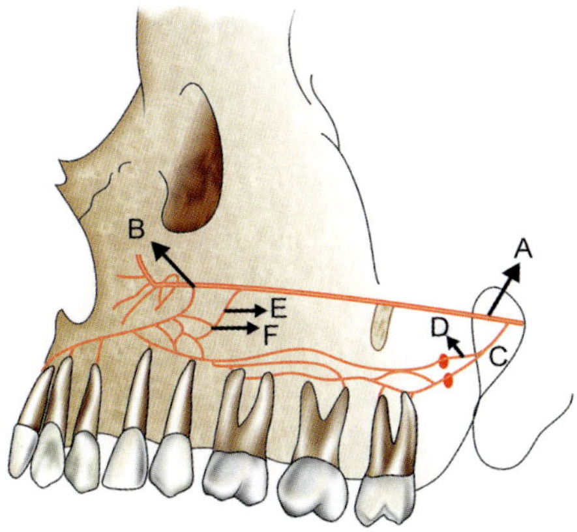

Fig. 11.4:[1] The superior alveolar nerves and associated dental plexus.
A = Trunk of maxillary division of the trigeminal nerve
B = Infraorbital nerve
C = Pterygopalatine fossa
D = Posterior superior alveolar nerves
E = Middle superior alveolar nerves
F = Anterior superior alveolar nerves.

An anterior superior alveolar branch leaves the infraorbital nerve first inside the infraorbital foramen and is distributed through bony canals to the incisor and canine teeth. All three superior alveolar nerves join in a plexus above the process, from the plexus, dental branches are given off to each tooth root and interdental branches to the bone periodontal membrane and gingiva. The distribution being similar to that described for the arteries.

Nerve Supply

The sensory nerve supply to the jaws and teeth is derived from the maxillary and mandibular branches of the fifth cranial or trigeminal nerve, whose ganglion the trigeminal is located at the apex of the petrous portion of the temporal bone (Fig. 11.4).

REFERENCES

1. Berkovitz KB, Holland GR, Moxham BJ. Oral Anatomy, Histology and Embryology. 4th edition. Elsevier. 2009.
2. Woelfel JB, Scheid RC. Dental Anatomy. Williams & Wilkins. 1997.
3. Ash, Nelson. Wheelers Dental Anatomy, Physiology & Occlusion. 8th edition. Elsevier. 2003.

CHAPTER

12

Occlusion

The alignment and occlusion of the dentition are extremely important in masticatory function. The basic activities of chewing, swallowing, and speaking depend greatly not only on the position of teeth in the dental arches but also on the relationship of opposing teeth as they are brought into occlusion. Tooth positions are determined not by chance, but by numerous controlling factors such as arch width and tooth size. They are also determined by various controlling forces, such as those provided by the surrounding soft tissues.

Occlusion is defined as "Any contact between the incising or masticatory surfaces of the maxillary and mandibular teeth".—GPT[1]

"Occlusion is the static relationship of the teeth and is basic to all aspects of dentistry".—JPO[1]

TERMINOLOGIES OF OCCLUSION COMMONLY USED IN DENTISTRY[1]

Ideal Occlusion: An ideal occlusion may be defined as one that has no structural, functional, or neurobehavioral characteristics that tend to interfere with occlusal stability.

Physiologic Occlusion: It is an occlusion that deviates in one or more way from ideal yet it is well adapted to that particular environment, is esthetic and shows no pathologic manifestations or dysfunctions.

Balanced Occlusion: An occlusion which balances and has equal contacts maintained throughout the entire arch during all excursions of the mandible.

Functional Occlusion: It is defined as an arrangement of teeth, which will provide the highest efficiency during all the excursive movements of the mandible which are necessary during function.

Therapeutic Occlusion: An occlusion that has been modified by appropriate therapeutic modalities in order to change a non-physiological occlusion to one that is at least physiological occlusion if not ideal.

Traumatic Occlusion: Traumatic occlusion is an abnormal occlusal stress, which is capable of producing or has produced an injury to the periodontium.

Trauma from Occlusion: It is defined as periodontal tissue injury caused by occlusal forces through abnormal occlusal contacts.

It is generally considered that occlusion deals with the static relationship of opposing teeth. The solutions to problems as such as bruxism, orthodontic relapse, denture instability, and periodontal trauma require concepts of occlusion that extend well beyond static arrangements of teeth, occlusal contacts and jaw position.

Concepts of Occlusion: The concepts of occlusion vary with almost every specialty of dentistry. Few concepts of occlusion include functional criteria and because the dentofacial complex is highly mobile, ideas of occlusal stability and homeostasis are often misunderstood and seldom mentioned as a part of a concept of occlusion were in the past often based on complete dentures and because of the problems of instability of denture bases the concept of "Balanced Occlusion" was developed to consider bilateral contacts in all functional excursions to prevent tipping of the denture bases. Occlusion is an important factor which governs the retention and stability of the complete denture in vivo. It is important for one to know the principles of occlusion before arranging artificial teeth.

VARIOUS CONCEPTS OF OCCLUSION WERE PUT FORWARD[1]

Spherical Concept of Occlusion (*Monson*)

According to this concept, the anteroposterior and mesiodistal inclines of the artificial teeth should be arranged in harmony with a spherical surface.

Organic concept of Occlusion: Here, the shapes of the teeth are altered to have cusps suitable for the patient. The movement of the condyle determines the direction of the ridges and grooves of the teeth, and the mandibular movements determine other factors like cusp height, fossa, and depth of the fissure and concavity of the lingual surfaces. The organic or organized occlusion, the aim is to relate the occlusal surfaces of teeth, so that the teeth are in harmony with the muscles and joints during function. The muscles and joints determine the mandibular position of occlusion without any tooth guidance, in function the teeth are supposed to have a positive role and do not influence or determine the path of mandibular movement. (In normal occlusion, tooth factors determine mandibular movements, e.g. incisal guidance).

Neurocentric concept of Occlusion: According to this concept, the plane of occlusion should be flat and parallel to the residual alveolar ridge. This concept is similar to the monoplane occlusion used to set non-anatomic teeth. The term neurocentric denotes an occlusion that eliminates the anteroposterior and buccolingual inclines in order to direct the forces to the posterior teeth.

Development of the Dentitions[2,3,4]

Functional disturbances of the masticatory system may have their beginning during the development of occlusion, a time when the *substrate* for tongue and swallowing habits, chewing patterns, tooth clenching and bruxism may be established. The alignment of the dentition in the dental arches occurs as a result of complex multidirectional forces acting on the teeth during and after eruption. As the teeth erupt, they are directed into a position where opposing forces are in equilibrium.

PRIMARY DENTITION[3,4]

It is during this period in the development of the orofacial complex that oral motor behavior reflects learning related to the advent of the teeth. Human oral functions that are acquired or modified during the natural progression from neonatal through infancy to adulthood are in part related to the development of occlusion, both of the deciduous and permanent teeth. Masticatory skill is influenced by the reflex mechanism of the oral facial area, sensory and higher center. The jaw positions and posturing of the mandible occurs along with the development of the muscle matrix and the active growth of the facial skeleton.

Primary Occlusion[2,3,4]

The maxillary and mandibular primary teeth when in occlusion is such that each tooth, with the exception of the mandibular central incisor and the maxillary second molar, occludes with two teeth of the opposing jaw. The primary teeth should be in normal alignment and occlusion shortly after the age of 2, with all the roots fully formed by the time the child is 3 years old. The rapid development of the jaws is sufficient to create an interdental space, or, diastema, between some of them. The separation of anterior teeth begins usually between the ages of 4 and 5 years. The canines and molars are supposed to keep their positive contact relation during all the jaw growth. Because the teeth do not hold their relative positions for long, they are worn off rapidly on incisal ridges and occlusal surfaces. If the primary teeth are in good alignment, the occlusion is most efficient during the time relatively for a short time. The normal jaw growth allows the eruption and occlusion of the first permanent molars immediately distal to the primary second molars. The child is approximately 6 years of age.

Eruption Chronology of Primary Teeth[3,4]

The significance of local environmental factors on the development of occlusion considered in its broader sense is relatively unknown. Thus, learning of

Table 12.1: The chronology of eruption of the primary teeth

	Tooth										Emergence of Teeth (Months)			
UPPER	+i1	E, F=									10 (8–12)			
	i2	D, G									11 (9–13)			
	c	C, H									19 (16–22)			
	m1	B, I									16 (13–19)(14–18)			
	m2	A, T									29 (25–33)			
						Maxillary teeth								
Right														
		A	B	C	D	E	F	G	H	I	J			*Left*
		T	S	R	Q	P	O	N	M	L	K			
						Mandibular teeth								
LOWER	i1	P, O									8 (6–10)			
	i2	Q, N									13 (10–16)			
	c	R, M									20 (17–23)			
	m1	S, L									16 (14–18)			
	m2	T, K									27 (23–31) (24–30)			

+ i1, central incisor; i2, lateral incisor; c, canine; m1, first molar; m2, second molar.
Universal numbering system for primary dentition which was adopted by American Dental Association (1975).

mastication may be highly dependent on the stage of development (type and number of teeth present) of the occlusion, maturation of the neuromuscular system, and such factors as diet. The chronology of eruption of the primary teeth is shown in Table 12.1.

CONTACT RELATIONS

The degree of bruxism present in the child will determine the contact relations of the teeth. The factors that determine the contact relations at the time of eruption of teeth include position of the tooth germ, presence of permanent teeth, and development of the condyles, cuspal inclines, and neuromuscular influences. The cusp fossa and temporomandibular joint relationship and usually only tooth to tooth observations have been made, namely, the mesiolingual cusp of the maxillary molar occludes in the central fossa of the deciduous mandibular molar.

Primary Arch Form[3,4]

The arch form and width has been established largely for both the primary and permanent dentitions by the age of 9 months. This observation may be untrue in view of the apparent difference in facial appearance between the child of that age and a young adult with a permanent dentition. Substantially there is increased anterior-posterior dimension of the jaws, which is necessary for the incorporation of the permanent molars into the occlusion. The alveolar bone and basal bone determine the shape of the dental arches.

Interdental Spacing[3,4]

Interdental spacing tends to decrease slightly with age. The size and spacing between primary teeth has a relationship to the position of the permanent teeth and the size of the dental arches.

Primary Molar Relationships[1,2,3,4] (Fig. 12.1)

Moyer's described the primary molar relationship as the *flush terminal plane, mesial step* and *distal step* (Fig. 12.2). The mesiodistal diameter of the mandibular second primary molar is greater than the maxillary second molar. This difference in dimension of the two teeth results in the distal surfaces of these two molars being in the same plane; a flush terminal plane is located at the end of the deciduous dentition. If a "step" occurs because of carious lesions or other disturbance it has been reported that a tendency to interfere with the development of normal occlusal relations of the permanent first molars is evident. Also the natural wearing away of the cusps in the deciduous dentition allows the mandible to assume a more forward position during a period when the mandible is growing more rapidly than the maxilla. In the absence of cuspal interferences, there is some evidence that the permanent incisors erupt with less vertical overlap and the permanent molars erupt into a more favorable occlusion.

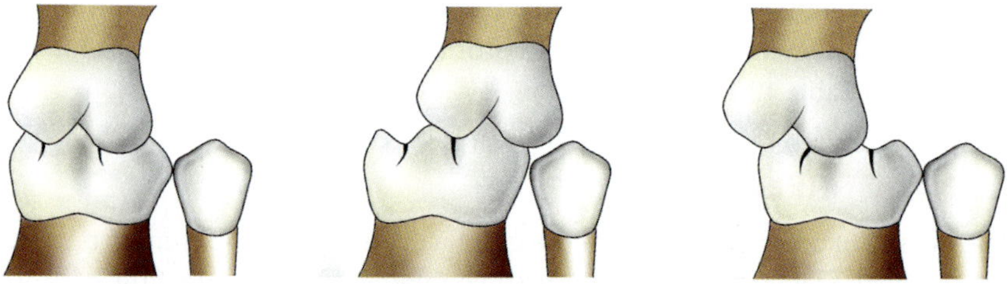

Fig. 12.1:[4] A, Angle class I molar relationship. B, Class II molar relationship. C, Class III molar relationship

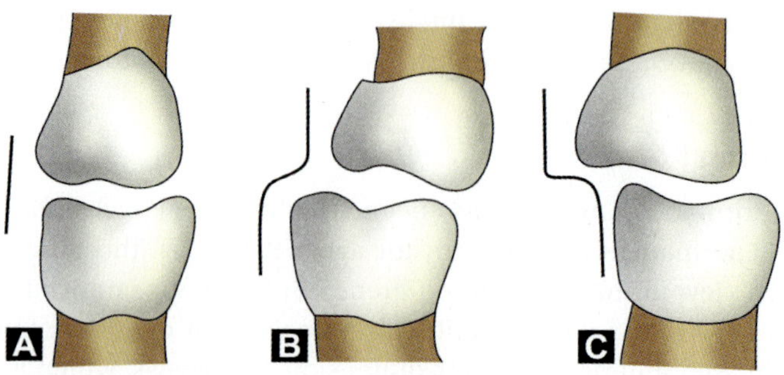

Figs 12.2:[4] Terminal plane relationship in the primary dentition: (A) Flush; (B) Distal step; and (C) Mesial step

Occlusion in Primary Dentition[1,2,3,4]

In a 3-year-old child, if development is normal, the spacing of the teeth is rather uniform. This biological change opens up contacts in the arch between teeth and increases occlusal wear.

The normal occlusion is as follows:

- Mesial surfaces of maxillary and mandibular central incisors are in line with each other at the median line.
- The maxillary central incisor occludes with the mandibular central incisor and the mesial third of the mandibular lateral incisor. The mandibular anterior teeth strike the maxillary anterior teeth lingually above the level of the incisal ridges.
- The maxillary lateral incisor occludes with the distal two thirds of the mandibular lateral incisor and that portion of the mandibular canine which is mesial to the point of its cusp.
- The maxillary canine occludes with that portion of the mandibular canine distal to this cusp tip and the mesial third of the mandibular first molar (that portion mesial to the tip of the mesiobuccal cusp).
- The maxillary first molar occludes with the distal two thirds of the mandibular first molar and the mesial portion of the mandibular second molar, which portion is represented by the mesial marginal ridge and the mesial triangular fossa.
- The maxillary second molar occludes with the remainder of the mandibular second molar, the distal surface of the maxillary molar projecting slightly over the distal portion of the mandibular second molar.

Mixed (transitional) Dentition[3,4]

The transition from primary or permanent dentition begins about 6 years of age with the emergence of the mandibular permanent central incisor or the first permanent molars at 6 to 7 years of age.

Arch Dimensions and Tooth Size[3,4]

The growth of the jaw provides space for the teeth to erupt and emerge into the mouth. Forward rotation of the maxillomandibular complex, which is the more usual pattern, influences the magnitude of tooth eruption, as well as the ultimate anteroposterior position of the incisors. Lingual position of the mandibular incisors related to the mandible often accompanies forward rotation during growth placement of incisors with rotation reflect a major influence on changes in arch length.

The premolar segment is very important portion of the dental arch in the development of occlusion of the permanent dentition. The erupting premolars are significantly smaller in mesiodistal dimension than the primary molars, which they replace. The arch perimeter of the permanent dentition, as measured from the mesial of the mandibular first molars, decreases an average of about 4 mm.

When a discrepancy is evident between the aggregate mesiodistal dimension of the teeth and the size of the bony supporting arches crowding or protrusion can occur.

Arch Width[3,4]

Arch width is measured between corresponding lingual points on the teeth in the same arch. Maxillary intermolar width, e.g. can be as much as 6 mm less in crowded dentitions than in uncrowded dentitions. According to a study if a transpalatal width is evident in a narrow dental arch (less than 31 mm) in the early mixed dentition it is unlikely that the child will reach adequate arch dimensions through normal growth mechanism.

Overbite[4]

Overbite is the amount of vertical overlap between the maxillary and mandibular central incisors. This relationship can be described either in millimeters or more often as a percentage of how much the upper central incisors overlap the crown of the lower incisors. The overbite in the primary dentition normally varies between 10% and 40%. When the incisal edges of the incisors are at the same level, the condition is described as "edge to edge or over overbite" (Figs 12.3 and 12.4A). When there is a lack of overlap, the condition is described as open bite and qualified in millimeters (Fig. 12.5).

Overjet[4]

Overjet is the horizontal relationship or the distance between the most protruded maxillary central incisor. This relationship is expressed in millimeters. If the maxillary incisors are lingual to the mandibular incisor, the relationship is described as an underjet. The normal range of overjet in the primary dentition varies between 0 and 4.0 mm (Fig. 12.4B).

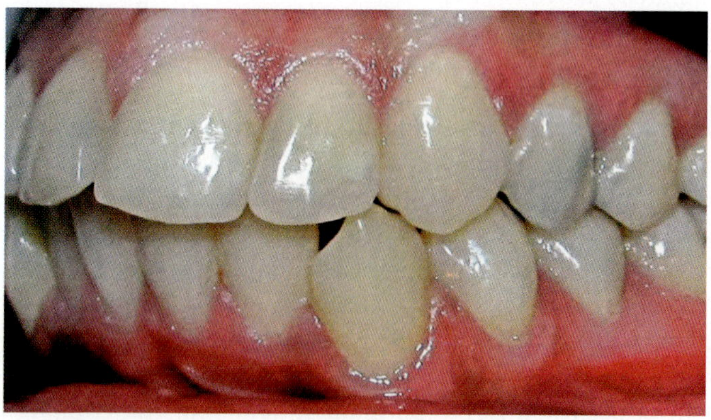

Fig. 12.3: Photograph of overbite

(*Courtesy:* Dr Lakshmi Krishnan, Post Graduate Student, Department of Oral Pathology, Vydehi Institute of Dental Sciences, Bangalore)

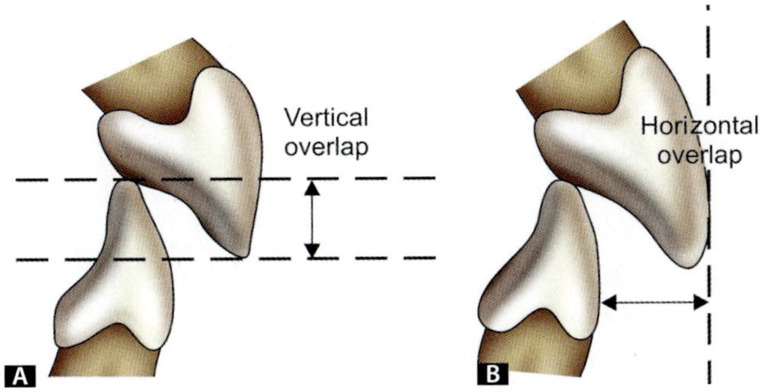

Figs 12.4: (A) Overbite; (B) Overjet

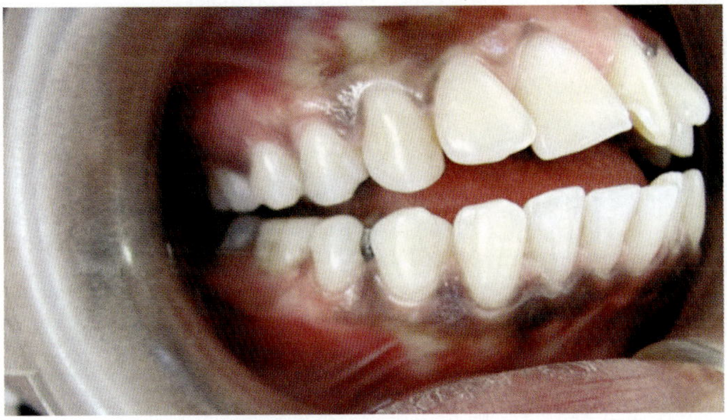

Fig. 12.5: Photograph showing anterior open bite

(*Courtesy:* Dr Lakshmi Krishnan, Post Graduate Student, Department of Oral Pathology, Vydehi Institute of Dental Sciences, Bangalore)

Spacings[3,4]

In the primary dentition stage, a child may have generalized spaces between the teeth, localized spaces, no spaces or a crowded dentition. The presence of spacing in the primary dentition stage is a common occurrence. Generalized spacings occur in almost $^2/_3$ of the individuals in the primary dentition stage.

In addition to the generalized spacings, localized spacings are often present and as referred to as primate spaces. Such spaces are present in 87% of the maxillary arches usually between the lateral incisors and canines. The primate spaces are also present in 78% of the mandibular arches, usually between the canines and first primary molars.

The leeway spaces in general the sum of the mesiodistal width of the primary canine and the primary first and second molars is larger than the sum of their succedaneous teeth, namely, the permanent canine and first and second premolars. This difference is called the leeway space and is present in both the maxillary and mandibular arches (Fig. 12.6). The most favorable dental arch pattern is when leeway space is excessive (i.e. the combined size of unerupted canine and premolars is smaller than the available arch space).

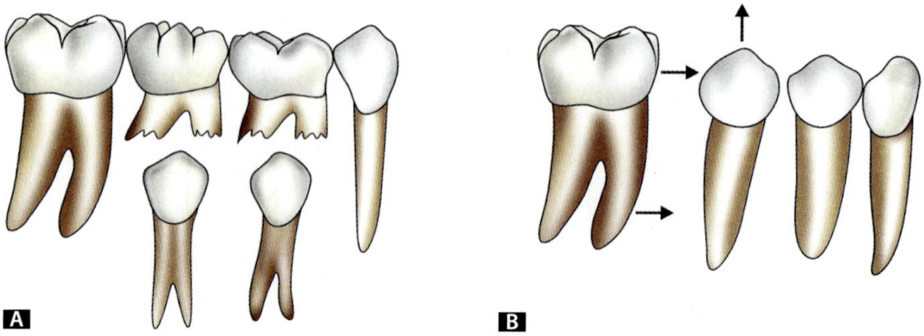

Figs 12.6A and B: Leeway space. Difference in mesiodistal dimensions between primary teeth (A) and permanent teeth (B). Arrows indicate the mesial movement of the permanent molars after loss of primary molars and eruption of the second permanent premolar

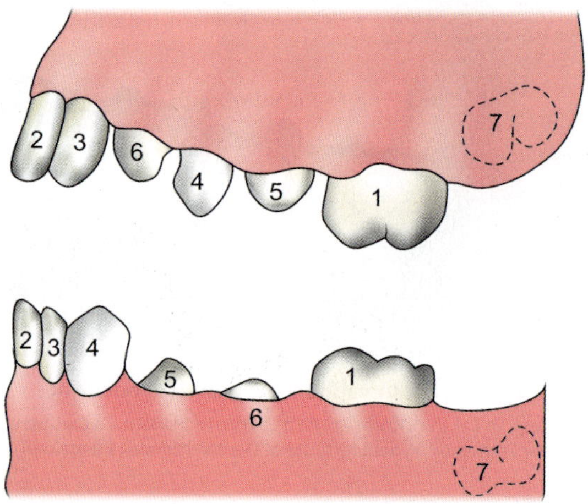

Fig. 12.7: Favorable eruption sequence of permanent teeth

The leeway space is larger in the mandibular arch than in the maxillary arch. On the average, the unerupted canine and premolars are 1.8 mm smaller per side, is the lower arch. In the upper arch, the leeway space is average only—0.9 mm per side. On the average, it is about 1.8 mm (0.9 mm on each side of the arch) in the maxillary arch and about 3.4 mm (1.7 mm on each side of the arch) in the mandibular arch. This excess space available after the exchange of the deciduous molars and canines is utilized for mesial drift to the mandibular molars to establish class I molar relation.

The Permanent Dentition[3,4]

The eruption sequence of the permanent dentition is more variable than the primary dentition. The eruption sequences for maxillary arch are 6-1-2-4-3-5-7-8 and 6-1-2-4-5-3-7-8 (Fig. 12.7). The common sequences for mandibular arch are (6-1)-2-4-3-5-7-8 and (6-1)-2-4-3-5-7-8 (Fig. 12.7).

Table 12.2: Chronology of permanent teeth

Tooth		Eruption (years)
C1 +	8, 9 ≠	7–8
L1	7, 10	8–9
C	6, 11	11–12
P1	5, 12	10–11
P2	4, 13	10–12
m1	3, 14	9–10
m2	2, 15	12–13
m3	1, 16	17–21

Maxillary Teeth

Right	1	2	3	4	5	6	7	8	9	10	11	12	13	14	15	16	Left
	32	31	30	29	28	27	26	25	21	23	22	21	20	19	18	17	

Mandibular Teeth

Tooth		Eruption (years)
C1	24, 25	6–7
L1	23, 26	7–8
C	22, 27	9–10
P1	21, 28	10–12
P2	20, 29	11–12
m1	19, 30	6–7
m2	18, 31	11–13
m3	17, 32	17–21

+C1, central incisor; L1, lateral incisor; C, canine; m1, first molar, m2, second molar
Universal numbering system for permanent dentition see Chapter 2.

If the second molars erupt before the premolars are fully erupted, the arch perimeter is reduced and this might lead to malocclusion (Table 12.2).

Dental arch form:[3,4]

The basic pattern of tooth position is the arch. Different forms of arch are V-shaped, ellipsoid, rotund and horseshoe shaped. Discrepancies in arch form between the maxillary and mandibular arches generally result in poor occlusal relationships. Figure 12.12 shows the normal intercuspation of teeth.

Types of cusps:[1] There are two types of cusps 1. Centric holding cusps 2. Non-supporting cusps.

Centric holding cusps:[1] The facial cusps of mandibular and palatal cusps of maxillary posterior teeth are called the centric holding cusps. They occlude into the central fossae and marginal ridges of opposing teeth.

Non-supporting cusps: The maxillary buccal and mandibular lingual cusps are called non-supporting cusps. They contact and guide the mandible during lateral excursions and shear food during mastication, also known as shearing or guiding cusps.

Curvatures of Occlusal Planes

The occlusal surfaces of the dental arches do not generally conform to a flat plane. It was noted that the cusps and incisal ridges of the teeth to display a curved alignment when the arches were observed from a point opposite the first molars.

Imaginary compensatory curves such as Curve of Spee, Curve of Wilson and Curve of Monson was introduced.

Curve of Spee[1,3,4]

It refers to the anteroposterior curvature of the occlusal surfaces beginning at the tip of the lower cuspid and following the cusp tips of the bicuspids and molars continuing as an arc through the condyle. If the curve were extended, it would form a circle of about 4" diameter.

The curve results from variations in axial alignment of the lower teeth. The long axis of each tooth is aligned nearly parallel to its individual arc of closure around the condylar axis. This requires a gradual progressive increased mesial tilting of teeth toward molars, which creates the Curve of Spee. This curvature is within the sagittal plane only.

Curve of Wilson[1,3,4]

This compensatory curve contacts the buccal and lingual cusp tips of the mandibular posterior teeth. The Curve of Wilson is mediolateral on each side of the arch. It results from inward inclination of the lower posterior. This curve helps so that the teeth are aligned parallel to the direction of medial pterygoid for optimum resistance to masticatory forces and the elevated buccal cusps prevent food from moving the occlusal table.

Curve of Monson[1,3,4]

The Curve of Monson is obtained by extending the Curve of Spee and Curve of Wilson to all cusps and incisal edges. Monson visualized the plane to be three-dimensional spherical curvature involving both the right and left condyles. That the center of sphere with an 8 inch diameter was the vector for converging lines of masticatory forces passing through the center of the teeth and that the occlusal surfaces of the molar teeth were congruent with the surface of a sphere of some dimension.

Inclination and Angulation of the Roots of the Teeth[4] (Figs 12.8 to 12.11)

Uses of knowing root angles:

1. To direct the X-ray beam to obtain true normal projections of the roots of the teeth.
2. To direct occlusal forces in restorations along the long axis of the teeth.
3. To control orthodontic forces for proper angulations of the teeth.
4. To place dental implants with the right angulations.

The mesiodistal and faciolingual axial inclinations of the teeth are usually described in terms of angles between the long axis of a tooth and a line drawn perpendicular to a horizontal plane, or to the median plane.

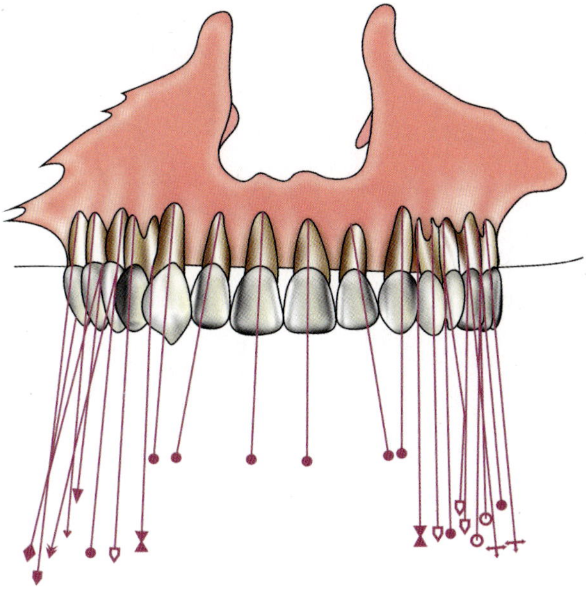

Fig. 12.8: Front view

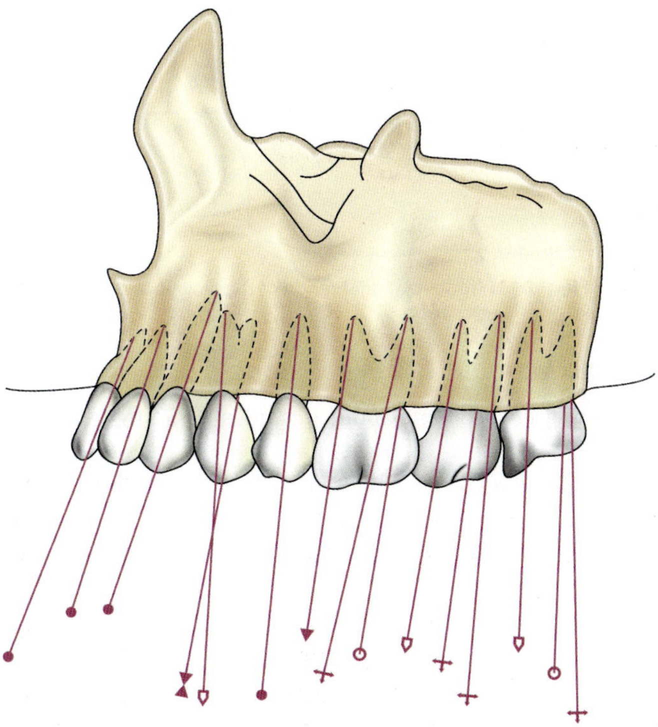

Fig. 12.9: Lateral view

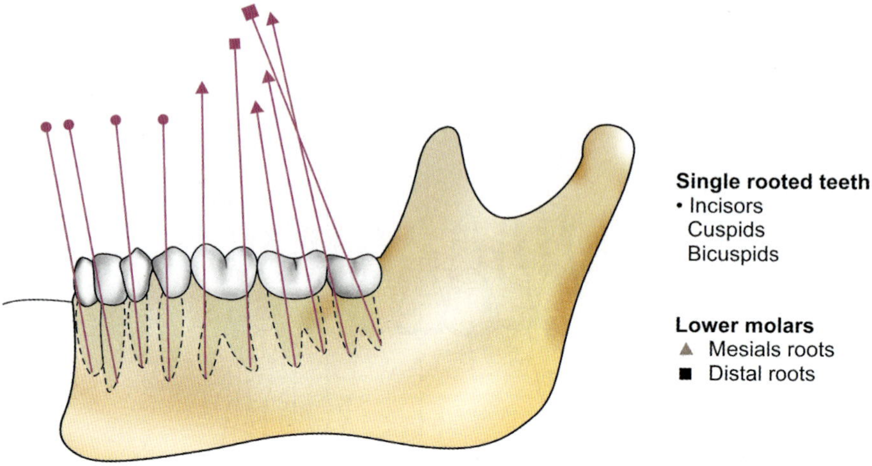

Fig. 12.10: Lateral view

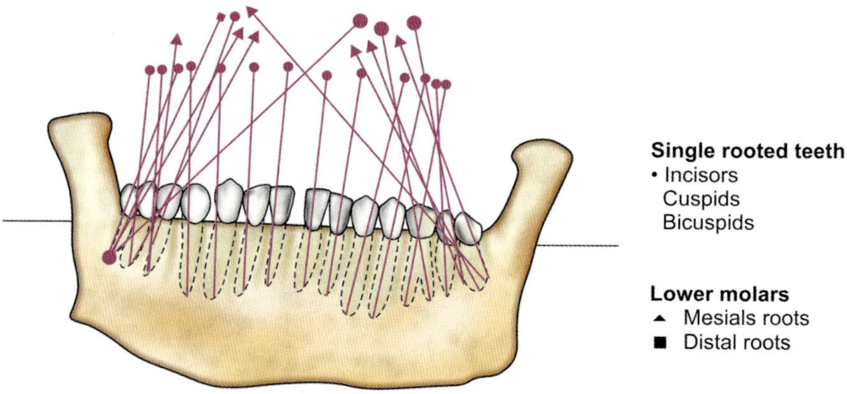

Fig. 12.11: Front view, orientation of the crowns and roots

Cusp, Fossa and Marginal Ridge Relations[3,4]

The centric holding cusp of one tooth occludes in a single fossa of a single opponent.

The contact of the lingual cusps of the maxillary premolars do not necessarily make contact in the fossa of the mandibular but occlude with the marginal ridges of the premolars and molars. Figures 12.13 and12.14 shows the occlusal landmarks.

Centric Relation and Centric Occlusion[1,3,4]

Centric relation is the relation of the mandible to the maxilla when the mandibular condyles are in the most superior and retruded position in their glenoid fossa with the articular disk properly interposed. Centric relation is also called ligamentous position or terminal hinge position.

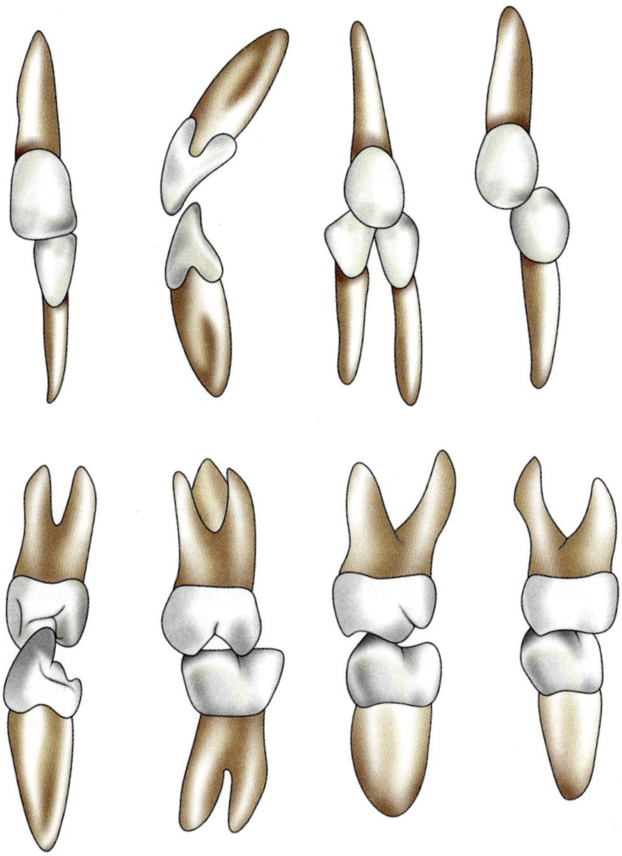

Fig. 12.12: Normal intercuspation of maxillary and mandibular teeth

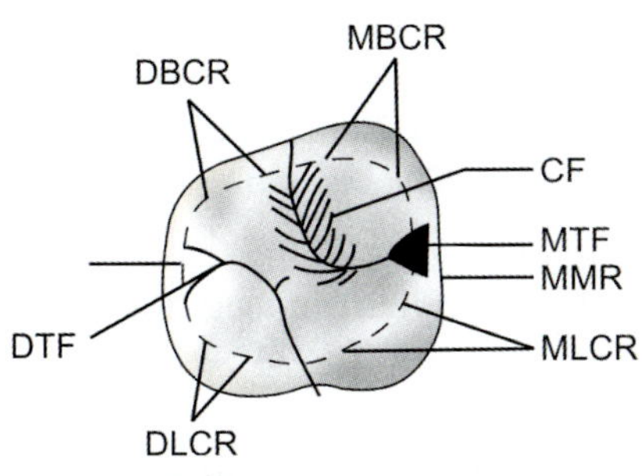

Fig. 12.13: Maxillary left first molar, occlusal landmarks. MBCR, mesiobuccal cusp ridge; CF, central fossa (shaded area); MTF, mesial triangular fossa (shaded area); MMR, mesial marginal ridge; MLCR, mesiolingual cusp ridge; DLCR, distolingual cusp ridge; DTF, distal triangular fossa (shaded area); DMR, distal marginal ridge; DBCR, distobuccal cusp ridge

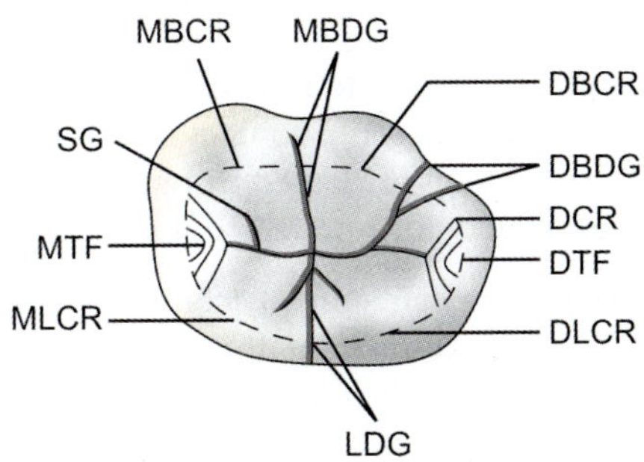

Fig. 12.14: Mandibular right first molar, occlusal aspect. DBCR, Distobuccal cusp ridge; DBDG, distobuccal developmental groove; DCR, distal cusp ridge; DTF, distal triangular fossa (shaded area); DLCR, distolingual cusp ridge; LDG, lingual developmental groove; MLCR, mesiolingual cusp ridge; MTF, mesial triangular fossa (shaded area); SG, a supplemental groove; MBCR, mesiobuccal cusp ridge; MBDG, mesiobuccal developmental groove

Often the contacts are either on the oblique ridge of the maxillary molar or the mesial cusp ridge of the maxillary first premolar. In the centric relation position the condyle-disk assemblies are positioned on the anterior slope of the mandibular fossae. This movement from the premature contact in centric occlusion is called a slide in centric.

Centric occlusion is that position of the mandibular condyle when the teeth are in maximum intercuspation.

If the occlusal interferences in centric relation contact are removed by selective grinding, the ability to close into maximum intercuspation (Fig. 12.12) without interference at any place between centric relation and centric occlusion is called 'freedom in centric' the adverse neuromuscular responses that may occur to retrusion and closure of the jaw in the presence of occlusal interferences to maximum intercuspation in centric relation can be detected electromyographically and by the clinician.

Centric contacts:[1,4] The areas of the teeth that contact the opposing teeth is termed as centric contacts. It is classified as posterior centric contacts and anterior centric contact.

Posterior centric contacts:[1,4] It consists of the facial and lingual contacts. The facial contact of posterior centric contacts involve the mandibular facial cusp tips contacting with the central fossae and mesial marginal ridges of the opposing maxillary teeth. The lingual posterior centric contacts involve the maxillary lingual cusp tips contacting the central fossae and distal marginal ridges of the opposing mandibular arch.

Anterior centric contacts:[1,4] Anterior teeth have only one range of centric contacts and are in line with the facial range of posterior centric contacts.

Posterior centric contacts result in axially directed forces as convex cusp tips occlude on opposing tooth areas that are perpendicular to the force. However, centric contacts often occur on inclines are called poded centric contacts. The contacts occuring on inclines should be balanced by an equal contact on an opposing incline to resolve the forces in an axial direction. If the contact occurs on two inclines, the contact is termed bi-poded contact. Contacts that occur on three inclines are called tri-poded contacts. Contacts that occur on four inclines are called quadri-poded contacts.

Eccentric occlusion:[1] Eccentric occlusion refers to contact of teeth that occur during movement of the mandible. Eccentric occlusion is of two types: 1. Functional occlusion, 2. Non-functional occlusion.

Functional occlusion:[1,4] Also called as working side occlusion, refers to tooth contacts that occur in the segment of the arch toward which the mandible moves. It is of two types: a. Lateral functional occlusion; b. Protrusive functional occlusion.

Lateral functional occlusion: This includes tooth contacts that occur on canines and posterior teeth on the side toward which the mandible moves. The lateral functional occlusion can be of two types:

1. Canine guided occlusion
2. Grouped lateral occlusion.

Canine guided occlusion: During lateral mandibular movement, the opposing upper and lower canines of the working side contact thereby causing disclusion of all posterior teeth on the working and balancing sides. Canine guided occlusion is usually seen in young persons with unworn dentition. In a canine guided occlusion, the mandibular canine cusp tip tracks from the centric contact point at the mesial marginal ridge toward the cusp tip of the maxillary canine.

Grouped lateral occlusion: In addition to canine guidance, certain other posterior teeth on the working side also contact during lateral movement of the mandible. Such a type of contact during lateral movement is called grouped lateral occlusion.

Protrusive functional occlusion: This includes eccentric contacts that occur when the mandible moves forward. Ideally the six mandibular anterior teeth contact along the lingual inclines of the maxillary anterior teeth while the posterior disocclude.

Non-functional or balancing occlusion:[1,4] These are tooth contacts that occur in the segment away from which the mandible moves. For example if the mandible is moved to the left side, contacts occur on the right side of the arch.

Disclusion:[1,4] The term disclusion is used to describe disocclusion or separation of non-functional posterior teeth during eccentric motions of the jaw. Disclusion of posterior teeth is brought about by condylar guidance and incisal guidance.

Condylar gudiance: It refers to the downward movement of both the condyles along the slopes of the articular eminence during protrusive movements leading to seperation of the posteriors. In case of lateral movements, the condyle on the non-functioning side translates forward along the eminence while the condyle on the functioning side pivots in its fossa leading to disclusion of posteriors on the non-functional side.

Anterior Guidance/Incisal Guidance

It refers to anterior tooth functions which separate the posterior teeth during eccentric motion of the jaw. During protrusive and lateral movements of the mandible, the lower anterior teeth track downward from their area of centric contact toward the incisal edges of maxillary teeth while discluding the non-functional posterior teeth.

Condylar guidance has its greatest influence on discluding the most distal posterior teeth, while the incisal guidance provides discluding effect on the more mesial teeth. The condylar guidance is a fixed anatomic factor that cannot be controlled by a dental practitioner while the incisal guidance can be controlled by modifying the form and arrangement of anterior teeth.

Occlusal stability:[4] Occlusal stability refers to the tendency of the teeth, jaws, joints and muscles to remain in an optimal functional state. The stability of the occlusion and the maintenance of tooth position are dependent on all of the forces that act on the teeth. Occlusal forces, eruptive forces, lip and cheek pressure, periodontal support, and tongue pressure are all involved in maintaining the position of the teeth.

Many factors (caries, periodontal disease, occlusal trauma, bruxism) may upset the delicate balance of an already marginally stable occlusion. An ideal occlusion may be defined as one that has no structural, functional, or neurobehavioral characteristics that tend to interfere with occlusal stability. Signs of bruxism may include loss of tooth structure, increased tooth mobility, root resorption, or decreased tooth mobility and increased density and thickness of the supporting tissues.

Neurobehavioral Aspects of Occlusion:[4] The neurobehavioral aspects of occlusion relate to function and parafunction of the stomatognathic system. Function includes a variety of actions or human behavior such as chewing, sucking, swallowing, speech, and respiration. Parafunction refers to action such as bruxism (e.g., clenching and grinding of the teeth). All these functions require highly developed sensory-motor mechanisms. The coordination of occlusal contacts, jaw motion, and tongue movement during mastication requires a very intricate control system involving a number of guiding influences from the teeth and their supporting structures. Temporomandibular joint (TMJ's) masticatory muscles and higher centers in the central nervous system.

On an individual clinical basis, however, the responses of a patient to occlusal therapy may be reflected in oral behavior outside the range of normal. The presence of several classes of teeth, powerful musculature and a most delicate positional control system indicates that it is important to understand the strategy underlying such sensitive control mechanisms.

Oral Motor Behavior[4]

The term oral motor behavior is a convenience of speech by which it is possible to refer with a brief phrase to observable actions involving orofacial structures, including simple actions like mandibular rest position and much more complex movements such as mastication. Although many of the actions or responses are common to all individuals, the response of a particular individual to stimulus may involve an inner experiential aspect of emotion in which the sensory experience may not fall into the usual acceptable range of pleasant or unpleasant. The advantage of viewing occlusion as human behavior is that the clinician has a better understanding of functional disturbances such as TMJ and muscle disorders and the recognition that how patients feel and respond to their occlusion is an important aspect of diagnosis and dental treatment.

REFERENCES

1. Nallaswamy D. Textbook of Prosthodontics. 1st edition. Jaypee Brothers. 2003.
2. McNeill C. Science and Practice of Occlusion. Quintessence Publishing Co, Inc.
3. Woelfel JB, Scheid RC. Dental Anatomy. Williams & Wilkins. 1997.
4. Ash, Nelson. Wheelers Dental Anatomy, Physiology & Occlusion. 8th edition. Elsevier. 2003.

CHAPTER

13

Spotters in Dental Anatomy Practical

IDENTIFICATION FEATURES OF NATURAL TEETH

PERMANENT TEETH

Permanent Maxillary Central Incisor

1. Mesial outline is straight, distal outline is convex from labial aspect.
2. Incisal outline is straight.
3. Mesioincisal angle is sharp, distoincisal angle is curved.
4. Cervical third of labial surface shows convexity.
5. The characteristic feature of this tooth from mesial or distal aspect is that when a line drawn through the center of the tooth, the line will bisect the tooth into two equal halves. That is the line touches the root apex, crest of curvature of cervical line and the incisal edge.
6. Linguoincisal ridge is present.

Permanent Maxillary Lateral Incisor

1. Mesiodistal width and length of crown is less.
2. Both mesioincisal and distoincisal angles are curved.
3. Incisal ridge is curved.
4. The complete labial surface is convex.
5. The root apex is inclined distally.
6. Lingual fossa is very deep.
7. The characteristic feature of this tooth from mesial or distal aspect is that when a line drawn through the center of the tooth, the line will bisect the tooth into two equal halves. That is the line touches the root apex, the crest of curvature of cervical line and the incisal edge.

Permanent Mandibular Central Incisor

1. The crown and root appear narrower.
2. The mesial outline of the crown is straight and it is continuous with the outline of the root.
3. Both mesioincisal and distoincisal angles are sharp.
4. The characteristic feature of this tooth is that the incisal ridge is straight and is perpendicular to the long axis of the tooth.
5. The labial outline inclines lingually in a cervical direction, so that the incisal edge is placed lingually when viewed from mesial aspect or distal aspect.
6. The cingulum and marginal ridges are poorly developed.

Permanent Mandibular Lateral Incisor

1. The crown appears slightly larger than the central incisor.
2. The mesioincisal angle is sharp.
3. The characteristic feature is that the incisal ridge slopes distally in a cervical direction. So the distal contact area is placed more cervically than the mesial contact area.
4. The incisal ridge is curved from the incisal aspect and is not perpendicular to the long axis of the tooth.
5. The cingulum and marginal ridges are poorly developed.

Permanent Maxillary Canine

1. Presence of mesial and distal slope. The mesial slope is short and straight than the distal slope which is long and curved. The cusp tip is placed mesially.
2. The labial ridge is present which curves mesially starting from the center of cervical line to the cusp tip.
3. The root is the longer and slender.
4. Buccolingually the crown appears bulky.
5. Cingulum is very prominent. A lingual ridge is continuous from cingulum to the cusp tip.
6. The cusp tip from the mesial or distal aspect is placed labially.
7. Distal portion from occlusal aspect appears to be stretched to make contact with the first premolar.

Permanent Mandibular Canine

1. Both the mesial slope and distal slope are straight even though the distal slope is longer.
2. The mesioincisal and distoincisal angle is sharp.
3. The mesial outline is straight and is continuous with the outline of the root.
4. The labial ridge is straight and thin from cusp tip to the center of cervical line.

5. The cusp tip is lingually placed from mesial or distal aspect.
6. Labiolingually the cervical third thickness is very thin from mesial or distal aspect.
7. Lingual ridge is confined only to the incisal third of crown.
8. Poorly developed cingulum is seen.

Permanent Maxillary First Premolar

1. The lingual cusp is shorter by 1 mm than the buccal cusp.
2. This is the only tooth which has mesial slope longer than the distal slope.
3. This tooth has 2 roots: buccal and lingual root.
4. The characteristic feature of this tooth is that, presence of mesial marginal developmental groove on the mesial aspect which is the extension of central developmental groove from occlusal aspect.
5. The second characteristic feature is presence of mesial developmental depression on the mesial aspect of the crown. It crosses the cervical line and ends at the bifurcation of root.
6. The shape of occlusal aspect is hexagonal and all the line angles are more angular.
7. The cusp tips are confined to the width of root trunk and the distance between the cusp tips is less.
8. Buccal ridge is present on buccal cusp.

Permanent Maxillary Second Premolar

1. Both the buccal and lingual cusp are of same height.
2. The buccal cusp appears broader.
3. The mesial slope is straight and shorter than the distal slope which is long and curved. So the buccal cusp tip is placed mesially.
4. All the line angles are rounded.
5. A single root is present.
6. There is no mesial marginal developmental groove and no mesial developmental depression is present on mesial aspect.
7. The distance between the two cusp tips is more wider.
8. The shape of occlusal outline is oval shaped.
9. Numerous supplemental grooves are present on occlusal aspect which make them appear wrinkled.
10. The grooves on occlusal aspect are more deeper.

Permanent Mandibular First Premolar

1. The buccal cusp is large and the lingual cusp is small or rudimentary.
2. The buccal cusp tip is more pointed.
3. The mesial slope is shorter than the distal slope.

4. At the cervical third of buccal aspect, the mesial and distal outline converges toward the cervical line.
5. The buccal ridge extends from cusp tip to cervical line which is broader.
6. Since the lingual cusp is small much of the occlusal part can be seen from lingual aspect.
7. The characteristic feature of this tooth is presence of mesiolingual developmental groove within the mesiolingual depression.
8. The buccal outline inclines lingually when viewed mesial or distal aspect.
9. The shape of occlusal outline is diamond shaped.

Permanent Mandibular Second Premolar

Two cusp type:

1. The buccal cusp length is slightly shorter. The lingual cusp about 1 mm shorter than the buccal cusp.
2. The buccal cusp tip is more pointed with a broader buccal ridge.
3. At the cervical third of buccal aspect, the mesial and distal outline converges cervically.
4. The buccal outline inclines lingually in a cervical direction from mesial or distal aspect.
5. The occlusal aspect is oval in shape.
6. All the line angles are round.
7. A single root is present.

Three cusp type:

1. Has three cusps—the buccal, mesiolingual and distolingual cusp.
2. The length of lingual cusps is shorter by 1 mm than the buccal cusp.
3. The cusp tip is pointed with broader buccal ridge.
4. The mesiolingual cusp is longer and broader than the distolingual cusp.
5. The mesiolingual cusp tip is more pointed than the distolingual cusp tip.
6. A lingual groove is present in between the lingual cusps.
7. The shape of occlusal aspect is square shaped.
8. The characteristic feature from occlusal aspect is presence of Y-shaped groove.

Permanent Maxillary First Molar

1. Five cusps and three roots are present. The cusps are mesiobuccal, distobuccal, mesiolingual, distolingual and fifth cusp (Cusp of Carabelli). The roots are mesiobuccal, distobuccal and lingual root.
2. The mesiolingual cusp is the largest, smallest is distobuccal and the lingual root is longest.
3. Buccal groove and lingual groove are present.

4. The distance between the three roots is greater.
5. The bifurcation level is different for all the three aspects, i.e. root trunk length on buccal aspect is 4 mm, mesial aspect is 3 mm and on distal aspect is 5 mm.
6. The occlusal outline shape is rhomboidal, i.e. it is wider lingually and mesially.
7. The presence of oblique ridge.
8. Transverse groove of oblique ridge is present.

Permanent Maxillary Second Molar

1. Four cusps and three roots are present. The cusps are mesiobuccal, distobuccal, mesiolingual and distolingual cusp. The roots are mesiobuccal, distobuccal and lingual root.
2. No fifth cusp is evident.
3. Line angles are more obtuse.
4. Occlusal outline form is rhomboidal.
5. Distally the crown convergence is greater.
6. Numerous supplemental grooves are present on the occlusal surface and are much deeper comparatively.
7. The distance between the three roots is reduced.

Permanent Maxillary Third Molar

1. Three cusps and three roots are seen. The mesiobuccal, distobuccal and lingual cusp; roots are mesiobuccal, distobuccal and lingual root.
2. The distance between the roots are highly reduced and may be fused sometimes.
3. The level of bifurcation of roots is more toward the apices of roots.
4. Distolingual cusp is less distinct.
5. Both crown and root are poorly developed—a small crown and root.
6. The occlusal outline shape is heart-shaped.
7. Numerous deeper supplemental grooves are seen on the occlusal surface.

Permanent Mandibular First Molar

1. Five cusps and two roots are present. The cusps are mesiobuccal, distobuccal, mesiolingual, distolingual, and distal cusp. The roots are mesial and distal root.
2. Mesiobuccal and distobuccal grooves are present on the buccal surface. The distobuccal groove is longer than mesiobuccal groove.
3. The buccal cusp tips are flat and the lingual cusp tips are pointed and are highly placed than the buccal cusps.
4. Cervical ridge is prominent on the buccal surface.
5. The occlusal outline form is hexagonal.

6. The developmental grooves on the occlusal surface are the central developmental groove, the mesiobuccal developmental groove, the distobuccal developmental groove and the lingual developmental groove.

Permanent Mandibular Second Molar

1. Four cusps and two roots are present. The cusps are mesiobuccal, distobuccal, mesiolingual and distolingual cusp. The roots are mesial and distal root.
2. Only buccal developmental groove is present on the buccal surface of the crown.
3. The buccal cusp tips are flat and the lingual cusp tips are pointed and are slightly placed higher than the buccal cusps.
4. The occlusal outline form is rectangular.
5. The central developmental groove, buccal developmental groove, and lingual developmental grooves are present.
6. The distance between the two roots is reduced.
7. Numerous supplemental grooves radiate from the central developmental groove and are much deeper.

Permanent Mandibular Third Molar

1. The number of cusps varies from five or more cusps. The roots present are mesial and distal root and they may be fused.
2. The buccal cusps are short and rounded. The lingual cusps height is lesser than the buccal cusp height.
3. The root apices are more pointed.
4. The occlusal outline form is rectangular.
5. The grooves are less distinct. Numerous supplemental grooves which are much deeper towards central part of the occlusal surface are seen.

DECIDUOUS TEETH

Deciduous Maxillary Central Incisor

1. The mesiodistal diameter is greater than the cervicoincisal length.
2. Prominent cervical ridge is present on the cervical third of the crown labially and lingually.
3. Prominent cingulum and marginal ridges are present. The cingulum extends till the incisal ridge dividing the lingual fossa into mesial and distal fossa.
4. The mesiodistal width is greater than the labiolingual width when viewed from incisal aspect.
5. The root length is much longer in proportion to the crown length.

Deciduous Maxillary Lateral Incisor

1. The crown is smaller and has a prominent cervical ridge on the cervical third of the crown labially and lingually.
2. The cervicoincisal length of the lateral crown is greater than its mesiodistal width.
3. The distoincisal angles of the crown are more rounded than those of the central incisor.
4. The root length is highly longer in comparison with the crown length.

Deciduous Mandibular Central Incisor

1. The mesial and distal outline of the crown taper evenly from the contact areas.
2. The incisal ridge is straight.
3. The labial surface is flat.
4. The mesiodistal width is almost equal to the length of the crown. This gives an appearance of permanent maxillary lateral incisor.
5. The incisal third and middle third is flat and cervical third is slightly convex lingually.
6. Cervical bulges of the crown is prominent labially and lingually.
7. The incisal ridge bisects the crown labiolingually when viewed from incisal aspect.

Deciduous Mandibular Lateral Incisor

1. The outlines of mandibular lateral incisor resembles central incisor.
2. Cervical bulges of the crown are prominent labially and lingually.
3. The incisal ridge slopes downward distally in a cervical direction.
4. The distal contact area is placed at a lower level than the mesial contact area.
5. The cingulum is more prominent and lingual surface concavity is much deeper.

Deciduous Maxillary Canine

1. The cusp is long, well-developed and sharp.
2. Mesiodistally cervical constriction is greater.
3. The mesial and distal contact areas are at the same level.
4. The marginal ridges, cingulum and incisal cusp ridges merge with each other.
5. The lingual ridge divides shallow lingual fossa into mesiolingual and distolingual fossae.
6. The mesial cusp slope is longer than the distal cusp slope.
7. The occlusal form is diamond shaped with prominent line angles.

Deciduous Mandibular Canine

1. The crown and root length is slightly shorter and the labiolingual width is also less compared with the maxillary canine. The neck is thicker.
2. The distal cusp slope is longer than the mesial cusp slope.
3. The cervical bulge on the crown labially and lingually is less pronounced.
4. The line angles are prominent from the occlusal aspect.
5. The mesial and distal contact areas are at the same level.

Deciduous Maxillary First Molar

1. Four cusps and three roots are present. The mesiobuccal, distobuccal, mesiolingual and distolingual cusp. Mesiolingual being the largest cusp.
2. This tooth of lesser dimensions somewhat resembles permanent maxillary premolars.
3. The crown narrows toward the cervix.
4. The roots are slender, long and spread widely. The bifurcation is nearly toward the cervical line.
5. From mesial aspect, the dimension at the cervical third is greater than the dimension at the occlusal third.
6. A prominent convexity is evident on the buccal outline of the cervical third. This convexity is characteristic of this tooth.
7. The occlusal outline is rectangular in form.
8. The central developmental groove, mesial developmental grooves with supplemental grooves within the mesial pit and distal developmental grooves are seen.
9. Oblique ridge may be present extending from triangular ridge of mesiolingual cusp and distobuccal cusp.

Deciduous Maxillary Second Molar

1. Five cusps and three roots are seen. The mesiobuccal, distobuccal, mesiolingual, distolingual and fifth cusp (cusp of Carabelli), the roots are mesiobuccal, distobuccal and lingual root.
2. The crown is larger and roots are much longer and heavier than those of the deciduous maxillary first molar.
3. A buccal developmental groove is seen on the buccal surface and the crown is narrow at the cervix in comparison with its mesiodistal measurement at the contact areas.
4. The point of bifurcation between the buccal roots is close to the cervical line of the crown.
5. A lingual developmental groove is seen on the lingual aspect. From mesial aspect, the crown resembles typical of permanent molars.

6. The crest of curvature at the cervical third lingually is more prominent than on the buccal surface, from this point the tooth resembles permanent maxillary first molar.
7. The occlusal outline is rhomboidal in form and resembles that of permanent maxillary first molar.
8. The mesial and distal triangular fossa, central fossa and distal fossa are seen. The grooves are central develepmental groove, buccal developmental groove, lingual developmental groove and distal developmental grooves.
9. The oblique ridge is prominent and connects the mesiolingual cusp with the distobuccal cusp.

Deciduous Mandibular First Molar

1. Two buccal cusps, the mesiobuccal and the distobuccal cusp, two lingual cusps, the mesiolingual and distolingual cusps. Roots are mesial and distal root.
2. A developmental depression is present in between the buccal cusps, instead of a developmental groove.
3. The roots are slender, long, flaring and the bifurcation is toward the cervical line.
4. The mesial portion is longer than the distal portion.
5. An outstanding feature is that the mesial marginal ridge is so well developed that it resembles of a small cusp lingually.
6. An extreme curvature buccally is noted at the cervical third when viewed from mesial aspect.
7. The mesial root drop straight down from the crown, tapering only slightly at the apical third and the distal root is rounder and shorter and tapers more apically.
8. The occlusal outline is rhomboidal in form. The mesiolingual cusp is the largest.
9. Ridges are cusp ridges and triangular ridges of all cusps and marginal ridges. The central developmental groove with buccal and lingual developmental groove are present. The pits present are mesial pit and central pit.

Deciduous Mandibular Second Molar

1. This tooth resembles permanent mandibular first molar but of smaller dimensions.
2. Five cusps and two roots. The cusps are mesiobuccal, buccal, distobuccal, mesiolingual and distolingual cusp. The roots are mesial and distal root.
3. All the three buccal cusps are equal in dimensions which is characteristic and this arrangement presents a straight buccal surface.
4. The roots are long, slender and have a characteristic flare at the middle and apical thirds.

5. The crest of contour buccally from mesial aspect is more prominent.
6. The mesial marginal ridge is high, a characteristic that makes the mesiobuccal cusp and the mesiolingual cusp appear short.
7. The occlusal outline form is rectangular. Grooves seen are central developmental groove, buccal developmental groove, lingual developmental groove. Cusp ridges, triangular ridges and marginal ridges are seen. The mesiodistal width of crown is greater than the buccolingual width.

DENTITION CASTS

IDENTIFICATION OF DENTITION CASTS

To identify a dentition cast, first whether it is maxillary or mandibular cast, what type of dentition whether it is permanent, deciduous or mixed dentition cast. Then the teeth present should be identified (not the number of teeth present) and then the dental age of cast should be determined by the last tooth erupted (know the sequence of eruption). The identification is as follows for some of the available casts in our department.

1. Maxillary Permanent Dentition Cast

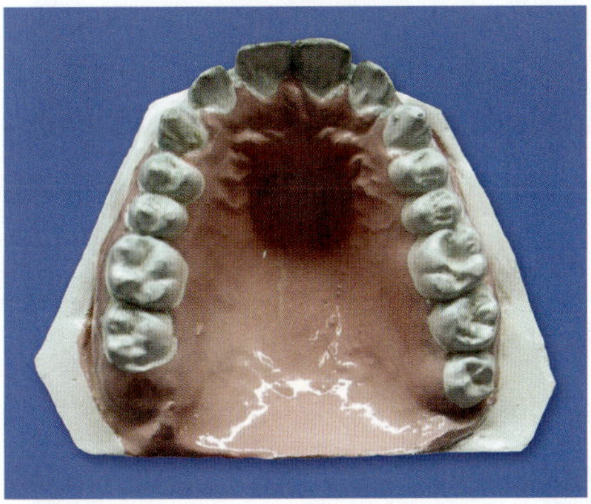

Teeth present:

17 16 15 14 13 12 11	21 22 23 24 25 26 27 28
Dental age of the cast; 17–21 years	

2. Mandibular Permanent Dentition Cast

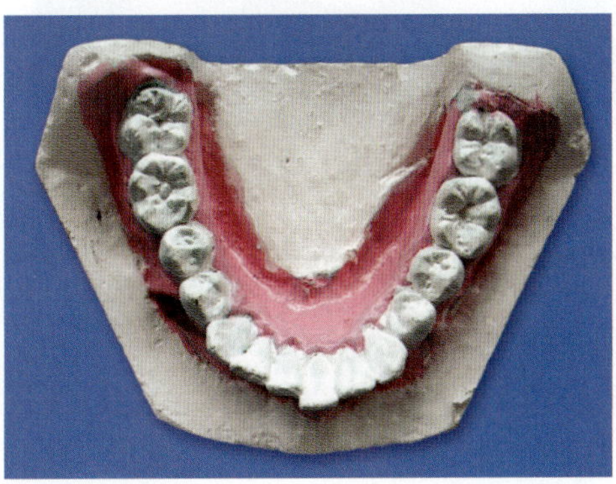

Teeth present:

47	46	45	44	43	42	41	31	32	33	34	35	36	37

Dental age of the cast: 11–13 years

3. Maxillary Mixed Dentition Cast

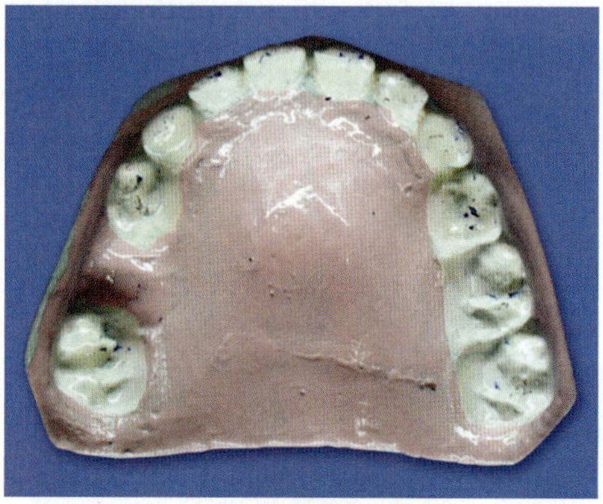

Teeth present:

16	54	53	52	51	61	62	63	64	65

Dental age of the cast: 7–8 years

4. Mandibular Mixed Dentition Cast

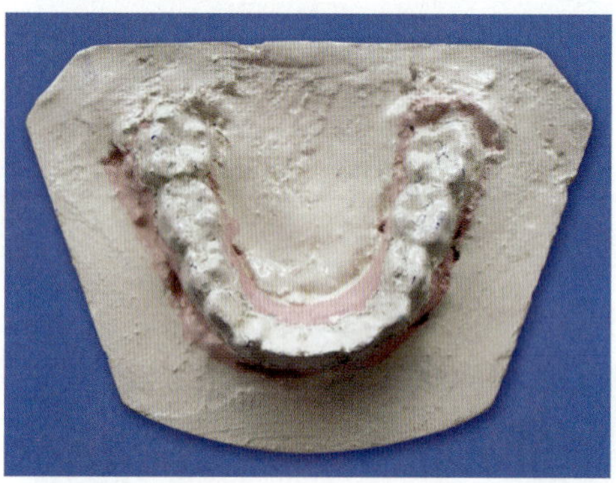

Teeth present:

46	85	84	43	42	41	31	32	33	74	75	36

Dental age of the Cast: 9–10 years

5. Maxillary Deciduous Dentition Cast

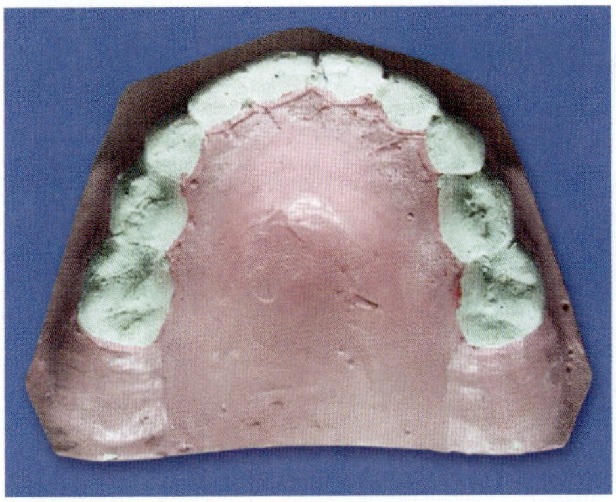

Teeth present:

16	54	53	52	51	61	62	63	64	65	26

Dental age of the cast: 29 months

6. Maxillary Mixed Dentition Cast

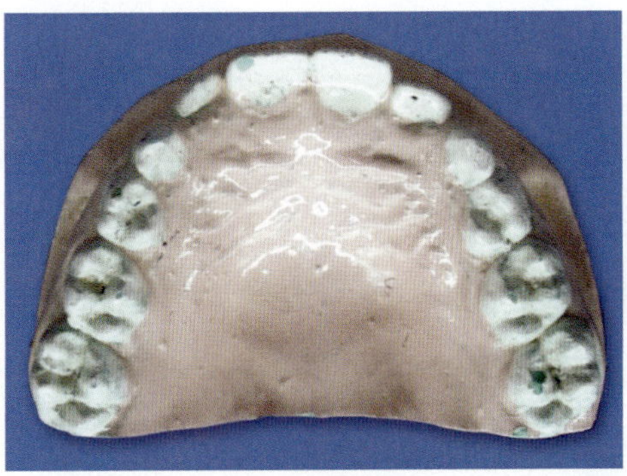

Teeth present:

16	55	54	53	12	11	21	22	63	64	65	26

12 and 22 are erupting

Dental age of the cast: 8–9 years

7. Mandibular Mixed Dentition Cast

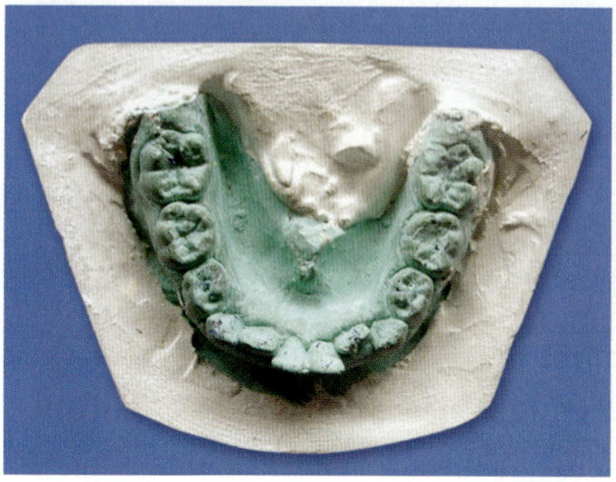

Teeth present:

46	85	84	83	42	41	31	32	73	74	75	36

Dental age of the cast: 7–8 years

8. Maxillary Mixed Dentition Cast

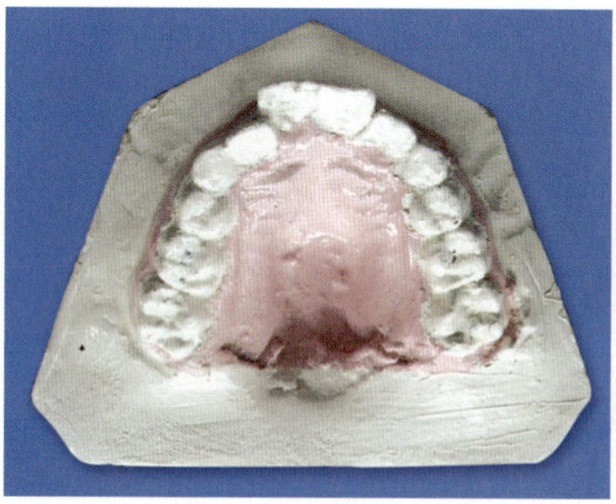

Teeth present:

16	55	54	53	12	11	21	22	63	64	65	26

Dental age of the cast: 8–9 years

9. Maxillary Mixed Dentition Cast

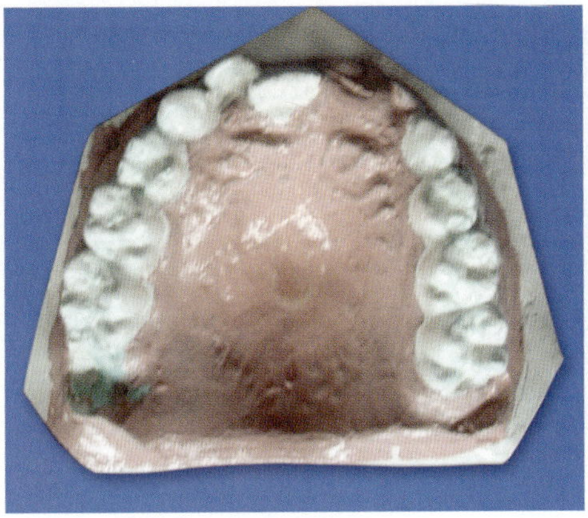

Teeth present:

16 55 54 53 12 11	22 63 64 65 26
21 and 22 are erupting.	

Dental age of the cast: 8–9 years

10. Maxillary Mixed Dentition Cast

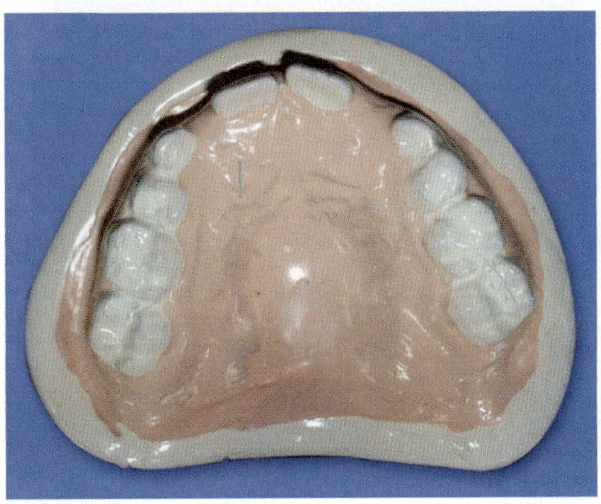

Teeth present:

16 55 54 53 11	21 63 64 65 26

Dental age of the cast: 7–8 years

11. Mandibular Mixed Dentition Cast

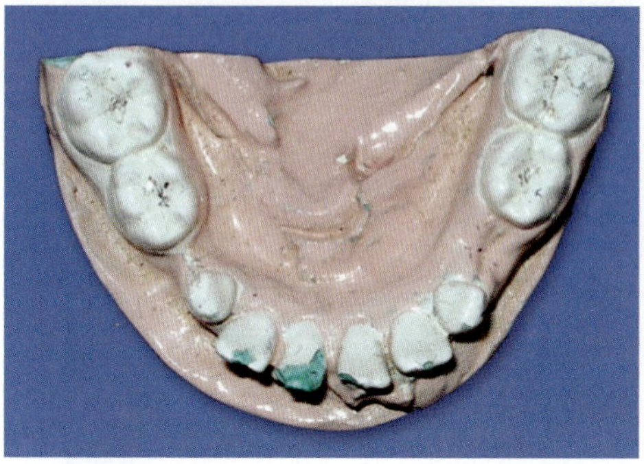

Teeth present:

46 85 83 42 41	31 32 73 75 36

Dental age of the cast: 7–8 years

12. Maxillary Mixed Dentition Cast

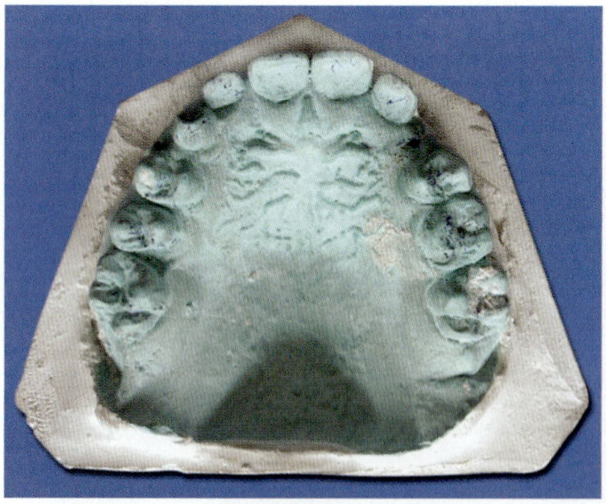

Teeth present:

16 15 14 53 12 11	21 22 24 65 26

Dental age of the cast: 10–12 years

13. Maxillary Mixed Dentition Cast

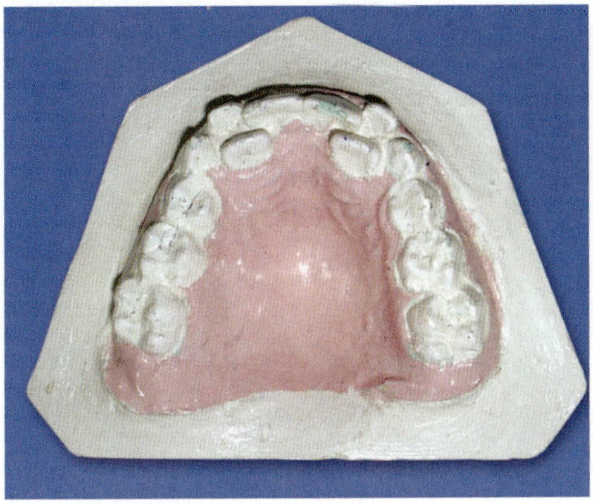

Teeth present:

16	55	54	53	52	12	11	21	22	62	63	64	65	26

12 and 22 are palatally erupted. 52 and 62 are retained.

Dental age of the cast: 8–9 years

14. Mandibular Mixed Dentition Cast

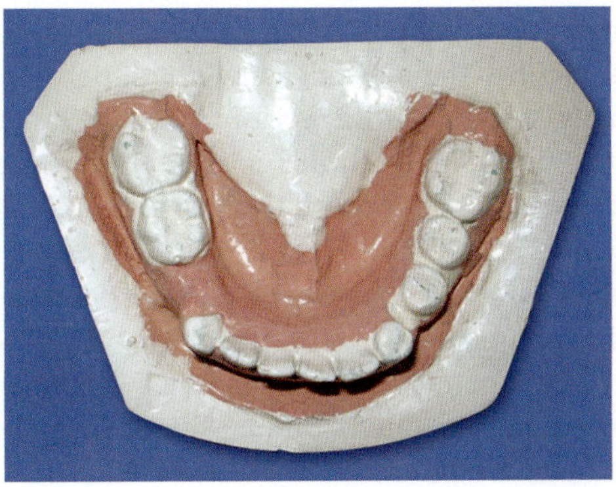

Teeth present:

46	85	43	42	41	31	32	33	34	35	36

Dental age of the cast: 11–12 years

15. Maxillary Mixed Dentition Cast

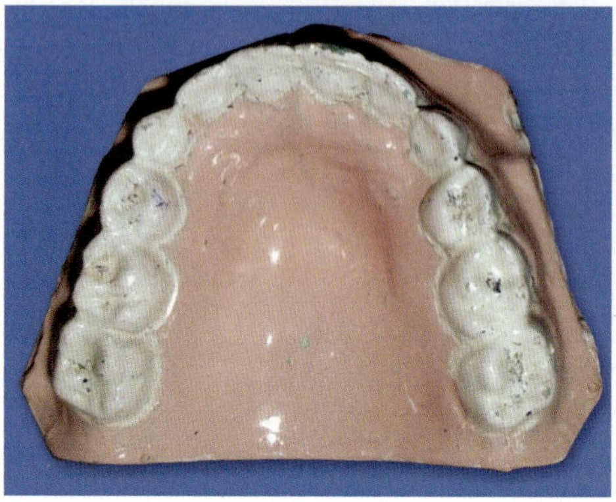

Teeth present:

16	55	54	53	52	51	61	62	63	64	65	26

Dental age of the cast: 6–7 years

Some TIPS to identify teeth in the dentition cast:

- To identify permanent incisors, look for mamelons, check for cervico-incisal length and mesiodistal width of crown.
- The common confusion is usually whether the present tooth is permanent canine or deciduous canine. The mesiodistal width of permanent canine will be almost similar to permanent central incisors. Even the length of crown will be almost equivalent to permanent central incisors. The cusp tip of permanent canine is more pointed, whereas the cusp tip of deciduous canine will be flat or attrited.
- For the premolar, usually the cusp tips will be pointed. For deciduous molars, the cusp tips will be attrited or flat. The deciduous first molar resembles permanent second premolar, but with flat cusp tips. Whereas the deciduous second molar resembles permanent first molar but of a smaller size (for both maxillary and mandibular teeth).
- Counting the number of teeth may help in identifying whether it is deciduous or permanent dentition cast for some extent. But in the mixed dentition cast the number of teeth present might mislead. So the knowledge of morphology of teeth is necessary to identify a tooth and then decide whether it is permanent, deciduous or mixed dentition cast.

Index

Page numbers followed by *f* refer to figure and *t* refer to table.

D

M

N

O

P